P9-CFI-288

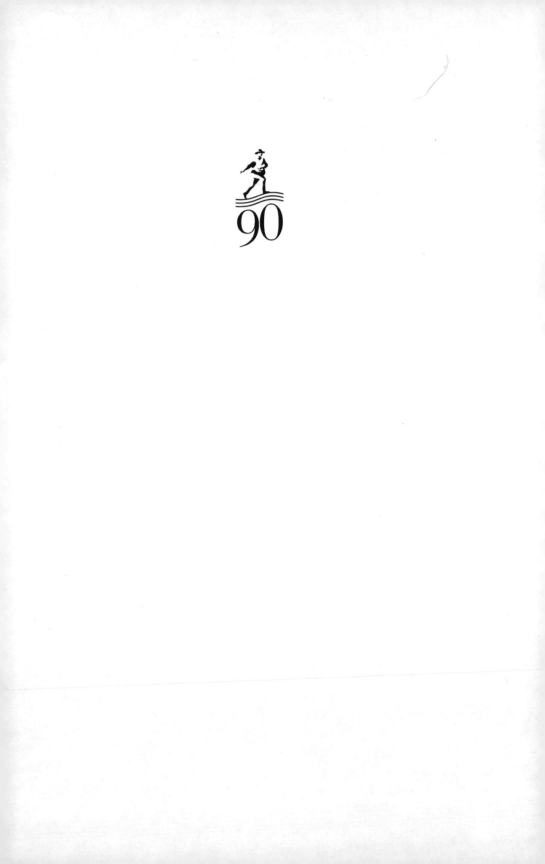

THE BIG
FAT
SURPRISE

Why Butter, Meat, and Cheese
Belong in a Healthy Diet

NINA TEICHOLZ

SIMON & SCHUSTER

New York   London   Toronto   Sydney   New Delhi

Iosco - Arenac District Library
East Tawas, Michigan

Simon & Schuster
1230 Avenue of the Americas
New York, NY 10020

This publication contains the opinions and ideas of its author. It is sold with
the understanding that the author and publisher are not engaged in rendering
health services in the book. The reader should consult his or her own medical and
health providers as appropriate before adopting any of the suggestions in this book
or drawing inferences from it.

The author and publisher specifically disclaim all responsibility for any liability, loss
or risk, personal or otherwise, which is incurred as a consequence, directly or indirectly,
of the use and application of any of the contents of this book.

Copyright © 2014 by Nina Teicholz

All rights reserved, including the right to reproduce this book or portions thereof in
any form whatsoever. For information address Simon & Schuster Subsidiary Rights
Department, 1230 Avenue of the Americas, New York, NY 10020.

First Simon & Schuster hardcover edition May 2014

SIMON & SCHUSTER and colophon are registered trademarks of Simon & Schuster, Inc.

For information about special discounts for bulk purchases, please contact
Simon & Schuster Special Sales at 1-866-506-1949 or business@simonandschuster.com.

The Simon & Schuster Speakers Bureau can bring authors to your live event.
For more information or to book an event contact the Simon & Schuster Speakers Bureau
at 1-866-248-3049 or visit our website at www.simonspeakers.com.

Interior design by Ruth Lee-Mui
Jacket design and photograph by Elixir Design INC.

Manufactured in the United States of America

10 9 8 7 6 5 4 3 2 1

Library of Congress Cataloging-in-Publication Data is available.

ISBN 978-1-4516-2442-7
ISBN 978-1-4516-2444-1 (ebook)

Permissions appear on page 455.

613.284
Te

For Gregory

Contents

Illustrations

THE BIG
FAT
SURPRISE

Introduction

I remember the day I stopped worrying about eating fat. It was long before I started poring over thousands of scientific studies and conducting hundreds of interviews to write this book. Like most Americans, I was following the low-fat advice set forth by the US Department of Agriculture (USDA) in its food pyramid, and when the Mediterranean diet was introduced in the 1990s, I added olive oil and extra servings of fish while cutting back further on red meat. In following these guidelines, I was convinced that I was doing the best I could for my heart and my waistline, since official sources have been telling us for years that the optimal diet emphasizes lean meats, fruits, vegetables, and grains and that the healthiest fats come from vegetable oils. Avoiding the saturated fats found in animal foods, especially, seemed like the most obvious measure a person could take for good health.

Then, around 2000, I moved to New York City and started writing a restaurant review column for a small paper. It didn't have a budget to pay for meals, so I usually ate whatever the chef decided to send out to me. Suddenly I was eating gigantic meals with foods that I would have never before allowed to pass my lips: pâté, beef of every cut prepared in every imaginable way, cream sauces, cream soups, foie gras—all the foods I had avoided my entire life.

Eating these rich, earthy dishes was a revelation. They were complex and remarkably satisfying. I ate with abandon. And yet, bizarrely, I found myself losing weight. In fact, I soon lost the 10 pounds that had dogged me for years, and my doctor told me that my cholesterol numbers were fine.

I might have thought no more about it had my editor at *Gourmet* not asked me to write a story about trans fats, which were little known at the time and certainly nowhere near as notorious as they are today. My article received a good deal of attention and led to a book contract.

The deeper I dug into my research, however, the more I became convinced that the story was far larger and more complex than trans fats. Trans fats seemed to be merely the latest scapegoat for the country's health problems.

The more I probed, the greater was my realization that *all* our dietary recommendations about fat—the ingredient about which our health authorities have obsessed most during the past sixty years—appeared to be not just slightly offtrack but completely wrong. Almost nothing that we commonly believe today about fats generally and saturated fat in particular appears, upon close examination, to be accurate.

Finding out the truth became, for me, an all-consuming, nine-year obsession. I read thousands of scientific papers, attended conferences, learned the intricacies of nutrition science, and interviewed pretty much every single living nutrition expert in the United States, some several times, plus scores more overseas. I also interviewed dozens of food company executives to understand how that behemoth industry influences nutrition science. The results were startling.

There's a popular assumption that the profit-driven food industry must be at the root of all our dietary troubles, that somehow food companies are responsible for corrupting nutrition recommendations toward their own corporate ends. And it's true, they're no angels. In fact, the story of vegetable oils, including trans fats, is partly about how food companies stifled science to protect an ingredient vital to their industry.

Yet I discovered that on the whole, the mistakes of nutrition science could not primarily be pinned on the nefarious interests of Big Food. The source of our misguided dietary advice was in some ways more disturbing, since it seems to have been driven by experts at some of our most trusted institutions working toward what they believed to be the public *good*.

Part of the problem is easy to understand. These researchers ran up against an enduring problem in nutrition science, which is that much of it turns out to be highly fallible. Most of our dietary recommendations are based on studies that try to measure what people eat and then follow them for years to see how their health fares. It is, of course, extremely difficult to trace a direct line from a particular element in the diet to disease outcomes many years later, especially given all the other lifestyle factors and variables at play. The data that emerge from these studies are weak and impressionistic. Yet in the drive to fight heart disease (and later obesity and diabetes), these weak data have had to suffice. And this compromise by researchers appears to have driven many of nutrition policy's failures: well-intentioned experts, hastening to address growing epidemics of chronic disease, simply overinterpreted the data.

Indeed, the disturbing story of nutrition science over the course of the last half-century looks something like this: scientists responding to the skyrocketing number of heart disease cases, which had gone from a mere handful in 1900 to being the leading cause of death by 1950, hypothesized that dietary fat, especially of the saturated kind (due to its effect on cholesterol), was to blame. This hypothesis became accepted as truth before it was properly tested. Public health bureaucracies adopted and enshrined this unproven dogma. The hypothesis became immortalized in the mammoth institutions of public health. And the normally self-correcting mechanism of science, which involves constantly challenging one's own beliefs, was disabled. While good science should be ruled by skepticism and self-doubt, the field of nutrition has instead been shaped by passions verging on zealotry. And the whole system by which ideas are canonized as fact seems to have failed us.

Once ideas about fat and cholesterol became adopted by official institutions, even prominent experts in the field found it nearly impossible to challenge them. One of the twentieth century's most revered nutrition scientists, the organic chemist David Kritchevsky, discovered this thirty years ago when, on a panel for the National Academy of Sciences, he suggested loosening the restrictions on dietary fat.

"We were jumped on!" he told me. "People would spit on us! It's hard to imagine now, the heat of the passion. It was just like we had desecrated the American flag. They were so angry that we were going against the suggestions of the American Heart Association and the National Institutes of Health."

This kind of reaction met all experts who criticized the prevailing view on dietary fat, effectively silencing any opposition. Researchers who persisted in their challenges found themselves cut off from grants, unable to rise in their professional societies, without invitations to serve on expert panels, and at a loss to find scientific journals that would publish their papers. Their influence was extinguished and their viewpoints lost. As a result, for many years the public has been presented with the appearance of a uniform scientific consensus on the subject of fat, especially saturated fat, but this outward unanimity was only made possible because opposing views were pushed aside.

Unaware of the flimsy scientific scaffolding upon which their dietary guidelines rest, Americans have dutifully attempted to follow them. Since the 1970s, we have successfully increased our fruits and vegetables by 17 percent, our grains by 29 percent, and reduced the amount of fat we eat from 43 percent to 33 percent of calories or less. The share of those fats that are saturated has also declined, according to the government's own data. (In these years, Americans also began exercising more.) Cutting back on fat has clearly meant eating more carbohydrates such as grains, rice, pasta, and fruit. A breakfast without eggs and bacon, for instance, is usually one of cereal or oatmeal; low-fat yogurt, a common breakfast choice, is higher in carbohydrates than the whole-fat version, because removing fat from foods nearly always requires adding carbohydrate-based "fat replacers" to make up for lost texture. Giving up animal fats has also meant shifting over to vegetable oils, and over the past century the share of these oils has grown from zero to almost 8 percent of all calories consumed by Americans, by far the biggest change in our eating patterns during that time.

In this period, the health of America has become strikingly worse. When the low-fat, low-cholesterol diet was first officially recommended to the public by the American Heart Association (AHA) in 1961, roughly one in seven adult Americans was obese. Forty years later, that number was one in three. (It's heartbreaking to realize that the federal government's "Healthy People" goal for 2010, a project begun in the mid-1990s, for instance, was simply to return the public back to levels of obesity seen in 1960, and even that goal was unreachable.) During these decades, we've also seen rates of diabetes rise drastically from less than 1 percent of the adult population to more than 11 percent, while heart disease remains the leading cause of death for both men and women. In all, it's a tragic picture for a nation that has, according to the government, faithfully been following all the official dietary guidelines for so many years. If we've been so good, we might fairly ask, why is our health report card so bad?

It's possible to think of the low-fat, near-vegetarian diet of the past half-century as an uncontrolled experiment on the entire American population, significantly altering our traditional diet with unintended results. That may sound like a dramatic assertion, and I never would have believed it myself, but one of the most astonishing things I learned over the course of my research was that for thirty years after the low-fat diet had been officially recommended and we were taking its supposed benefits for granted, it had not been subjected to a large-scale, formal scientific trial. Finally, there was the Women's Health Initiative (WHI), a trial that enrolled 49,000 women in 1993 with the expectation that when the results came back, the benefits of a low-fat diet would be validated once and for all. But after a decade of eating more fruits, vegetables, and whole grains while cutting back on meat and fat, these women not only failed to lose weight, but they also did not see any significant reduction in their risk for either heart disease or cancer of any major kind. WHI was the largest and longest trial ever of the low-fat diet, and the results indicated that the diet had quite simply failed.

Now, in 2014, a growing number of experts has begun to acknowledge the reality that making the low-fat diet the centerpiece of nutritional advice for six decades has very likely been a bad idea. Even so, the official solution continues to be more of the same. We are still advised to eat a diet of mostly fruits, vegetables, and whole grains with modest portions of lean meat and low-fat dairy. Red meat is still virtually banned, as are whole-fat milk, cheese, cream, butter, and, to a lesser extent, eggs.

A line of argument in favor of eating these whole-fat animal foods has sprung up among cookbook authors and "foodies," who can't believe that all the things their grandparents ate could really be so bad for them. There are also the Paleo eaters, who swap information on Internet blogs and survive on little else *but* red meat. Many of these recent animal foods devotees have been inspired by the doctor whose name is most closely associated with the high-fat diet: Robert C. Atkins. As we will see, his ideas have endured to a surprising extent and have been the subject of a great deal of scholarship and scientific research in recent years. But newspapers still carry alarming headlines about how red meat causes cancer and heart disease, and most nutrition experts will tell you that saturated fat is absolutely to be avoided. Hardly anyone advises otherwise.

In writing this book, I had the advantage of approaching the field as a scientifically minded outsider free from affiliation with or funding from any entrenched views. I've reviewed nutrition science from the dawn of the field in the 1940s up until today to find the answer to the questions: Why are we avoiding dietary fat? Is that a good idea? *Is* there a health benefit to avoiding saturated fat and eating vegetable oils instead? Is olive oil truly the key to a disease-free long life? And are Americans better off having attempted to rid the food supply of trans fats? This book does not offer recipes or specific dietary recommendations, but it does arrive at some general conclusions about the best balance of macronutrients for a healthy diet.

In my research I specifically avoided relying upon summary reports, which tend to pass along received wisdoms and, as we'll see, can unwittingly perpetuate bad science. Instead, I've gone back to read all the original studies myself and in some cases have sought out obscure data that were never intended to be found. This book therefore contains many fresh and often alarming revelations about flaws in the foundational work of nutrition as well as the surprising ways in which it was both ill-conceived and misinterpreted.

What I found, incredibly, was not only that it was a mistake to restrict fat but also that our fear of the saturated fats in animal foods—butter, eggs, and meat—has never been based in solid science. A bias against these foods developed early on and became entrenched, but the evidence mustered in its support never amounted to a convincing case and has since crumbled away.

This book lays out the scientific case for why our bodies are healthiest on a diet with ample amounts of fat and why this regime necessarily includes meat, eggs, butter, and other animal foods high in saturated fat. *The Big Fat Surprise* takes us through the dramatic twists and turns of fifty years of nutrition science and lays out the evidence, so that a reader can fully understand the evidence to see for him- or herself how we arrived at our present understanding. At its heart, this book is a scientific investigation, but it is also a story about the strong personalities who corralled colleagues into believing their ideas. These ambitious, crusading researchers launched the entire American population, and subsequently the rest of the world, on the low-fat, near-vegetarian diet, a regime that ironically may have directly exacerbated many of the ills it was intended to cure.

For all of us who have spent much of our lives believing and following this diet, it is of vital importance to understand how and what went wrong, as well as where we might go from here.

Major Sources of Different Types of Fat

Saturated

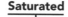

- *Cocoa butter*
- *Dairy (cheese, milk, cream)*
- *Eggs*
- *Palm oil*
- *Coconut oil*
- *Meats*

Unsaturated

Monounsaturated
- *Olive oil*
- *Lard*
- *Chicken and duck fat*

Created through chemical processing
- *Hydrogenated oils
  (trans fats)*

Polyunsaturated "omega 6s"
- *Corn oil*
- *Cottonseed oil*
- *Soybean oil*
- *Safflower oil*
- *Peanut oil*
- *Canola oil*

"omega 3s"
- *Fish oils*
- *Flaxseed*

1

The Fat Paradox:
Good Health on a High-Fat Diet

In 1906, Vilhjalmur Stefansson, the son of Icelandic immigrants to America and a Harvard-trained anthropologist, chose to live with the Inuit in the Canadian Arctic. He was the first white man these Mackenzie River Inuit had ever seen, and they taught him how to hunt and fish. Stefansson made a point of living exactly like his hosts, which included eating almost exclusively meat and fish for an entire year. For six to nine months, they ate nothing but caribou, followed by months of exclusively salmon, and a month of eggs in the spring. Observers estimated that some 70 to 80 percent of the calories in their diet came from fat.

It was clear to Stefansson that fat was the most favored and precious food to all the Inuit whom he observed. The fat deposits behind the caribou eye and along the jaw were most prized, followed by the rest of the head, the heart, the kidney, and the shoulder. The leaner parts, including the tenderloin, were fed to the dogs.

"The chief occasion for vegetables . . . with most Eskimos, was famine," wrote Stefansson in his controversial 1946 book, *Not by Bread Alone*. Recognizing how shocking a statement this would be, Stefansson added,

"If meat needs carbohydrate and other vegetable additives to make it wholesome, then the poor Eskimos were not eating healthfully." Worse, they spent months in the near complete darkness of winter idly, unable to hunt, with "no real work" to do, he observed. "They should have been in a wretched state. . . . But, to the contrary, they seemed to me the healthiest people I had ever lived with." He witnessed neither obesity nor disease.

Nutrition experts of the early twentieth century did not emphasize the importance of eating fruits and vegetables nearly as much as they do today, but even in his day, Stefansson's assertions were considered hard to believe. Eager to prove his revelations upon his return home from the Arctic, he therefore devised a rather drastic experiment. In 1928, he and a colleague, under the supervision of a highly qualified team of scientists, checked into Bellevue Hospital in New York City and vowed to eat nothing but meat and water for an entire year.

"A storm of protests" met the two men as they entered the hospital. Stefansson wrote, "Eating meat raw, our friends chorused, would make us social outcasts." (In fact the meat would be cooked.) Others feared that Stefansson and his colleague would certainly die.

After some three weeks on the diet, during which they underwent a constant battery of hospital tests, the still-healthy men were released to their homes under close supervision. During the ensuing year, Stefansson fell ill only once—when experimenters encouraged him to eat only lean meat without the fat. "The symptoms brought on at Bellevue by an incomplete meat diet (the ration of lean without fat)" came on fast: "diarrhoea and a feeling of general baffling discomfort," he recalled, and were quickly cured by a meal of fat sirloin steaks and brains fried in bacon fat.* At the end of a year, both men felt extremely well and were found to be in perfect health. Half a dozen papers published by the scientific oversight committee recorded the fact that scientists could find nothing wrong with them. The men were expected to contract scurvy, at the very least, since cooked meat is not a source of vitamin C. Yet they did not, probably because they ate

---

*A ratio of three parts fat to one part lean meat seemed to be the ideal balance, and indeed, that was the formula followed by Stefansson during his yearlong experiment. "All meat" was therefore a misnomer; the diet was actually mostly fat.

the whole animal, including the bones, liver, and brain, which are known to contain that vitamin, rather than just the meat. For calcium, they chewed bones, just as the Inuit did. Stefansson followed this diet not only for the year of the experiment but for pretty much his entire adult life. He remained active and in good health until he died at the age of eighty-two.

Across the globe half a century later, George V. Mann, a doctor and professor of biochemistry who had traveled to Africa, had a similarly counterintuitive experience. Although his colleagues in the United States were lining up in support of an increasingly popular hypothesis that animal fats cause heart disease, in Africa Mann was seeing a totally different reality. He and his team from Vanderbilt University took a mobile laboratory to Kenya in the early 1960s in order to study the Masai people. Mann had heard that the Masai men ate nothing but meat, blood, and milk—a diet, like the Inuits', comprised of almost entirely animal fat—and that they considered fruits and vegetables fit to be eaten only by cows.

Mann was building upon the work of A. Gerald Shaper, a South African doctor working at a university in Uganda, who had traveled farther north to study a similar tribe—the Samburus. A young Samburu man would drink from 2 to 7 liters of milk each day, depending on the season, which worked out on average to well over a pound of butterfat. His cholesterol intake was sky-high, especially during periods when he would add 2 to 4 pounds of meat to his daily diet of milk. Mann found the same with the Masai: the warriors drank 3 to 5 liters of milk daily, usually in two meals. When milk ran low in the dry season, they would mix it with cow blood. Not shirking the meat, they ate lamb, goat, and beef regularly, and on special occasions or on market days, when cattle were killed, they would eat 4 to 10 pounds of fatty beef per person. For both tribes, fat was the source of more than 60 percent of their calories, and all of it came from animal sources, which meant that it was largely saturated. For the young men of the warrior ("murran") class, Mann reported that "no vegetable products are taken."

Despite all of this, the blood pressure and weight of both these Masai and the Samburu peoples were about 50 percent lower than their American counterparts—and, most significantly, these numbers did not rise with age. "These findings hit me very hard," said Shaper, because they forced him to realize that it was not biologically normal for cholesterol, blood pressure, and other indicators of good health automatically to worsen with aging, as everyone in the United States assumed. In fact, a review of some twenty-six papers on various ethnic and social groups concluded that in relatively small homogenous populations living under primitive conditions, "more or less undisturbed by their contacts with civilization," an increase in blood pressure was not part of the normal aging process. Was it possible that we in the Western world were the anomaly, driving up our blood pressure and generally ruining our health by some aspect of our diet or modern way of life?

True, the Masai were free from the kind of emotional and competitive stresses that gnaw away at the citizens of more "civilized" countries and which some people believe contribute to heart disease. The Masai also got more exercise than desk-bound Westerners: these tall, slender shepherds would walk for many miles each day with their cattle, searching for food and water. Mann thought that perhaps all this exercise might be protecting the Masai from heart disease.* But he also acknowledged that subsistence was "easy" and "labor light," and that the elders, who "seem sedentary," were not dying from heart attacks, either.

If our current belief about animal fat is correct, then all the meat and dairy these tribesmen were eating would have caused an epidemic of heart disease in Kenya. However, Mann found exactly the opposite—he could identify almost no heart disease at all. He documented this by performing electrocardiograms on four hundred of the men, among whom he found no evidence of a heart attack. (Shaper did the same test on one hundred of the Samburu and found "possible" signs of heart disease in only two cases.) Mann then performed autopsies on fifty Masai men and found only one case with "unequivocal" evidence of an infarction. Nor did the Masai suffer from other chronic diseases, such as cancer or diabetes.

---

*Mann was one of the first researchers to investigate the potential benefits of exercise for prevention of heart disease. The advantages of running do not appear to be un-equivocal, however; prominent running enthusiast Jim Fixx died of a massive heart attack while running in 1984, for instance. And the fabled ancient Greek soldier, Pheidippides, who ran the first marathon to deliver a message of victory from the Battle of Marathon to Athens, is said to have expired on the spot.

NINA TEICHOLZ

On the surface, these stories from Africa and the Arctic (and New York City) seem paradoxical, given what we think we know about animal fats and heart attack risk. Good health and high consumption of animal fats should be mutually exclusive, according to the prevailing consensus that these fats, especially red meat, cause coronary disease and possibly cancer. These beliefs have become so ingrained as to seem self-evident to us.

Instead of animal products, we're supposed to eat plants, according to the advice we've been living with for decades now—that a nearly vegetarian diet is the healthiest. The American Heart Association and the USDA, as well as pretty much every expert group on the planet, recommend obtaining the day's calories mainly from fruits, vegetables, and whole grains while minimizing animal fats of all kinds. Red meat is not advised. As Mark Bittman, lead food columnist for the *New York Times*, wrote, "To eat 'better,' . . . the core of the answer is known to everyone: Eat more plants." The first point on the USDA dietary guidelines is: "Increase vegetable and fruit intake." Or as Michael Pollan, in a hugely popular book, *In Defense of Food*, declares in his opening line, "Eat food. Not too much. Mostly plants."

What, then, should we think about the Inuit and Masai, who appeared quite healthy on a high-fat diet of nearly zero plants? Stefansson and Mann, who observed them, were highly respected researchers whose studies followed scientific standards and were published in reputable journals. They were not marginal characters seeking out freaks of nature; Stefansson and Mann were simply grappling with some atypical observations.

The practice of good science requires that when we observe something that doesn't fit a hypothesis, these observations need to be reckoned with somehow. Is there a flaw in the observations themselves? If not, does the hypothesis need to change in some way to accommodate them? The types of close observations made by Stefansson and Mann can't just be brushed away or ignored—although that was exactly what other researchers did at the time. Critics just couldn't imagine that these accounts could be true.

For half a century, nutrition experts have been dedicated to the hypothesis that fat, especially saturated fat, causes heart disease (plus obesity and cancer). Any evidence to the contrary has been difficult, if not impossible, for experts to acknowledge—even though there has been plenty of it. A careful look at the vast body of scientific observations about diet and health shows a surprising and unexpected picture, and one that does not seem to support a solid argument against saturated fat.*

Indeed, Steffanson and Mann represent but two of the many "paradoxical" stories that we could tell. As it turns out, many healthy human populations have survived mainly on animal foods historically and into the present day. It's easy to find examples. In the early 1900s, for instance, Sir Robert McCarrison, the British government's director of nutrition research in the Indian Medical Service and perhaps the most influential nutritionist of the first half of the twentieth century, wrote that he was "deeply impressed by the health and vigour of certain races there. The Sikhs and the Hunzas," notably, suffered from "none of the major diseases of Western nations such as cancer, peptic ulcer, appendicitis, and dental decay." These Indians in the north were generally long-lived and had "good physique[s]," and their vibrant health stood "in marked contrast" to the high morbidity of other groups in the southern part of India who ate mainly white rice with minimal dairy or meat. McCarrison believed he could rule out causes other than nutrition for these differences, because he found that he could reproduce a similar degree of ill-health when feeding experimental rats a diet low in milk and meat. The healthy people McCarrison observed ate some meat but mostly "an abundance" of milk and milk products such as butter and cheese, which meant that the fat content of their diet was mainly saturated.

Meanwhile, the Native Americans of the Southwest were observed between 1898 and 1905 by the physician-turned-anthropologist Aleš Hrdlička, who wrote up his observations in a 460-page report for the Smithsonian Institute. The Native Americans he visited were eating a diet of predominantly meat, mainly from buffalo, yet, as Hrdlička observed, they seemed to be spectacularly healthy and lived to a ripe old age. The incidence of centenarians among these Native Americans was, according

---

*Saturated fats are found mainly in animal foods. "Saturated" refers to the type of chemical bonds in the individual fatty acids and will be discussed later in the chapter. (See the Glossary.)

to the 1900 US Census, 224 per million men and 254 per million women, compared to only 3 and 6 per million among men and women in the white population. Although Hrdlička noted that these numbers were probably not wholly accurate, he wrote that "no error could account for the extreme disproportion of centenarians observed." Among the elderly he met of age ninety and up, "not one of these was either much demented or helpless."

Hrdlička was further struck by the complete absence of chronic disease among the entire Indian population he saw. "Malignant diseases," he wrote, "if they exist at all—that they do would be difficult to doubt—must be extremely rare." He was told of "tumors" and saw several cases of the fibroid variety, but never came across a clear case of any other kind of tumor, nor any cancer. Hrdlička wrote that he saw only three cases of heart disease among more than two thousand Native Americans examined, and "not one pronounced instance" of atherosclerosis (buildup of plaque in the arteries). Varicose veins were rare. Nor did he observe cases of appendicitis, peritonitis, ulcer of the stomach, nor any "grave disease" of the liver. Although we cannot assume that meat eating was responsible for their good health and long life, it would be logical to conclude that a dependence on meat in no way *impaired* good health.

In Africa and Asia, explorers, colonialists, and missionaries in the early twentieth century were repeatedly struck by the absence of degenerative disease among isolated populations they encountered. The *British Medical Journal* routinely carried reports from colonial physicians who, though experienced in diagnosing cancer at home, could find very little of it in the African colonies overseas. So few cases could be identified that "some seem to assume that it does not exist," wrote George Prentice, a physician who worked in Southern Central Africa, in 1923. Yet if there were a "relative immunity to cancer" it could not be attributed to the lack of meat in the diet, he wrote:

> The negroes, when they can get it, eat far more meat than the white people. There is no limit to the variety or the condition, and some might wonder whether there is a limit to the quantity. They are only vegetarians when there is nothing else to be had. . . . Anything from a fieldmouse to an elephant is welcomed.

Perhaps all this is true, but no savvy heart disease researcher can read these historical observations without raising a standard and reasonable objection, namely, that the meat from today's domesticated animals is far more fatty—and a greater proportion of that fat is saturated—than was the meat from wild animals roaming around a hundred years ago. Experts argue that the meat from wild animals contained a higher proportion of polyunsaturated fats, which are the type found in vegetable oils and fish.* If wild animals contained less saturated fat, the argument goes, then early carnivorous populations would have consumed less of this fat than people eating meat from domesticated animals today.

It is true that American beef from a cow raised on grain does have a different fatty-acid profile from an ox hunted in the wild. In 1968, the English biochemist Michael Crawford was the first to look at this question in detail. He had the Uganda Game Department send him the muscle meat from various kinds of exotic animals: the eland, hartebeest, topi, and warthog, plus a giraffe and a few others. He compared these meats to those of domesticated cows, chickens, and pigs in England and reported that the meat of the wild animals contained ten times more polyunsaturated fats than did the flesh of domesticated ones. Thus, on its surface, his paper seemed to confirm that modern-day people should not consider their domesticated meat to be anywhere near as healthy as hunted meat from the wild. And for the past forty-five years, Crawford's paper has been widely cited, forming the general view of the subject.

What Crawford buries in his data, however, is that the *saturated* fat content of the wild and domesticated animal meats hardly differed at all. In other words, the factor that was supposedly dangerous in red meat was no higher in the English cows and pigs than it was in Uganda's beasts. Instead, the domesticated animals turned out to be higher in *mono*unsaturated fats,

---

*This objection reflects a reality about meat—that it contains a mixture of different kinds of fats. Half the fat in a typical cut of beef, for example, is unsaturated, and most of that fat is the same type (monounsaturated) that is found in olive oil. Half of chicken fat is unsaturated, and 60 percent of lard is unsaturated. (Asserting that animal fats are synonymous with saturated fats is, therefore, a simplification, although because saturated fats are found *mainly* in animal foods, I will also resort to the same simplification in this book, for the sake of brevity.)

which is the kind found predominantly in olive oil. So whatever the differences between wild and domesticated animal meat, saturated fat was not the issue.

An additional flaw in these studies was that they assumed early human beings ate mainly the muscle flesh of animals, as we do today. By "meat," they mean the muscle of the animal: the loins, ribs, flank, chuck, and so on. Yet focusing on the muscle appears to be a relatively recent phenomenon. In every history on the subject, the evidence suggests that early human populations preferred the fat and viscera (also called offal or organ meat) of the animal over its muscle meat. Stefansson found that the Inuit were careful to save fatty meat and organs for human consumption while giving leaner meat to the dogs. In this way, humans ate as other large, meat-eating mammals do. Lions and tigers, for instance, first ravage the blood, hearts, kidneys, livers, and brains of the animals they kill, often leaving the muscle meat for vultures. These viscera tend to be much higher in fat, especially saturated fat (half of the fat in a deer kidney is saturated, for instance).

Preferentially eating the fattest part of the animal and selecting animals at the fattest point in their life cycle appear to have been consistent hunting patterns among humans throughout history. For the Bardi tribe of northwest Australia, for example, researchers found that fat was "the determining criteria" when hunting fish, turtles, and shellfish. The Bardi people had developed an extraordinary knowledge of the proper season and technique of hunting in order to satisfy what researchers deemed their "obsession with fatness," including the ability to detect the fatness of a green turtle at night from nothing more than the smell of its breath when it popped up for air. Flesh that lacked fatness was considered "rubbish" and "too dry or tasteless to be enjoyed."

Meat consumed without fat was commonly understood to lead to weakness. The Inuit avoided eating too much rabbit, because, as an observer in the Arctic wrote, "if people had only rabbits . . . they would probably starve to death, because these animals are too lean." And in the winter of 1857, a party of trappers exploring Oregon's Klamath River who came to be stranded "tried the meat of horse, colt and mules, all of which were in a starved condition, and of course not very tender, juicy." They consumed an enormous amount of meat, from five to six pounds per man each day, but "continued to grow weak and thin" until, after twelve days, "we were able to perform but little labor, and were continually craving for fat."

Even Lewis and Clark reported this problem during their travels in 1805: Clark returned from a hunting party with forty deer, three buffalo, and sixteen elk, but the haul was considered a disappointment because most of the game "were too lean for use." That meant plenty of muscle meat but not enough fat.

The anthropological and historical record is full of such accounts of humans consistently devising hunting strategies that capitalized on finding animals during the season when they were at their fattest and then eating the fattest parts of the animal.

Now that we tend to eat only the lean meat—and to trim off the fat of even that—these stories seem exotic and unbelievable to us in the modern day; it's hard to square these ideas with our own conception of a healthy diet. How could populations eat a diet so apparently unhealthy by our contemporary standards, so dependent on the very things we blame for our own ills, and yet not suffer from the diseases that are such a burden to us today? It hardly seems possible that nutrition experts could have overlooked this information about diet and heart disease. Yet the scientific literature supporting our current dietary recommendations makes no attempt to grapple with it.

Nevertheless, we have to assume that there is an explanation for this paradox that has somehow been overlooked. After all, our modern, advanced knowledge is strictly based in science, endorsed and promoted by the most prestigious and influential institutions and government agencies in the world—right? Surely more than half a century of scientific "evidence" couldn't be wrong, could it?

2

Why We Think Saturated Fat Is Unhealthy

The idea that fat and saturated fat are unhealthy has been so ingrained in our national conversation for so long that we tend to think of it more as "common sense" than a scientific hypothesis. But, like any of our beliefs about the links between diet and disease, this one, too, began as an *idea*, proposed by a group of researchers, with its origin fixed at a moment in time.

The hypothesis that saturated fat causes heart disease was developed in the early 1950s by Ancel Benjamin Keys, a biologist and pathologist at the University of Minnesota. At his lab, he ran experiments looking for early indications of disease, and in the 1950s, no health issue seemed more urgent than the problem of heart disease. Americans felt themselves to be in the midst of a terrible epidemic. A sudden tightening of the chest would strike men in their prime on the golf course or at the office, and doctors didn't know why. The disease had appeared seemingly out of nowhere and had grown quickly to become the nation's leading cause of death.*

Thus, when Keys first proposed his ideas about dietary fat, the back-

---

*Death rates from heart disease have declined since the late 1960s, presumably due to more advanced medical care. However, it's not clear whether the underlying incidence rates of heart disease themselves have declined. And the disease is still a lead-

drop was a tense and fearful nation thirsting for answers. At the time, the prevailing view held that human arteries slowly narrowed as an inevitable accompaniment of aging and that modern medicine could do little about it. Keys, by contrast, thought that heart attacks could be avoided, based on the simple logic that there had not always been such an epidemic. In this way, he was like George Mann, whose observations decades later of the Masai in Africa led him to realize that heart attacks were not an inevitable part of human experience. Keys argued that the US Public Health Service should expand its role beyond just *containing* diseases like tuberculosis to *preventing* diseases before they struck. In offering an actionable solution, Keys sought to shed the "defeatist attitude about heart disease."*

Keys himself was an inveterate nonconformist. Born in 1904, he grew up in Berkeley, California, and was fiercely independent from an early age. As a teenager, Keys hitchhiked from Berkeley to Arizona and worked for three months in a cave collecting bat dung for a commercial fertilizer company. Similarly, having grown impatient with college after just one year, he left and hired himself out as a manual laborer on a boat to China. Later, his closest colleague at the University of Minnesota, Henry Blackburn, would describe him as being "direct to the point of bluntness, critical to the point of skewering, and possessing a very quick, bright intelligence." By all accounts, Keys also had an indomitable will and would argue an idea "to the death." (Less admiring colleagues called him "arrogant" and "ruthless.") He earned a PhD in biology at Berkeley in just three years and then went on to earn a second doctorate in physiology at Kings College, London.

In 1933, Keys spent ten days in the highlands of the Andes measuring the effect of altitude on his blood, and those days changed his life. In ob-

---

ing cause of death for men *and* women in America, killing some 600,000 people each year (Lloyd-Jones et al. 2009).

*Heart disease is an umbrella term used to describe a number of diseases affecting the heart, such as reduced blood supply to the organs (ischaemic heart disease), deterioration of the heart muscle (cardiomyopathy), inflammation of the heart muscle (inflammatory heart disease), and weakening of the whole circulatory system due to high blood pressure (hypertensive heart disease). The kind of heart disease that primarily preoccupied researchers of this period was atherosclerosis, which involves the buildup of plaque in the arteries.

serving how the thin air intimately affected the workings of his own body, Keys discovered a passion for human physiology. An interest in how nutrition affects the body came later, during World War II, when he conducted pioneering studies on starvation and developed K rations for soldiers. The K stood for Keys.

He then set his formidable mind and ambition to the study of heart disease, and it should come as no surprise that he revolutionized the field.

From the start, one of the main factors in the discussion of heart disease has been cholesterol, the yellow, waxy substance that is a necessary part of all body tissues. It is a vital component of every cell membrane, controlling what goes in and out of the cell. It is responsible for the metabolism of sex hormones and is found at its highest concentration in the brain. In addition to these crucial roles, however, researchers found that cholesterol is a primary component of atherosclerotic plaques, so it was assumed to be one of the main culprits in the development of coronary disease. The buildup of this plaque, which was understood to narrow the arteries until it cuts off blood flow, was thought at the time to be the central cause of a heart attack.

Although the development of heart disease turned out to be far more complex, this compelling early imagery of cholesterol accumulation established it as the brightest evil star in the firmament of public health. As Jeremiah Stamler, one of the original and most influential researchers in the field, wrote, cholesterol was "biological rust" that can "spread to choke off the flow [of the blood], or slow it just like rust inside a water pipe so that only a dribble comes from your faucet." Indeed, we still talk about cholesterol as "clogging up the arteries," like hot grease down a cold drainpipe. This vivid and seemingly intuitive idea has stayed with us, even as the science has shown this characterization to be a highly simplistic and even inaccurate picture of the problem.

The first set of clues that appeared to implicate cholesterol as *causing* heart disease came from late-nineteenth-century reports that certain children with abnormally high cholesterol in the blood (known as "serum cholesterol") had an exceptionally high risk for heart problems. (One unfortunate girl had a heart attack and died by the age of eleven, according to an early report.) These children also had large, lumpy fatty deposits on their hands or ankles, called *xanthomas*.

By the early 1940s, researchers had determined that these children had a rare genetic condition that was unrelated to their diets. However, the fact that older people with high serum cholesterol also got these xanthomas, especially on their eyelids, led researchers to believe that high serum cholesterol might ultimately be the cause of these waxy accumulations under the skin. Researchers made the assumptions that the visible deposits on the *outside* of the body must be just like the invisible, insidious ones building up on the *inside* of the arterial wall and that these buildups must lead to heart attacks. These were both leaps of faith, really, but nonetheless plausible. Not everyone agreed with this chain of reasoning (an obvious objection was that the children's genetic disease might be operating by a different mechanism from a chronic one developing over a lifetime), but these concerns did not impede the cholesterol hypothesis from moving forward.

Early evidence suggestively linking cholesterol to heart disease also came from animals. In 1913, the Russian pathologist Nikolaj Anitschkow reported that he could induce atherosclerotic-type lesions in rabbits by feeding them huge amounts of cholesterol. This experiment became quite famous and was widely replicated on all sorts of animals, including cats, sheep, cattle, and horses, leading to the widespread view that cholesterol in the *diet*—such as one finds in eggs, red meat, and shellfish—must cause atherosclerosis. Contemporaries noted that rabbits, along with most of the animals used in follow-up experiments, are all herbivores. They therefore do not normally eat animal foods and are not biologically designed to metabolize them. By contrast, when the experiment was replicated on dogs (which eat meat as humans do), the animals demonstrated an ability to regulate and excrete extra cholesterol. The canine comparison seemed like a better model for humans, yet the original rabbit experiment had already riveted heart disease researchers, and cholesterol fixed itself as the principal suspect in the development of heart disease.*

By 1950, elevated serum cholesterol was broadly viewed as a probable

---

*Researchers later discovered that many of these experiments were flawed because researchers did not know to take steps to prevent oxidation of the cholesterol they

cause of heart disease, and many experts believed that it would be safer for anyone with high blood cholesterol to try to nudge it lower.

One of the early ideas for how people might lower cholesterol was simply to consume less of it. The notion that cholesterol in the diet would translate directly into higher cholesterol in the blood just seemed intuitively reasonable, and was introduced by two biochemists from Columbia University in 1937. The assumption was that if we could avoid eating egg yolks and the like, we could prevent cholesterol from accumulating in the body. The idea is now lodged firmly in our minds: Indeed, how many brunch guests will demur at the sight of a plate of shirred eggs with a murmur about "too much cholesterol"?

It was Ancel Keys himself who first discredited this notion. Although in 1952 he stated that there was "overwhelming evidence" for the theory, he then found that no matter how much cholesterol he fed the volunteers in his studies, the cholesterol levels in their blood remained unchanged. He found that "tremendous" dosages of cholesterol added to the daily diet—up to 3,000 milligrams per day (a single large egg has just under 200 mg)—had only a "trivial" effect and by 1955, he had already decided that "this point requires no further consideration."

Many other studies have reinforced this conclusion. In one case, when Uffe Ravnskov, a Swedish doctor, upped his consumption of eggs from one to eight per day (about 1,600 mg of cholesterol) for nearly a week, he made the remarkable discovery that his total cholesterol level went *down*. This, he later recorded in a book chapter called "Egg Consumption and Cholesterol Values in One Skeptical Swedish Doctor." In fact, eating two to three eggs a day over a long period of time has never been shown to have more than a minimal impact on serum cholesterol for the vast majority of people. Remember that Mann would later find the Masai to have extremely low serum cholesterol on average, despite a diet composed entirely of milk, meat, and blood. In 1992, one of the most comprehensive analyses of this subject concluded that the vast majority of people will react to even a great

---

fed the animals. (Once cholesterol is oxidized, plaque is more likely to be produced.) (Smith 1980).

deal of cholesterol in the diet by ratcheting down the amount of cholesterol the body itself produces.* In other words, the body seeks to keep its internal conditions constant. In the same way that the body excretes sweat to lower body temperature, the process of homeostasis is constantly returning the internal conditions of the body—cholesterol levels included—to a state where all biological systems can function optimally.

Responding to this evidence, health authorities in Britain and most other European nations in recent years have rescinded their advisories to cap dietary cholesterol. The United States, however, has continued recommending a limit of 300 mg per day for healthy people (the equivalent of one and a half eggs). Moreover, the Food and Drug Administration (FDA) continues to allow food products to advertise themselves as "cholesterol-free," so consumers walking down the supermarket aisle between shelves of cholesterol-free Cheerios and cholesterol-free salad dressings could easily get the impression that cholesterol in our food is an enduring health concern.

Yet if foods high in cholesterol do not cause the high serum cholesterol that some people experience, then what does? Having determined that cholesterol in the diet could be "disregarded" as a cause, Keys suggested that researchers focus on other elements of the diet. Quite a few scientists starting in the early 1950s were already investigating how different nutrients affected not only cholesterol but other aspects of blood chemistry. In previous years, the focus of heart disease research had been on proteins and carbohydrates, but an explosion of new methods for separating out fatty acids, especially a 1952 invention called gas-liquid chromatography, made it possible to test different kinds of fats (also called "lipids") and their effect on human biology. The "sleepy old field of lipid research suddenly took off for the moon," wrote E. H. "Pete" Ahrens of Rockefeller University in New York City, who was one of the leading "lipidologists" of his day. A swarm of researchers entered the field; funds for research swelled each year, and, as Ahrens described it, "lipid research hit the Big Time."

---

*This study was the first to correct for methodological problems that had distorted previous studies on cholesterol, such as the lack of baseline cholesterol scores against which changes could be properly measured.

A Fatty Acid Is a Chain of Carbon Atoms Surrounded by Hydrogen Atoms

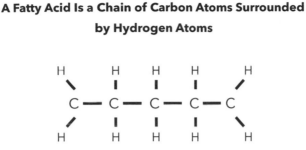

In the 1950s, Ahrens set up the first gas-liquid chromatography lab in the United States and embarked on some of the pioneering experiments looking at various kinds of dietary fat. It's useful to understand a bit about the basic chemical structure of fats. They are, basically, made up of chains of carbon atoms surrounded by hydrogen atoms.

These chains can be of various lengths and can also have different types of chemical bonds holding them together. It is the *type* of bond that makes a fatty acid "saturated" or "unsaturated." A bond is a chemical term referring to the way that two atoms are linked together. A double bond is like a double handshake between atoms and has two practical implications: first, the bond is less stable, since one hand can be freed up at any moment to take on more atoms, and second, the bond causes a kink along the carbon-atom chain, so that it does not lie neatly against its neighbors. These squiggly molecules with double bonds in them therefore pack together loosely, forming oils. A single double bond in a chain makes it a "monounsaturated" fatty acid, which is the principal kind found in olive oil. More than one double bond makes a "polyunsaturated" fat, which characterizes the "vegetable" oils and includes canola, safflower, sunflower, peanut, corn, cottonseed, and soybean oils.

Saturated fatty acids, by contrast, contain no double bonds, only single bonds. The molecules cannot take on any new atoms because they are already "saturated" with hydrogen atoms. These fats are also straight chains and can pack together densely—making them solids at room temperature, like butter, lard, suet, and tallow.

Lipid scientists in the 1950s were intensely focused on how these different kinds of fats affect various aspects of the blood, especially cholesterol

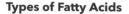

Types of Fatty Acids

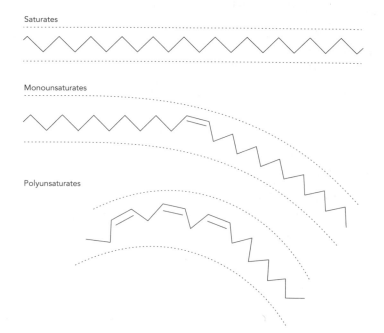

Saturates

Monounsaturates

Polyunsaturates

levels, when eaten. At the Institute for Metabolic Research in Oakland, California, for instance, researchers first discovered in 1952 that replacing animal fats with vegetable fats would dramatically lower total cholesterol. A team at Harvard University found that the serum cholesterol levels of vegetarians were lower in those who ate no dairy products compared to those in people who ate eggs and milk. A Dutch study of vegetarians found the same.

Ahrens at Rockefeller University was a particularly meticulous researcher. He made every effort to control all aspects of the trials he conducted, keeping his patients hospitalized on a metabolic ward and feeding them liquid-formula diets to avoid the nutritional complications that accompanied real foods. He found that the saturated fats in butter and coconut oil raised serum cholesterol more than did any other fats, followed by palm oil, lard, cocoa butter, and olive oil. The lowest levels of serum cholesterol in his subjects were found on diets of peanut, cottonseed, corn, and safflower oils. Later on, using more advanced techniques, Ahrens found that cholesterol didn't go up and down quite so consistently in response to different dietary fats; there was far more heterogeneity than he had originally thought. The discovery of this "heterogeneity" of human responses, as Ahrens wrote at the end of his career, was one of his most "gratifying contributions" to the field. But in the 1950s, researchers were convinced that these cholesterol reactions were strictly uniform, and they focused on saturated fats as the ones driving up cholesterol levels most severely.

Although Keys would become the most influential researcher in the field of diet and disease, he was actually a little late to the game in singling out *types* of fats. He agreed more with researchers who thought that the *total* amount of dietary fat better determined heart disease risk than the *type* of fat. Keys conducted his own work on this topic in ethically questionable experiments on male schizophrenic patients at a nearby Minnesota hospital. He fed them diets in which the fat content ranged from 9 percent to 24 percent and discovered that the lower-fat diets performed slightly better in lowering cholesterol. These experiments were hardly definitive: a series of two- to nine-week tests involving a total of only sixty-six people.* And Keys would soon change his mind about the findings. Nonetheless, in a style that foreshadowed how Keys would rise to the apex of the nutrition world, he promoted these tentative early results as if there were already little room for doubt: "No other variable in the mode of life besides the fat calories in the diet is known which shows anything like such a consistent relationship to the mortality rate from coronary or degenerative heart disease," he told his colleagues at a gathering to discuss atherosclerosis in 1954.

Keys confidently drew a direct line of causation from fat in the diet to serum cholesterol in the blood to heart disease. In a 1952 presentation at Mt. Sinai in New York (later published in a paper that received enormous attention), Keys formally introduced this idea, which he called his "diet-heart hypothesis." His graph showed a close correlation between fat intake and death rates from heart disease in six countries.†

It was a perfect upward curve, like a child's growth chart. Keys's graph

---

*In a deviation from normal scientific standards, Keys did not report details of these trials, such as the number of men involved and the duration of each intervention.

†The other argument that Keys presented for his diet-heart hypothesis in these early years was that *trends* in the consumption of dietary fat seemed to mirror the growing heart disease epidemics in Germany, Norway, and the United States.

suggested that if you extended the curve back down to zero fat intake, your risk of heart disease would nearly disappear.

This connect-the-dot exercise in 1952 was the acorn that grew into the giant oak tree of our mistrust of fat today. All of the ailments that have been ascribed to eating fat over the years—not just heart disease but also obesity, cancer, diabetes, and more—stem from the implantation of this idea in the nutrition establishment by Ancel Keys and his perseverance in promoting it. Now, as you eat a salad with a lean chicken breast for lunch and choose pasta over steak for dinner, those choices can be traced back to him. The influence of Keys on the world of nutrition has been unparalleled.

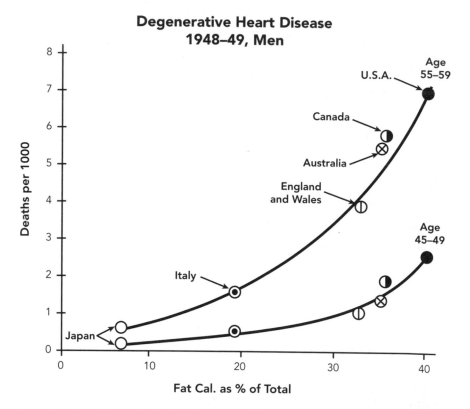

Keys's 1952 Chart:

Fat Calories vs. Deaths from Degenerative Heart Disease

Source: Ancel Keys, "Atherosclerosis: A Problem in Newer Public Health," *Journal of Mt. Sinai Hospital, New York* 20, no. 2 (July–Aug 1953): 134.

The 1952 chart that Keys used to promote his idea that dietary fat causes heart disease

Does Fat Make You Fat?

In addition to causing atherosclerosis, Keys thought that fat must *make* people fat. Because fat contains a little more than 9 calories per gram, whereas protein and carbohydrates contain only about 4 calories per gram, nutrition experts have long reasoned that a low-fat diet enables weight loss due to its reduced calorie content.* In other words, if we *eat* fat, we will *be* fat.

Probably no one has explained this prevailing attitude about fat better than Jerry Seinfeld when he described being in a supermarket. "You're looking at the label "Fat content. . . . People just see Fat Content. It has *fa-a-a-t*! There's *fat* in it. It's gonna be in *meeeee*!"

Has there ever been a more unfortunate homonym? One word means two very different things: the fat we eat and the fat on our bodies. It's so hard for our brains to fully grasp that there are two entirely separate definitions of fat. A lurking fear of dietary fat as fattening goes back to the 1920s in America, as staying slender was an important part of new middle-class fashions and lifestyles; also, life insurance companies started basing their premiums on people's height and weight. Cutting back on calories was one of several competing theories at this time about how people should lose weight, and since fat packed more calories, many doctors advised their patients to cut back on this part of the diet. Since then, fat in all forms has simply come to be commonly understood as something to be avoided. A large number of experiments have since confirmed that restricting fat does nothing to slim people down (quite the reverse, actually), yet even so, the idea that there could be such a thing as a "slimming fat" will probably always seem to us like an oxymoron.

Regarding dietary fat and heart disease, Keys recognized early on that international examples posed a serious threat to his hypothesis. His early papers devoted a good deal of space to arguing against evidence coming in from around the world that wasn't doing his hypothesis any favors: the

---

*Keys was never concerned about obesity, however, and thought it was unrelated to the development of heart disease, although this link has since proven to be quite strong (Keys in *Symposium on Atherosclerosis*, 1954, 182–184).

Masai in Africa, the Eskimos in the Arctic, even the Navajo Indians in his own country. He had preliminary reports from a few countries such as Finland and Japan where the data *did* seem to be in line with his ideas. And one of his early strokes of genius was to realize that this kind of international evidence could be powerfully employed to support his ideas. Thus, while his rivals toiled in academic labs, Keys found a way to go adventuring and would bring back an impressive sweep of global data.

Keys began taking trips all over the world in the early 1950s. He and his wife, Margaret, traveled to South Africa, Sardinia, Sweden, Spain, and Italy, and everywhere they went, they measured the locals' cholesterol while assessing the fat content of their diets. The couple visited a remote logging camp in Finland, where heart disease was rampant among young men. In Japan, they measured the cholesterol levels of rural fisherman and farmers, and they did the same for Japanese immigrants living in Honolulu and Los Angeles.

Keys was particularly fascinated by the countries around the Mediterranean, because he heard that heart disease rates in the region were exceptionally low, and in 1953, he traveled first to Naples and then to Madrid to find out for himself. After measuring serum cholesterol levels and performing electrocardiographs on a small sample of men, he concluded that the general population in these cities did, indeed, have rates of heart disease far lower than those typically found in the United States. More broadly, Keys speculated that because rates of coronary mortality varied so much by country, the disease could not be attributed to genetics, or even the natural process of aging. It must instead be due to diet, Keys decided. Mann would later draw the same conclusion based on his observations of Masai warriors, but Keys had very different ideas about what part of the diet was to blame: "only the factor of fat appears important so far," he wrote.

The plaque-riddled state of American arteries was "dominated by the long-time effects of a rich fatty diet, and innumerable fat-loading meals," said Keys in 1957. As proof, he pointed to the young Finnish loggers, who snacked on "slabs of cheese the size of a slice of bread on which they smeared butter . . . and they washed it down with beer. It was an object lesson for the coronary problem."

Although he had observed only a small number of men on these early travels and had no particular method for measuring their diets, Keys wrote with assurance that total fat was "clearly" a "major factor" in the development of heart disease. This was, of course, what he had been looking for, so it is perhaps predictable that it is what he found.

On his travels, Keys made professional alliances worldwide and persuaded researchers to test his idea. These colleagues subsequently collected data from South Africa to Sweden, and all the evidence they accumulated appeared to confirm his hypothesis that high-fat diets and relatively high serum cholesterol went hand in hand. Again, the numbers of people observed were minuscule, but Keys deftly knit together these skimpy data from far and wide into a picture that looked convincing.

Keys found further ammunition for his hypothesis from a compelling observation made during World War II, which is that deaths from heart disease dropped dramatically across Europe during wartime and rebounded soon afterward. These events led Keys to presume that the food shortages—particularly of meat, eggs, and dairy—were very likely the cause. There were, however, other explanations: for instance, sugar and flour were also scarce during the war; people breathed fewer car-exhaust fumes due to gasoline shortages and got more exercise by cycling or walking to get around. Other scientists noted these alternative explanations for the decline in heart disease, but Keys dismissed them outright.

By the mid-1950s, Keys was beginning to back away from his idea that *total* fat was the principal cause of heart disease, although he didn't acknowledge this explicitly. Instead, his papers start talking more about the *type* of dietary fat as the critical factor in raising cholesterol. Keys came to this conclusion after conducting a few small, short-term experiments on those same schizophrenic patients at a Minnesota hospital in 1957 and 1958. He found that serum cholesterol would go up after the men ate saturated fat and down after the vegetable oils, just as Ahrens and others had found earlier.

Thus, as Keys announced in a cluster of papers in top medical journals in 1957,* total serum cholesterol could be reduced by cutting back on

---

*Keys asserted these claims in no fewer than twenty papers in top scientific journals in 1957 and 1958.

saturated fats. Keys was quite sure of his new findings—so much so that he published a specific mathematical formula by which he claimed the *exact* amount that serum cholesterol could be calculated to rise or fall in a population, depending upon the amount of saturated fat, polyunsaturated fat, and cholesterol eaten. This was the famous "Keys equation," which gained enormous influence in the nutrition research community, probably because it was a relief for people looking for answers to have a just-so formula for the mass of humanity. Unlike Ahrens, who urged his colleagues to be modest about their knowledge in the face of the enormous complexity of human biology (and who, as we've seen, ultimately argued for the *diversity* of biological reactions), Keys reduced this complexity to a sure and confident explanation. He still believed that people shouldn't eat too much fat *overall*, but once he landed upon the idea that saturated fat was the real dietary evil, he began advocating for this theory above all others. If people just stopped eating eggs, dairy products, meats, and all visible fats, he argued, heart disease would "become very rare." Keys advised a "sharp reduction" in dietary fats, especially those naturally occurring in animal foods—and a switch to vegetable oils instead.

The Polyunsaturated President: Eisenhower's Heart Attack

Keys's ideas were thrust into the national spotlight on September 23, 1955, when President Dwight D. Eisenhower suffered the first of several heart attacks. The president's personal doctor, Paul Dudley White, flew to his bedside in Denver, Colorado. White, a cardiologist, was one of the original observers of the heart disease epidemic as it was starting up in the early 1900s. He wrote a classic 1931 textbook on the disease and was one of six founders of the AHA. He had also worked closely with President Harry Truman to set up the National Heart Institute (NHI) as part of the National Institutes of Health (NIH) in 1948. Now a renowned Harvard professor, White's influence in the field was nearly boundless.

Keys had long shown a talent for cultivating powerful people; to win the job of developing those famous K rations, for instance, he had secured an appointment, from 1939 to 1943, as a special assistant to the secretary of defense. White was another clearly desirable ally, and in recent years Keys had persuaded him to come along on some of his and Margaret's international travels to measure fat and cholesterol. No doubt it was during those trips—to Hawaii, Japan, Russia, and Italy—that White began to be persuaded by Keys's ideas.

The day after Eisenhower's heart attack, White held a press conference and gave the American public a clear and authoritative lecture on heart disease as well as the preventative steps that could be taken to avoid it: stop smoking, reduce stress, and on the dietary front, cut down on saturated fat and cholesterol. In the following months, White continued to report to the nation on the president's health at press conferences and in the pages of the *New York Times*. In a front page *Times* article that White was allowed to guest write, Keys is the only researcher he mentions by name (calling his work "brilliant"), and his is the only dietary theory that is quoted at length. If a middle-aged American man learned nothing else from the entire presidential episode, it was that the country's top doctors believed the public should cut back on dietary fat. Eisenhower himself became obsessed with his blood-cholesterol levels and religiously avoided foods with saturated fat; he switched to a polyunsaturated margarine, which came on the market in 1958, and ate melba toast for breakfast—until he died of heart disease in 1969.*

Keys, meanwhile, was busy promoting his graph and other data apparently showing the link between deaths from heart disease and fat consumption to scientific audiences around the world. A "rich fatty diet, and innumerable fat-loading meals" were the "probable" cause for the development of coronary disease in the "majority of cases," he wrote in 1957.

Keys had developed a sizable following among his nutrition colleagues, yet at least one scientist in his audience, Jacob Yerushalmy, was not impressed. Yerushalmy was the founder of the Biostatistics Department at the University of California, Berkeley; he saw Keys speak at a World Health Organization (WHO) conference in Geneva in 1955. Yerushalmy thought that the data seemed a little fishy. Right there in Geneva, for instance, the

---

*Eisenhower was a four-pack-a-day cigarette smoker, which might have contributed to his heart disease, although he had stopped five years before his first heart attack.

local population consumed a great deal of fat—animal fat—but did not die from heart disease very often. Like the so-called French paradox (those surprisingly healthy omelet eaters), one could also observe a Swiss paradox. In fact, if you looked at all the twenty-two countries for which national data were available in 1955, such "paradoxes" existed also for West Germany, Sweden, Norway, and Denmark; clearly these were not paradoxes but data points demanding an alternative explanation.

Yerushalmy and Hilleboe: Data from Twenty-Two Countries

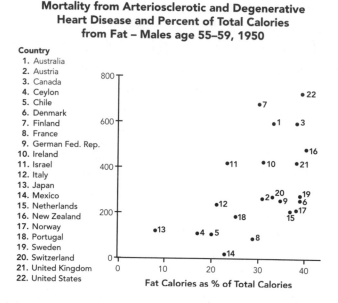

Mortality from Arteriosclerotic and Degenerative Heart Disease and Percent of Total Calories from Fat – Males age 55–59, 1950

Country
1. Australia
2. Austria
3. Canada
4. Ceylon
5. Chile
6. Denmark
7. Finland
8. France
9. German Fed. Rep.
10. Ireland
11. Israel
12. Italy
13. Japan
14. Mexico
15. Netherlands
16. New Zealand
17. Norway
18. Portugal
19. Sweden
20. Switzerland
21. United Kingdom
22. United States

Fat Calories as % of Total Calories

Source: Yerushalmy, J. and Herman E. Hilleboe, "Fat in the Diet and Mortality from Heart Disease: A Methodologic Note," *New York State Journal of Medicine* 57, no. 14 (July 1957): 2346.

Chart by critics of Keys showed *no* correlation of dietary fat with heart disease, when more countries beyond Keys's original six were added

Yerushalmy's objection was that Keys seemed to have selected only certain countries that fit his hypothesis. There were other factors that could equally well explain the trends in heart disease in all these countries, he asserted. In a 1957 paper, Yerushalmy listed some of them: the number of cars sold per capita, number of cigarettes sold, consumption of protein, and consumption of sugar. These were all associated with one common factor: wealth. So anything that accompanied a growing midcentury prosperity, including meat, sugar, car exhaust, and margarine, could be causing heart disease. As for fat, when Yerushalmy and his colleague, Herman E. Hilleboe, plotted the data for all twenty-two countries instead of just the six that Keys had selected, they observed that his correlation nearly disappeared. Only a random Jackson Pollock–like splatter of data points was left. That mess of data points did not go over so well with Keys.

"I remember the mood in the lab when that study came out," said Henry Blackburn, Keys's longtime right-hand man, who was retired from the University of Minnesota when I interviewed him.

"The mood. . . . Not good?" I asked.

"Mmmmm," said Blackburn. A long pause.*

By now, Keys had a number of critics, including George V. Mann, who would conduct the work on the Masai. Mann wrote of his hope that this confrontation with Yerushalmy would be a "crushing blow" to Keys's theory on fat and heart disease. But Keys came back swinging. He responded, in the *Journal of Chronic Diseases*, that Yerushalmy and Hilleboe's data were deeply flawed because national statistics were unreliable, and especially those collected by European governments during the volatile, postwar period. Too true! Even without a war raging, there are enormous differences among countries in how often doctors will write down "heart disease" as the cause on a death certificate. Such variations have always cast a great deal of doubt on these sorts of international comparisons. Just one example is an investigation from 1964, which found that American doctors, when presented with exactly the same health records as European doctors, diagnosed heart disease 33 percent more often than did British

---

*Blackburn later claimed that Yerushalmy and other critics had unfairly singled out this six-country chart from the evidence Keys presented to support his theory. However, in 1957, when Yerushalmy published his critique, the only evidence Keys had provided were observations about reduced rates of heart disease in Europe during World War II (which had other possible causes) and some unpublished data collected on the Finns and the Japanese. Rather than further substantiating his theory in the main 1957 paper in which he makes the case for his hypothesis, Keys instead devotes several pages to attacking theories that competed with his own, such as the possibility that protein, lack of exercise, or dietary cholesterol caused heart disease (Blackburn and Labarthe 2012, 1072; Keys 1957, 552–559).

doctors and 50 percent more often than Norwegian doctors. Keys was fully aware of this problem, but it didn't stop him from using the very same national statistics for his own charts, since, flawed or no, there were no other data available. However, at the time, no one questioned him on this double standard.

In his retort to Hilleboe, Keys also accused him of being biased in favor of "negative versus positive conclusions." "I doubt that Dr. Hilleboe really believes he has adequate evidence to state that there is *not* a causal relationship between dietary fat and the tendency to develop atherosclerosis in man," wrote Keys.

In other words, Keys wanted his hypothesis to be presumed right until proven wrong. Yet—and this is an important point—science is not like the justice system. Whereas Americans are presumed to be innocent until proven guilty, scientific knowledge is just the opposite: a hypothesis must not be presumed right until a pile of significant evidence grows up behind it, and even then, you can never be entirely sure. All that one can ever really say is that the preponderance of the evidence tends to support one idea over another. Keys's unwavering belief in his own hypothesis, even in its formative stages and even in the face of conflicting evidence, however, suggests he was willing to stray from these scientific principles to defend it.

In any case, it seems clear that the skeptical response by Keys's colleagues to his presentation at the 1955 World Health Organization conference in Geneva represented a humiliating but important moment for him: "*the* pivotal moment in Keys life," remembers Blackburn. After the confrontation in Geneva, "[Keys] got up from being knocked around and said, 'I'll show those guys' . . . and he designed the Seven Countries study."

The Seven Countries Study

Unlike the earlier international sampling that Keys had done on his travels with Margaret, the Seven Countries study was the first multicountry epidemiological undertaking in human history.* By standardizing the data

---

*In epidemiological, or "observational," studies, a group of subjects is profiled (their diets and smoking habits are measured, for instance), and investigators then watch

NINA TEICHOLZ

collection and using on-the-ground surveys of sample populations, Keys aimed to amass accurate and detailed data that could be compared across nations—unlike those slippery national statistics—and thus settle the debate about diet and coronary disease once and for all.

Keys launched the study in 1956 with an annual grant from the US Public Health Service of $200,000, then an enormous sum of money for a single project. He planned to follow in detail some 12,700 middle-aged men in mostly rural populations in Italy, Greece, Yugoslavia, Finland, the Netherlands, Japan, and the United States.

A number of critics have since pointed out that had Keys taken the critiques of Yerushalmy to heart, he might have selected a European country to *challenge* his fat hypothesis, like Switzerland or France (or Germany or Norway or Sweden). Instead, he chose only those nations (based on national statistics) that seemed likely to confirm it.

Since the early twentieth century, investigators have known the importance of avoiding bias on the part of the investigators by selecting subjects in a random way. This is called "randomization," and researchers follow protocols to achieve a random sampling. But Keys's selection criteria could not be called random; instead, as he wrote, he chose places that he thought showed some contrast in rates of diet and death, and even more importantly, places "where he found enthusiastic help," meaning both people and resources, to conduct the study, as Blackburn described to me. Attempting to explain why Keys did not seek out countries that would offer more challenges to his ideas, Blackburn said, "Keys just had a personal aversion to being in France and Switzerland."

The historical period of the Seven Countries study was also a problem. The years that it encompassed, from 1958 to 1964, were a time of transition in the Mediterranean region: Greece, Italy, and Yugoslavia were still recovering from World War II, which had brought about extreme poverty

them over a period of time. Older subjects are preferable, so that health outcomes such as heart attacks, cancer, or death can be observed without having to wait too long. These outcomes are then correlated to the variables originally measured, allowing researchers to see if there might be an association between, say, smoking and lung cancer.

and near-starvation, and Italy was also emerging from twenty-five years of suffering under a fascist government. Hardship led four million Italians to flee their country, and at least 150,000 Greeks to leave theirs.

These are facts that should give a researcher pause. Keys might have asked himself whether, in dipping into Europe of the 1960s, he might be getting an anomalous picture. The people he studied were in a moment of deprivation. They would have eaten a richer diet in childhood before the war, as would have their mothers during pregnancy. Since some researchers believe that the tendrils of heart disease might be laid down in the womb or are an accumulation of lifelong habits, then a 1960s' sampling was indeed a risky thing. It was clearly not reflective of a larger reality.

Within the limitations of these questionable choices, however, the study aimed for the highest possible standards. In the countries that Keys chose, his teams of researchers visited rural villages and selected middle-aged male laborers. They measured body weight, blood pressure, and cholesterol levels in addition to surveying the men about diet and smoking habits. For a small subset of these men, samples of the food they ate over the course of a week were collected and sent to labs for chemical analysis.

The Seven Countries study results first appeared in a 211-page monograph published by the AHA in 1970, followed by a book from Harvard University Press. Seven books and more than six hundred articles by the various members of the original study team followed. By 2004, according to one tally, there had been close to one million references to the Seven Countries study in the medical literature.

What Keys found, as he had hoped, was a strong correlation between the consumption of saturated fat and deaths from heart disease. In North Karelia, Finland, where the men worked hard as lumberjacks and farmers yet ate a daily diet high in dairy products and meat, deaths from heart disease were high: 992 men per 10,000 over the course of a decade. On Crete and Corfu, with plenty of olive oil and very little meat, the number was ridiculously low at 9. In Italy, the number was 290. Among railroad workers in the United States, it was 570.

Because Keys had carefully standardized the diagnoses of heart attacks and other manifestations of coronary disease across countries, one of the great accomplishments of his Seven Countries data was simply to demonstrate that people living in different nations really did suffer vastly different rates of heart attacks. For this reason, says Blackburn, the study was the first to demonstrate that "heart attacks might be prevented . . . that they were not a natural aging phenomenon, or genetically predetermined or acts of God."

The results seemed to show that although Finnish lumberjacks and Greek farmers were eating roughly the same total amount of fat, it was the *type* of fat that mattered. The more saturated fat one ate, according to the results, the greater the risk of having a heart attack. Saturated fat comprised only 8 percent of calories eaten by the Cretans, compared to 22 percent for the Finns. These findings appeared conclusive and seemed to offer a definitive answer to Keys's critics.

Or did they? Despite the celebrated results, there were some vexing problems with data points that failed to support his hypothesis. For instance, the Eastern Finns died of heart disease at rates more than three times higher than the Western Finns, yet their lifestyles and diets, according to Keys's data, were virtually identical. The islanders of Corfu ate even less saturated fat than did their countrymen on Crete, yet on Corfu rates of heart disease were far higher. Thus, within countries, the correlation between saturated fat and heart disease didn't hold up at all.

Fifteen years later, in 1984, Keys followed up with these populations in all seven countries and found that the outcomes had become even more paradoxical. By then the consumption of saturated fat could no longer explain differences in heart disease rates at all. And now, because heart disease accounted for only a third of all deaths, Keys took the logical step of looking at all causes of death, not just those from heart disease. After all, isn't this ultimately what we want to know? Not just what we can do to avoid a heart attack but what we can do to live longer? (If a low-fat diet spares people from heart disease but instead gives them cancer, for instance, then what's the point?)

Frustratingly for Keys, the data from the Seven Countries study showed that although a diet low in saturated fat appeared to be associated with fewer deaths from heart disease (within those countries, at least), that advantage did not extend to total mortality. People eating diets low in saturated fat had just as high a risk of dying as their fat-gorging counterparts.

The animal food minimalists simply died of other causes. In the study, the people who survived the longest overall lived in Greece and the United States, and their longevity showed no relationship to the amounts of fat or saturated fat they ate, nor to the cholesterol levels in their blood.

The nutritional data did not quite hold up, either. If you read Keys's study design very closely, you find that, of the 12,770 participants, the food they ate was evaluated for only 499 of them, or 3.9 percent. And there was no consistency among nations as to how the nutritional data were collected: in the United States, a one-day record sample was taken for 1.5 percent of the men, whereas in other nations, data were collected for up to seven days. Some food samples were collected cooked, some before they were cooked, some a mixture of the two.

I looked more closely into the dietary data on Greece, because it became the exemplar for the Mediterranean diet (see Chapter 7), and I found one of the most stunning and troubling errors. In that country, Keys had sampled the diets on Crete and Corfu more than once, in different seasons, in order to capture variations in the food eaten. Yet in an astonishing oversight, one of the three surveys on Crete fell during the forty-eight-day fasting period of Lent. How would this have affected the diet? "The Greek Orthodox fast is a strict one and means abstaining from all foods of animal origin, including fish, cheese, eggs and butter," wrote a contemporary observer. (In Italy, the expression "pari corajisima" (he/she looks like Lent) has long referred to a person who is ugly, unpleasant, and thin from malnourishment.) Since the foods avoided during Lent are the principal sources of saturated fat, a sampling of the diet during this holiday would obviously undercount that nutrient. A study conducted on Crete in 2000 and 2001 showed that saturated-fat consumption *halved* during Lent.

Keys did mention this problem in his monograph but immediately excused it, saying that "strict adherence [to Lent] did not seem to be common." He gave no further details and made no mention of the issue at all in his main paper on the Greek diet. Later, when two researchers from the University of Crete tracked down the original directors of the Greek section of the Seven Countries study, they were told that 60 percent of the study population in Crete was fasting during the survey, although "no attempt was made" in the study to differentiate between fasters and non-fasters. This was "a remarkable and troublesome omission," the researchers wrote in *Public Health Nutrition* in 2005, but that was forty years too late to correct the study's original impressions.

Surprised and alarmed by this discovery, I called up Daan Kromhout, who directed the nutritional component of the Seven Countries study. He is now a professor of public health research in the Netherlands and also serves as a senior advisor to his government on health policy. He was clearly somewhat chagrined about this Lent oversight but emphasized how little was known about food sampling at the time and how blindly they were groping forward in this entirely new field. "In an ideal situation, we should not have done that," he acknowledged. "But you can't do the ideal thing all the time." And this explanation would seem fair enough had not the Cretan data ended up being the cornerstone of our dietary advice for the past half-century.

Keys did not seem eager to report on his dietary data at all, and, indeed, I had trouble tracking down some of it. He published most of the data in a Dutch journal, *Voeding,* where he knew it would go unnoticed,* not in one of the mainstream British or American publications where he published most of his other Seven Countries papers. And one has to read between the lines to get a sense of all the many technical difficulties Keys encountered. In Greece alone, three different chemical methods were used to analyze fats in the food samples, and their results did not line up. ("It was not possible to make sure which system provided the most accurate results," as he put it.)

Yet in the Seven Countries report itself there is no indication that the data might be flawed in any way, and overall, it has been given a pass by researchers in the field for decades. When I tracked down papers, it became clear to me that Keys, in his ambition for the study, had done everything he could to bury its problems—problems so significant that had they been

---

*Keys wrote of his frustration regarding an earlier paper that he had published in *Voeding,* which got "no international attention," he said, because the journal, though respectable, had "very little circulation outside the Netherlands and even there [was] primarily read by nutritionists" (Keys in Kromhout, Menotti, and Blackburn 1994, 17).

known at the time, the Seven Countries study might never have been published.

Beyond these data issues, there was also a huge structural limitation to the Seven Countries study: it was an epidemiological investigation and therefore could show only an association, not causation. In other words, it could show that the two elements occurred together, but it could not establish any causal connection. Keys's study could, therefore, at the very best establish an *association* between a diet low in animal fats and minimal rates of heart disease; it could say nothing about whether that diet *caused* people to be spared the disease. Other aspects of diet and lifestyle also correlated with the low rates of heart disease seen in Keys's study, and these could not be ruled out as causes.

Sugar: An Alternative Explanation?

In 1999, when the Seven Countries study's lead Italian researcher, Alessandro Menotti, went back twenty-five years later and looked at data from the study's 12,770 subjects, he noticed an interesting fact: the category of foods that best correlated with coronary mortality was sweets. By "sweets," he meant sugar products and pastries, which had a correlation coefficient with coronary mortality of 0.821 (a perfect correlation is 1.0). Possibly this number would have been higher had Menotti included chocolate, ice cream, and soft drinks in his "sweets" category, but those fell under a different category and, he explained, would have been "too troublesome" to recode. By contrast, "animal food" (butter, meat, eggs, margarine, lard, milk, and cheese) had a correlation coefficient of 0.798, and this number likely would have been lower had Menotti excluded margarine. (Margarine is usually made from vegetable fats, but researchers at the time tended to lump it in with animal foods because it looked so much like butter.)

Ancel Keys was alert to the idea that sugar might be an alternative dietary explanation to his own as a cause of heart disease. From the late 1950s to the early 1970s, he held an ongoing debate in the scientific literature with John Yudkin, a professor of physiology at Queen Elizabeth College, London University, who at the time was *the* man behind the sugar hypothesis. "Keys was very opposed to the sugar idea," Daan Kromhout recalled in an interview, though he could not say why. Philosophers of science would say that the job of a scientist is to be as skeptical as possible about his or her own ideas, but Keys was evidently just the opposite. "He was so convinced that fatty acids were *the* thing in relation to atherosclerosis, he saw everything from that perspective," says Kromhout. "He was a very driven person and had his own point of view." About the views of others, Keys could be aggressively disparaging: Yudkin's idea that sugar causes heart disease is a "mountain of nonsense," he concluded at the end of a nine-page critique in *Atherosclerosis*. "Yudkin and his commercial backers are not deterred by the facts; they continue to sing the same discredited tune," he wrote later.

Keys specifically defended his Seven Countries study from the idea that sugar might explain some of the mortality differences he observed. In response to a letter by a Swedish researcher who raised the question in 1971, Keys ran some regression analyses showing that fat intake alone correlated perfectly with the variation in heart disease; sugar had no additional impact. But he did not run the reverse calculation, asking whether sugar alone had the same correlation (as Menotti later did). Keys published his numbers in a letter, not an article (which would have been peer-reviewed), and he did not provide the raw numbers, so his calculations could not be checked by others.

"Sugar was never discussed properly among us [Seven Countries study research leaders]," Menotti told me. "We didn't know how to treat it. We reported the facts and had some difficulty explaining our findings."

Was it the sugar or was it the fat? Even if diet could be precisely assessed, an epidemiologist can never know if a particular food or something else entirely might be the cause of heart disease observed many years later. The science of epidemiology was invented to study infectious diseases, which come on suddenly and can usually be traced back to a source, such as the water supply. Chronic diseases, by contrast, evolve over a much longer period of time, and it's just about impossible to measure the many thousands of factors over the course of a person's life that might contribute to a condition decades later. Epidemiology's single greatest success in solving a riddle of chronic disease was the discovery that cigarettes caused lung cancer. In that case, however, the difference between smoking and nonsmoking populations was huge: thirtyfold, whereas with saturated fats, Keys was observing only a twofold difference.* Also, the effect that Keys saw did not rise in lockstep with the gradual increase in saturated-fat consumption, which was another warning sign that his evidence was weak, since epidemiologists consider this kind of "dose-response relationship" to be crucially important in establishing reliable associations.

Despite these types of problems that routinely afflict nutritional epidemiology, decision-makers have nevertheless often used these findings as "proof," simply because they are often the only kind of data available. Clinical trials, which could establish *cause*, are far more complicated and expensive undertakings and are therefore conducted much less frequently. In the absence of trial data, as we'll see again and again over the last 50 years of nutrition history, epidemiological evidence has therefore been made to suffice. Even though it cannot, by its very nature, make claims about causation, it has repeatedly been employed in just this way. This practice of using epidemiological data as a basis for official dietary guidelines was pioneered by Keys himself. And it's not hard to understand the motivation. After a researcher has followed a population for ten to fifteen years, one can only imagine the desire to maximize the impact of one's findings in the arena of public health and, upon these laurels, win the acclaim and further funding for research that usually follow.

Keys, one of the original nutrition epidemiologists, was understandably keen for this acclaim. Burying any concerns about his data or its inherent limitations, Keys aggressively drove home his study's main "takeaway" point, that eating saturated fat leads to high cholesterol and that high cholesterol leads to heart disease. Now, with the Seven Countries study ostensibly supporting his claims, Keys could defend his idea even more commandingly. As *Time* magazine reported a Philadelphia physician saying, "Every time you question this man Keys, he says, 'I've got 5,000 cases. How many do you have?' " Scientists at the time knew, of course,

---

*These differences are expressed by epidemiologists as the "effect size," and very low numbers such as those Keys found continue to be the norm in most of the epidemiological findings on nutrition published today, including the alarming findings in 2012 linking red meat to chronic disease (Pan et al. 2012).

that an association did not prove causation, but the sheer magnitude of data amassed in Keys's study, especially in a field where so little research had yet been done, granted him an unusual degree of stature, and he did not hesitate in reaping the benefits of that special status.

It's not that no one questioned Keys along the way, of course. There were plenty of skeptics, including esteemed, influential scientists. Remember that Swedish egg-eating doctor, Uffe Ravnskov? On my own travels through the world of nutrition as I researched this book, he was the first "skeptic" I met. Whereas once a large and prominent group of scientists had opposed Keys and his hypothesis, the great majority of them had disappeared by the late 1980s. Ravnskov picked up their torch later, with the publication of a book called *Cholesterol Myths* in 2000.

At a conference that we were both attending near Copenhagen in 2005, he stood out in the crowd simply because he was willing to confront this gathering of top nutrition experts by asking questions that were considered long since settled.

"The whole pathway, from cholesterol in the diet, to cholesterol in the blood, to heart disease—has this pathway really been proven?" he stood up and asked, rightly though rhetorically, after a presentation one day.

"Tsh! Tsh! Tsh!" A hundred-plus scientists wagged their heads in unison.

"Next question?" asked an irritated moderator.

The incident illustrated, for me, the most remarkable aspect of the nutrition research community, namely its surprising lack of oxygen for alternative viewpoints. When I started out my research, I expected to find a community of scientists in decorous debate. Instead, I found researchers like Ravnskov, who, by his own admission, was a cautionary tale for independently minded scientists seeking to challenge the conventional wisdom. His predecessors from the 1960s onward hadn't been convinced by the orthodoxy on cholesterol; they'd just been silenced, worn out, or had come to the end of their careers. As Keys's ideas spread and became adopted by powerful institutions, those who challenged him faced a difficult—some might say impossible—battle. Being on the losing side of such a high-stakes debate had caused their professional lives to suffer. Many of them had lost jobs, research funding, speaking engagements, and all the many other perks of prestige. Although these diet-heart opponents included a number of researchers who were at the top of their fields, including, notably, an editor of the *Journal of the American Medical Association*, they were not invited to conferences and were unable to get prestigious journals to publish their work.* Experiments that had dissenting results, they found, were not debated and discussed but instead dismissed or ignored altogether. Even being subject to slander and personal ridicule were surprisingly not unusual experiences for these opponents of the diet-heart hypothesis. In short, they found themselves unable to continue contributing to their fields, which of course is the very essence of every scientist's hopes and ambitions.

To a surprising degree, in fact, the story of nutritional science is not, as we would expect, one of sober-minded researchers moving with measured, judicious steps. It falls, instead, under the "Great Man" theory of history, whereby strong personalities steer events using their own personal charisma, intelligence, wisdom, or wits. In the history of nutrition, Ancel Keys was, by far, the Greatest Man.

---

*The former editor of the *Journal of the American Medical Association* was Edward R. Pinckney, whose 1973 book, *The Cholesterol Controversy*, was followed in 1988 by a groundbreaking scientific critique of the evidence used to support the diet-heart hypothesis. This second effort is still the most thorough critical review of that science ever written, but he could not find a publisher (Pinckney and Pinckney 1973; Smith and Pinckney 1988).

NINA TEICHOLZ

3

The Low-Fat Diet Is
Introduced to America

The year 1961 was an important one for Ancel Keys and his diet-heart hypothesis. He managed three significant coups: one within the American Heart Association, the most powerful heart disease group in US history; another on the cover of *Time* magazine, the most influential magazine of its day; and the third at the National Institutes of Health, which was not only the leading scientific authority in the land but also the richest source of research funds. These three groups were the most important actors in the world of nutrition, and as a bias in favor of the diet-heart hypothesis settled in among them, they operated like a tag team, institutionalizing Keys's ideas and conveying them onward and upward for decades to come.

The AHA alone was like an ocean liner steaming the diet-heart hypothesis forward. Founded in 1924 at the outset of the heart disease epidemic, the group was a scientific society of cardiologists seeking to better understand this new affliction. For decades, the AHA was small and underfunded, with virtually no income. Then, in 1948, it got lucky: Procter & Gamble (P&G) designated the group to receive all the funds from its "Truth or Consequences" contest on the radio, raising $1,740,000, or $17 million in today's dollars. At a luncheon, P&G executives presented a check to the AHA president, and "suddenly the coffers were filled and there were funds available for research, public health progress and development of local groups—all the stuff that dreams are made of!" according to the AHA's official history. The P&G check was the "bang of big bucks" that "launched" the group. Indeed, one year later the group opened seven chapters across the country and collected $2,650,000 from donations. By 1960, it had more than three hundred chapters and brought in more than $30 million annually. With continued support from P&G and other food giants, the AHA would soon become the premiere heart disease group in the United States, as well as the largest not for profit group of any kind in the country.

The new funds in 1948 allowed the group to hire its first professional director, a former fund-raiser for the American Bible Society, who unfolded an unprecedented fund-raising campaign across the United States. There were variety shows, fashion shows, quiz programs, auctions, and collections at movie theaters, all meant to raise money and let Americans know that heart disease was the country's number one killer. By 1960, the AHA was investing hundreds of millions of dollars in research. The group had become the authoritative source of information about heart disease for the public, government agencies, and professionals alike, including the media.

Because diet was considered a probable cause of heart disease, the AHA in the late 1950s pulled together a committee of experts to develop some advice about what a middle-aged man ought to eat as a measure of defense. President Eisenhower was already following a "prudent" diet to battle his condition under the supervision of AHA founder Paul Dudley White. The fact that White's care had allowed Eisenhower to get back to work in the Oval Office was itself of great significance to the AHA, since it showed that the group had advice worth following. It helped, too, with fund-raising: after Eisenhower's heart attack, the AHA took in 40 percent more in donations than it did the year before.*

---

*Eisenhower was extremely supportive of the AHA throughout his presidency: he presented the AHA's annual "Heart of the Year Award" from the Oval Office, held opening ceremonies for the AHA's "Heart Fund Campaign" in the White House, attended AHA board meetings, and assumed the AHA post of Honorary Chairman of

NINA TEICHOLZ

The newly formed AHA nutrition committee acknowledged that the average doctor faced a great deal of pressure to *do* something: "People want to know whether they are eating themselves into premature heart disease," the committee wrote. It nevertheless resisted this pressure and published a cautious report. The evidence, it stated, could not even reliably say whether high cholesterol in any given person would predictably lead to a heart attack, so it was too soon to be telling Americans to make any "drastic" dietary change toward this end. (The committee did, however, recommend reducing fat to between 25 percent and 30 percent of calories for people who were overweight because this would be a good way to cut calories.) Committee members went so far as to rap diet-heart supporters like Keys on the knuckles for taking "uncompromising stands based on evidence that does not stand up under critical examination." The evidence, they concluded, did not permit such a "rigid stand." *

However, a significant shift in AHA policy came a few years later, when Keys, together with Jeremiah Stamler, a doctor from Chicago who became his ally, maneuvered themselves onto the nutrition committee. Although some critics noted that neither Keys nor Stamler had been trained in nutrition science, epidemiology, or cardiology, and although the evidence for Keys's ideas had not grown any stronger since the AHA's previous position paper on nutrition, the two men managed to convince their fellow committee members that the diet-heart hypothesis should prevail. The AHA committee swung around in favor of their ideas, and the resulting report in 1961 argued that "the best scientific evidence available at the present time" suggested that Americans could reduce their risk of heart attacks and strokes by cutting the saturated fat and cholesterol in their diets.

The report also recommended the "reasonable substitution" of saturated fat with polyunsaturated fats such as corn or soybean oil. This so-called "prudent diet" was still relatively high in fat overall. In fact, the

the Future. Members of his cabinet also served on the AHA board. The AHA's official historian concludes, "Thus, the top leaders of the United States government were active Heart campaigners" (Moore 1983, 85).
*Other theories at the time that mainstream scientists seriously considered as the cause of heart disease included vitamin B_6 deficiency, obesity, lack of exercise, high blood pressure, and nervous strain (Mann 1959, 922).

AHA would not stress the reduction of total fat until 1970, when Jerry Stamler steered the group in this direction. For the first decade, however, the group's focus was primarily on reducing the consumption of the *saturated* fats found in meat, cheese, whole milk, and other dairy products. The 1961 AHA report was the first official statement by a national group anywhere in the world recommending that a diet low in saturated fats be employed to prevent heart disease. It was Keys's hypothesis in a nutshell.

This was a huge personal, professional, and ideological triumph for Keys. The influence of the AHA on the subject of heart disease was—and still is—unparalleled. For scientists in the field, the chance to serve on the AHA nutrition committee is a highly sought-after plum, and from the start, the dietary guidelines published by that committee have been the gold standard of nutritional advice. These guidelines are influential not only in the United States but around the world. Thus Keys's ability to insert his own hypothesis into these guidelines was like splicing DNA into the group: it programmed the AHA's growth, and as it grew, the group has in turn served as both rudder and engine for Keys's diet-heart ship over the past half-century.

Keys himself thought that the 1961 AHA report he had helped write suffered from "some undue pussy-footing" because it had prescribed the diet only for high-risk people rather than the entire American population, but he need not have complained too much. Two weeks later, *Time* magazine featured the fifty-seven-year-old Keys on its cover, bespectacled and dressed in a white lab coat, with a heart drawn in behind him sprouting veins and arteries. *Time* called him "Mr. Cholesterol!" and quoted his advice to cut dietary fat from its current average of 40 percent of total calories down to a draconian 15 percent. Keys advised an even sterner cut for saturated fat—down from 17 percent to 4 percent. These measures were the "only sure way" to avoid high cholesterol, he said.

The article dwelled on the diet-heart hypothesis at length, as well as Keys's personal history: he was depicted as unbridled and sharp, but in a way that commands authority. He was the man with the harsh medicine: "People should know the facts," he said. "Then, if they want to eat themselves to death, let them." Keys himself, according to the article, seemed barely to follow his own advice; his "ritual" of dinner by candlelight and "soft Brahms" at home with Margaret included meat—steak, chops, and roasts—three times a week or less. (He and Stamler were also once spotted by a colleague at a conference tucking into scrambled eggs and "five or so rations" of bacon.) "Nobody wants to live on mush," Keys explained. In the *Time* article, there is only a brief mention of the reality that Keys's ideas were "still questioned" by "some researchers" with conflicting ideas about what causes coronary disease.

And here was the other engine moving the diet-heart hypothesis ship forward: the media. Most newspapers and magazines became persuaded by Keys's ideas early on. The *New York Times* gave that front-page space to Paul Dudley White, for instance, and picked up on Keys's views early on ("Middle Aged Men Cautioned on Fat" a headline read in 1959). Like the research community itself, the media was looking for answers to the heart disease epidemic, and dietary fat plus cholesterol made sense. Not only did Keys have a talent for publicity, but his fiery language and

Ancel Keys on the Cover of *Time*, January 13, 1961

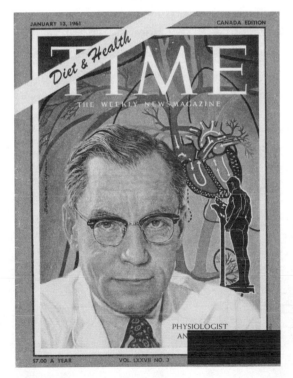

Ancel Keys launched the idea that saturated fat causes heart disease and was the twentieth century's most influential nutrition expert.

From *TIME* Magazine, January 13, 1961 © 1961, Time Inc. Used under license. *TIME* and Time Inc. are not affiliated with, and do not endorse products or services of, Licensee.

definitive-sounding solution were clearly more appealing to reporters than the dispatches from scientists such as Rockefeller's Pete Ahrens, who cautioned soberly about the lack of adequate scientific evidence. The media also took its cue from the AHA, and soon after that group issued its "prudent diet" guidelines, the *New York Times* reported that the "highest scientific body has lent its stature" to the view that reducing or altering the fat content of a person's diet could help prevent heart disease.

A year later, the *New York Times* gave an air of apparent inevitability to these new dietary patterns: "whereas people once thought of dairy products in terms of health and vitality, many people now associate them with cholesterol and heart ailments," stated one article entitled "Is Nothing Sacred? Milk's American Appeal Fades." The media was nearly unanimous in its support of Keys's hypothesis. Newspapers and magazines made his diet known nationwide, while women's magazines carried it into the kitchen with recipes to cut back on fat and meat. Influential health columnists also helped spread the word: the Harvard nutrition professor Jean Mayer wrote a syndicated column that appeared twice weekly in one hundred of the largest US newspapers, with a combined circulation of 35 million. (In 1965, he called the low-carbohydrate diet "mass murder.") And from the 1970s on, *New York Times* health writer Jane Brody became one of the greatest promoters of the diet-heart hypothesis. She reported faithfully on AHA pronouncements

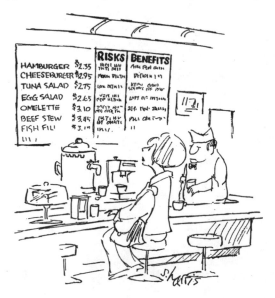

NINA TEICHOLZ

as well as any new studies linking fat and cholesterol to heart disease or cancer. One article she wrote in 1985 called "America Leans to a Healthier Diet" starts off featuring Jimmy Johnson, who "used to wake up to the smell of bacon in the pan," while his wife remembered saving the bacon grease to then fry the eggs; now, said Mr. Johnson, "just a bit ruefully: 'the smells are gone from breakfast, but we're all a lot better off for it.' "

Journalists could paint a vivid picture and reach a broad audience, but they were not saying anything different from what health officials themselves advised. For the media and nutrition experts alike, the chain of causation that Keys had proposed seemed to make eminent sense: dietary fat caused cholesterol to rise, which would eventually harden arteries and lead to a heart attack. The logic was so simple as to seem self-evident. Yet even as the low-fat, prudent diet has spread far and wide, the evidence could not keep up, and never has. It turns out that every step in this chain of events has failed to be substantiated: saturated fat has *not* been shown to cause the most damaging kind of cholesterol to go up; total cholesterol has *not* been demonstrated to lead to an increased risk of heart attacks for the great majority of people, and even the narrowing of the arteries has *not* been shown to predict a heart attack. But in the 1960s, these revelations were still a decade away, and official institutions, along with the media, were already gathering enthusiastically behind Keys's attractively simple idea. It seems they were convinced enough, moreover, that their eyes were already closing to evidence to the contrary.

It's worth looking at some of the evidence they were ignoring, because although some scientific observations—most prominently the Seven Countries study—seemed to support the diet-heart hypothesis, a great many studies from those early years proved to be surprisingly uncooperative. We'll take a tour through a handful.

Early Observations That Did Not Support Keys's Hypothesis

In the 1950s, at the behest of the US Public Health Service, the researcher William Zukel headed to the northeastern corner of North Dakota to examine people who had suffered a heart attack or coronary death. During a year, his team identified 228 such cases and obtained detailed diet and lifestyle histories for 162 of them. The heart patients were more likely to be smokers, but beyond that, Zukel could find no difference between the two groups in terms of the amount of saturated fat, unsaturated fat, or total calories consumed.*

In Ireland, researchers analyzed the diets of one hundred men under the age of sixty who had suffered a heart attack and compared them, over the course of several years, to a group of age- and sex-matched controls. These investigators could find no difference between the two groups in the amount or type of fat eaten. A similar study performed by the same team on fifty middle-aged women a year later had the same results. The authors published their findings in the widely read *American Journal of Clinical Nutrition* (AJCN). They noted that although Keys was proposing a link between saturated fat and heart disease (based, at that point, on international statistics), their own study "fails to support" this conclusion.

S. L. Malhotra, the chief medical officer of the Western Railway of Bombay, *did* find a dietary difference between men with and without heart disease, but not in a way that favored the diet-heart hypothesis. Malhotra studied the disease among more than one million male employees of the Indian railways in the mid-1960s, and during a five-year period he found the rate of heart disease among railroad sweepers in Madras, southern India, to be seven times higher than the rate for Punjabi railroad sweepers in the north—even though the latter were eating eight to nineteen times more fat (mostly from dairy products). The southerners ate very little fat,

---

*This type of investigation, where patients are asked about their diets retroactively, is called a "case-control" study. These studies are understood to suffer from "recall bias," whereby patients may inaccurately remember past consumption. Specifically in the case of heart disease patients, who, upon diagnosis, would normally be advised by their doctors to reduce the saturated fat (and probably total fat) content of their diets, those patients would likely bias their recollections in favor of having complied with this advice. Also, since all Americans have been advised to eat a low-fat diet since the 1960s, the control group might be biased in the same way. However, Zukel's study from the 1950s is unlikely to be distorted by these problems, because most practitioners did not start advising heart disease patients to eat a low-fat diet until the 1960s.

and what they did eat was unsaturated groundnut oil. Nonetheless, they died on average twelve years earlier than their counterparts in the north. Malhotra concluded his paper with the suggestion to "eat more fermented milk products, such as yogurt, yogurt sherbet, and butter." Malhotra published his findings in one of the most important journals in the field of epidemiology, but no one commented upon his work, and it has almost never been cited.

Around the same time, other investigators traveled to Roseto, Pennsylvania, to find out why the mostly Italian population living there had a "strikingly low" number of deaths from heart disease—less than half the rate of neighboring towns. It wasn't a lack of fat, as researchers quickly realized, since the local diet included copious amounts of animal fats, including prosciutto with fat an inch thick around the rim, and most meals cooked in lard. The majority of the 179 Roseto men observed ate large meals and drank a great deal of wine. They were also generally overweight, yet not a single one under fifty died of a heart attack from 1955 to 1961, the years of the survey.

This particular study came out in another widely read publication, *The Journal of the American Medical Association* (JAMA), in 1964, and received what Keys described, resentfully, as "extravagant worldwide publicity and apparently ready acceptance in some medical circles." A response, he felt, was clearly needed, and he supplied one in an extensive three-page critique, also in JAMA, in 1966. This was highly unusual, since questions about a study are usually confined to short "Letters to the Editor," and the space given to Keys no doubt reflected his outsized stature in the field. Keys observed that the study population was self-selected (and therefore not a random sample) and that the collection of dietary data did not accurately reflect a lifetime of eating patterns for many of the men who had immigrated from Italy.* Although the methodologies employed by the researchers were standard for their day, Keys concluded that the Roseto data "certainly cannot be accepted as evidence that calories and fats in the diet

---

*Keys was being hypocritical here, since his Seven Countries study had also collected data from people whose dietary patterns, due to World War II, had almost certainly changed dramatically over their lifetimes.

are not important." His article appears to have been successful in marginalizing the study—for it has been little mentioned since.

These sorts of findings, where fat consumption did not correlate well with heart disease risk, were a problem for Keys's hypothesis, but they kept popping up all over the world. In 1964, F. W. Lowenstein, a medical officer for the World Health Organization in Geneva, collected every study he could find on men who were virtually free of heart disease, and concluded that their fat consumption varied wildly, from about 7 percent of total calories among Benedictine monks and the Japanese to 65 percent among Somalis. And there was every number in between: Mayans checked in with 26 percent, Philippinos with 14 percent, the Gabonese with 18 percent, and black slaves on the island of St. Kitts with 17 percent. The *type* of fat also varied dramatically, from cottonseed and sesame oil (vegetable fats) eaten by Buddhist monks to the gallons of milk (all animal fat) drunk by the Masai. Most other groups ate some kind of mixture of vegetable and animal fats. One could only conclude from these findings that any link between dietary fat and heart disease was, at best, weak and unreliable.

Nearly all these studies were published in reputable scientific journals; some of them were discussed and debated—they were part of the nutrition "conversation"—but supporters of the diet-heart hypothesis always found reasons to dismiss them: the studies must have been misinterpreted, irrelevant, or based on untrustworthy data.

In general, a researcher always has a choice of which studies to select and which to reject in working toward a hypothesis. In this process, it's hard to overcome the essentially human instinct to select only those observations that conveniently support one's own hypothesis while rejecting those that do not. A large number of psychological studies have shown that people respond to scientific or technical evidence in ways that justify their preexisting beliefs. "Selection bias," as it's called, is the danger of becoming overly attached to one's own hypothesis or belief system.

Resisting these "idols of the mind," as the great seventeenth-century theorist Francis Bacon dubbed them, is exactly what the scientific method tries to do. A scientist must always try to disprove his or her own hypothesis. Or, as one of the great science philosophers of the twentieth century,

Karl Popper, described, "The method of science is the method of bold conjectures and ingenious and severe attempts to refute them."*

In seeing how these early studies from Roseto, Pennsylvania to North Dakota were overlooked or dismissed out of hand, it's hard, as a student of the history of the diet-heart hypothesis, not to conclude that selection bias has consistently been practiced for decades. Dozens of trials either were forgotten or had their findings distorted. The ones we have reviewed here were early and relatively small. As we'll see, the studies ignored or willfully misinterpreted later on were some of the biggest and most ambitious trials of diet and disease ever undertaken in the history of nutrition science.

Alternative Ideas and the Opposition

One of the hallmarks of selection bias is that people—even scientists trained to look for it—often don't realize that they, themselves, might be suffering from it. This is the innocent part of the explanation about what was at work among any number of researchers during these formative years of the diet-heart hypothesis. It can justifiably be said, however, that Keys was not on the lookout for his own biases. He considered the burden of proof to be on those opposing him. He made no attempts to refute his own ideas, as Popper advised. He promoted the "idol of his mind" without hesitation. It seemed obvious to Keys and his colleagues that his hypothesis should not only be accepted but also promoted for the entire US population, since the potential health benefits appeared to them to be so great. And they found the unintended consequences of reducing dietary fat to be hard to imagine.

One person who *could* foresee those consequences was Pete Ahrens.

---

*A particularly poetic examination of the difficulty in remaining objective about one's own ideas was written in 1897 by the famous geologist and president of the American Association for the Advancement of Science, T. C. Chamberlin. The moment you affix yourself to an idea, an "intellectual child springs into existence," and it is difficult to remain neutral. The mind lingers "with pleasure" on the facts that support the theory, and feels a "natural coldness" toward those that do not, he wrote (Chamberlin [1897] 1965).

Ahrens had emphasized from the beginning that Keys's ideas, first about total fat, and then saturated fat, were far from certain and that alternative explanations for heart disease were still plausible. (Ahrens was objecting already in 1957: "When unproved hypotheses are enthusiastically proclaimed as facts, it is timely to reflect on the possibility that other explanations can be given for the phenomena observed.") Ahrens's own research had opened up another line of inquiry, suggesting that the carbohydrates found in cereals, grains, flour, and sugar might be contributing directly to if not actually causing obesity and disease. And he correctly predicted that a fat-reduced diet would only increase our consumption of these foods.

While nearly everyone else was exclusively obsessed with serum cholesterol, Ahrens was instead interested in triglycerides, which are molecules made up of fatty acids circulating in the blood. As is common in science, new technologies tend to move fields forward, and Ahrens pioneered the use of silic acid chromatography to separate out triglycerides from blood samples. The highly controlled liquid-formula feeding experiments that he conducted from 1951 to 1964 consistently revealed that these triglycerides shot up whenever carbohydrates replaced fat in the diet. (A breakfast of cereal instead of eggs and bacon is a good example of a choice which would do just that.)

Teaming up with Margaret Albrink, a young doctor at Yale University, Ahrens compared the triglyceride and cholesterol levels of heart disease patients at New Haven Hospital with those of healthy employees of the nearby American Steel and Wire. They found that high triglyceride levels were far more common than high cholesterol in coronary patients; so they posited that triglycerides, *not* total cholesterol, were a better indicator of heart disease. Although this wasn't a popular line of inquiry, a handful of researchers confirmed his basic findings over the next decade.

Ahrens found that triglycerides would cloud up the blood with a milky white liquid, easily visible in a test tube, which he would display to lecture audiences. Then he would reveal the punch line: the cloudy blood belonged to someone on a high-carbohydrate diet, whereas a contrasting vial of clear blood plasma belonged to someone following a high-fat regimen. In a small minority of cases, the reverse would happen, but Ahrens believed that these people suffered from a rare genetic disorder. A majority of patients showed the clouding because of a "normal chemical process which occurs in all people on high carbohydrate diets," Ahrens wrote.

Ahrens also found that the blood cleared up when carbohydrates were reduced. Restricting overall calories had the same effect. Ahrens thought that perhaps this second, low-calorie effect explained why impoverished people in rural Japan following the war were found to have low triglycerides, despite eating a lot of rice.

Because high triglycerides are also usually found in diabetics and because people with diabetes are at higher risk for heart disease, Albrink sketched out a scenario whereby these two diseases had a common cause: excessive weight gain. Whatever caused people to get fat was spiking their triglycerides and also leading to heart disease and diabetes. The probable cause that Albrink had identified was carbohydrates. It was a grim scenario that today is supported by a growing stack of evidence, but in the early 1960s, when Albrink and Ahrens first proposed the idea, it was quite new.

The implications for diet, however, were entirely the opposite of what Keys was proposing. According to the Ahrens model, carbohydrates, not fat, were the cause of heart disease. Since a low-fat diet is inevitably one high in carbohydrates (cutting back on meat and dairy necessitates eating more grains and vegetables, simply because there are no alternatives), the two hypotheses were inimical.

Ahrens was concerned that the low-fat diet being prescribed to the American public would worsen their triglyceride levels and thus exacerbate the problem of obesity and chronic disease.

Yet, like the nutrition world's Cassandra, Ahrens never managed to carry the day, even though he was one of the most highly respected scientists in the field, to whom many influential researchers paid heed. He was indefatigable in pointing out the need for more and better evidence in support of reduced-fat diets. He continually cautioned colleagues against jumping to conclusions too quickly; but he was perhaps simply not aggressive enough.

Keys and his close colleagues enjoyed immense success in promoting their hypothesis because they were tireless advocates of their own ideas. And they employed another tactic, namely that they relentlessly disparaged the opposition. Indeed, they practiced what might be called the blood sport of nutrition science. Rolling over the opposition by force of will was a strategy that Keys and Stamler may not have invented, but they were certainly some of its most effective practitioners.

The Sharp Elbows of Nutrition Scientists

Jeremiah Stamler brought this sport to life for me when I met him in 2009. He was then aged eighty-nine and still remarkably spry. Stamler was a heart disease specialist at Northwestern University in Chicago and an important colleague of Keys's from the late 1950s on. I asked him about the crucial studies used to establish the diet-heart hypothesis; Stamler had been at the helm of most of them as well as being a key figure at the AHA and NIH. The substance of his contributions will be discussed later in the book, but for now it's relevant simply to note how readily his conversation turned to attacking his various opponents, an apparent reflection of nutrition science as a kind of political battlefield.

"But let's talk about Pete Ahrens," he volunteered. "Pete Ahrens! He was always a big roadblock on everything! I used to have *vigorous* discussions with Pete."

Mockingly, Stamler proceeded to channel Ahrens: *"No, We're researching this, give us another five years. We have to do balanced studies. We have to figure it out. We don't know."* Stamler and Keys, by contrast, sought, urgently, to move ahead with broad public health recommendations. They represented one side of a debate that has been the central issue in the field of nutrition: Were the correlations found by epidemiological studies sufficient as a basis for administering dietary advice to an entire population? Keys and Stamler believed the answer was yes. It wasn't that they thought the evidence was perfect, by any means, but they thought that in a world of difficult trade-offs, epidemiological data was adequate. Waiting for the results of a large clinical trial would take a decade or more, and in the meantime, men were dying of heart attacks. The dispassionate, cautionary tone that Ahrens took therefore made Stamler's blood boil. "He always opposed any statement. I would say, 'Pete, what you're saying is that the present American diet is the *best* diet you can conceive of for the health of the

American people.' 'No! No!' 'But Pete, *please*, the *logic!*' Anyway, he's dead and gone now."

Listening to Stamler talk, I could almost picture his spear. "And Yudkin!" Stamler nearly bellowed to me, referring to the British doctor who promoted the rival sugar hypothesis. "I was part of shooting him down!" And of Michael Oliver, a prominent British cardiologist and critic of the diet-heart hypothesis, Stamler repeatedly said that he was a "scoundrel."

Like Stamler, Keys allowed virtually no oxygen for debate. It's astonishing, actually, to read his reaction to those who dared disagree with him. When Texas A&M professor Raymond Reiser wrote an extremely thorough and rigorous critique of the saturated-fat hypothesis for the *American Journal of Clinical Nutrition* in 1973, Keys began a *twenty-four*-page reply by saying that Reiser's analysis "reminds one of the distorting mirrors in the hall of jokes at the county fair." Keys's tone throughout is relentlessly sneering: "This is a typical distortion," he wrote, and "It would be difficult to pack more imprecision in a 16-word sentence"; "Resier pompously states . . . ," "He completely ignores . . . ," "Obviously, Reiser has no comprehension."

Reiser was one of quite a few critics who had reexamined the important studies at the foundation of the diet-heart hypothesis. And he made a number of crucial observations that have recently resurfaced: he listed the many methodological problems undermining those early studies and noted that certain types of saturated fatty acids, such as stearic acid, which is the main one found in meat, demonstrated no cholesterol-raising effect at all. Keys's response included rebuttals about specific problems, and although he agreed that stearic acid is "neutral," he defended the cholesterol-raising properties of other types of saturated fats. Replying to Keys, Reiser wrote a short letter to the journal—reluctantly, he said, because "I feel I must give some rebuttal to the accusation that I have tried to smear the scientists whose papers I reviewed and that I have deliberately lied."

Whatever the disagreements—and the complexity of science means that there will always be some—the aggressive style adopted by Keys and Stamler was beyond the norm. Few men could match them, and as time went on and the diet-heart hypothesis gained followers as well as institutional legitimacy, fewer and fewer tried.

George V. Mann

Along with Ahrens and Reiser, one of the few prominent scientists who made a public show of his skepticism was George Mann, the Vanderbilt biochemist who had gone to Africa to study the Masai. Mann's early career was punctuated by flashes of brilliance: he was one of the first scientists to raise the alarm about trans fats, in *1955,* and he speculated that the sudden breaking off of plaque in the arteries must be a more important factor in heart attacks than the slow clogging-up of the arteries. He was proven correct, but not until decades later.

In Africa, Mann had seen people thriving on diets of meat, blood, and milk whose total cholesterol levels were among the lowest in the world and who did not contract heart disease—nor, apparently, any other chronic diseases.

These findings so clearly undermined the diet-heart hypothesis that nutrition researchers made a substantial effort to disprove them. Several US universities pulled together a team of scientists who traveled to Kenya to look for flaws in Mann's data. To their chagrin, they reluctantly wound up confirming his findings instead. Then, scraping around for an explanation for these unexpected results, one set of researchers suggested that maybe the Masai over thousands of years had developed some gene with a freaky ability to reduce blood cholesterol. That theory was soon disproved, however, by the discovery of a group of Masai who had moved to nearby Nairobi. Their cholesterol numbers were fully a quarter higher than those of their kinsmen in the countryside, meaning they looked a lot more like Westerners. Environment had therefore clearly trumped genetic advantage, if there had ever been one.

Keys predictably attempted to relegate Mann's work to the sidelines. "The peculiarities of those primitive nomads have no relevance" to understanding heart disease in other populations, he wrote. Keys himself, in his Seven Countries study, had looked for dietary truth by comparing different peoples from around the globe, but, as he wrote later, these were mostly Europeans, whom he thought were a better reference point for Americans.

Keys used the same disparaging arguments to dismiss observations of Inuit in the Arctic. Like Mann, Vilhjalmur Stefansson had also seen for himself how good health and a high-fat diet could go hand in hand; the Inuit diet, as we've seen, was at least 50 percent fat. And in 1929 Stefansson conducted that yearlong experiment of eating only meat and fat. Optimistically, he expected that these efforts would lead to "a path of garlands for the high-fat regimens" laid down by admiring colleagues. He was thus unprepared for his fall from grace. "And what a fall!" he wrote. "The first cloud in the sky was no bigger than a man's hand, in fact no larger than a brief and friendly personal note from Dr. Ancel Keyes [sic]" in 1954.

Soon, Keys was publicly dismissing Stefansson's work as a venture that like Mann's, was exotic and irrelevant: Although "their bizarre manner of life excites the imagination," especially that "popular picture of the Eskimo . . . happily gorging on blubber," on "no grounds" was it possible to suggest that the case of the Inuit "contributes anything," and it "certainly did not demonstrate an exception to the diet-fat coronary heart disease hypothesis."

It was also possible to kill with kindness, which is the attitude that Fredrick J. Stare, a Keys supporter and the chairman of the department of nutrition at the Harvard School of Public Health, took toward Stefansson's work. Stare was friends with Stefansson and wrote an introductory comment for one of his books on the Inuit. But Stare belittled the substantive question that Stefansson's work posed and gave his readers little reason to consider it seriously. "Would it be good or bad for you?' he asked rhetorically. "Of course, if we all began eating more meat, there soon wouldn't be enough, particularly of the 'choice' cuts."* Continuing this jovial approach, without ever grappling with the implications of Stefansson's scientific work, Stare ends by recommending this "entertaining" book to the reader.

Stefansson died in 1962, eight years after the publication of that book, and his ideas subsequently disappeared from the nutritional mainstream.

---

*Stefansson acknowledged that one ancillary benefit to being pretty much the lone person in Hanover, New Hampshire, who desired fat was that it was considered a discard, obtained free from the butcher, whose other customers didn't consider those fatty scraps worth giving even to their dogs (Stefansson 1956, xxxi).

The Framingham Study

George Mann, who came to the field in the early 1960s, achieved a remarkable degree of success before he mired himself in controversy by studying the Masai. He was, in fact, an associate director for one of the most famous heart disease investigations ever undertaken: the Framingham Heart Study. Framingham is a small town near Boston, Massachusetts, that has been a virtual petri dish for the study of heart disease since 1948. Now on its third generation of research subjects, it began with some five thousand middle-aged men and women who took part in a survey of every factor researchers could think of that might play a role in the development of heart disease. Participants subjected themselves to comprehensive physicals, interviews, and follow-up tests every two years. It was the first large-scale attempt to find out whether risk factors such as cigarette smoking, high blood pressure, and genes might reliably predict death from heart disease.

In 1961, after six years of study, the Framingham investigators announced their first big discovery: that high total cholesterol was a reliable predictor for heart disease. This is considered one of the most significant findings in the history of heart disease research because before then, even though experts had come to assume serum cholesterol was bad, the evidence was only circumstantial.

The news had broad implications. For one, it solved a problem that had plagued heart disease research from the start, namely, that investigators needed something they could measure to assess heart attack risk before death. It may seem callous to say, but when trying to detect the cause of disease, death is the ideal end point to study. Researchers prefer to follow subjects, looking at what they eat, whether they smoke, and other factors, until they die. Death is the "event," or "hard end point," in the language of research; it is the indisputable data at the end of an experiment. (Heart attacks are also considered "hard" end points, but even these are subject to diagnostic uncertainty, as we've seen.) Looking back from the undeniable fact of death, researchers can then ask, "Was it how much bacon they ate, or the cigarettes, or something else?"

Waiting for subjects to die, however, means that researchers are bur-

dened with following a population over many years. Finding an "intermediary" or "soft" end point to measure before death has therefore been the
subject of a great science hunt. If an indicator could reliably predict heart
disease, researchers could run shorter experiments and measure those intermediary factors instead. The identification by Framingham of total cholesterol as a soft end point was therefore seen as a breakthrough for the field:
scientists could now presumably conclude that any food that raised total
cholesterol would also increase the risk of a heart attack. In all likelihood,
doctors could use this factor in helping patients to identify their coronary
risk as well.

The Framingham finding about cholesterol was thus highly important.
And above all, it seemed to erase any lingering doubts that researchers
might have had about the diet-heart hypothesis. William Kannel, the medical director of Framingham, was quoted in a local newspaper as saying,
"That blood cholesterol is somehow intimately related to coronary atherosclerosis is no longer subject to reasonable doubt."

However, thirty years later, in the Framingham follow-up study—when
investigators had more data because a greater number of people had died—
it turned out that the predictive power of total cholesterol was not nearly
as strong as study leaders had originally thought. For men and women
with cholesterol between 205 and 264 milligrams per deciliter (mg/dL),
no relationship between these numbers and heart disease risk could be
found. In fact, half of the people who had heart attacks had cholesterol levels below the "normal" level of 220 mg/dL. And for men aged forty-eight
to fifty-seven, those with cholesterol in the midrange (183–222 mg/dL)
had a *greater* risk of heart attack death than those with higher cholesterol
(222–261 mg/dL). Total cholesterol turned out not to be a reliable predictor for heart disease after all.

Because the Framingham leaders had been trumpeting total cholesterol
as the best possible risk factor for heart disease for so many years, they did
not take great pains to publicize these weaker follow-up numbers when
they came out in the late 1980s. (Soon they would be shifting the conversation over to cholesterol subfractions, known as high-density lipoprotein
[HDL] and low-density lipoprotein [LDL], which could now be measured

and whose predictive powers showed more promise, although even aspects of these subfractions turned out to be disappointing in the end, as we'll see in Chapters 6 and 10.)

The Framingham data also failed to show that *lowering* one's cholesterol over time was even remotely helpful. In the thirty-year follow-up report, the authors state, "For each 1% mg/dL drop of cholesterol there was an 11% *increase* in coronary and total mortality [italics added]." This is a shocking finding, the very opposite of the official line on cholesterol lowering. Yet this particular Framingham finding is never discussed in scientific reviews, even though many large trials have found similar results.

Other important findings from Framingham have also been ignored, including—notably—those on dietary risk factors, which were examined in the part of the study that Mann conducted. Together with a dietician, Mann spent two years collecting food-consumption data from one thousand subjects, and when he calculated the results in 1960, it was very clear that saturated fat was *not* related to heart disease. Concerning the incidence of coronary heart disease and diet, the authors concluded, simply, "No relationship found."

"That went over like a wet blanket with my superiors at NIH," Mann told me, "because it was contrary to what they wanted us to find." The NIH also generally favored the diet-heart hypothesis from the early 1960s on, and "they wouldn't allow us to publish that data," he says. Mann's re-

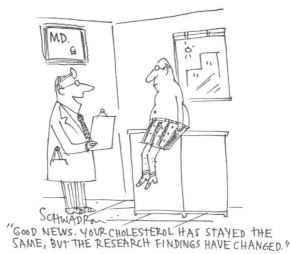

"GOOD NEWS. YOUR CHOLESTEROL HAS STAYED THE SAME, BUT THE RESEARCH FINDINGS HAVE CHANGED."

NINA TEICHOLZ

sults lay in an NIH basement for nearly a decade. (To withhold scientific information "is a form of cheating," Mann lamented.) And even when the findings eventually came out in 1968, they were so deeply buried that a researcher has to dig through twenty-eight volumes to find the news that variations in serum cholesterol levels could not be traced back to the amount or type of fat eaten.

Not until 1992, in fact, did a Framingham study leader publicly acknowledge the study's findings on fat. "In Framingham, Mass, the more saturated fat one ate . . . the *lower* the person's serum cholesterol . . . and [they] weighed the *least*," wrote William P. Castelli, one of the Framingham directors, and he published this admission not as a formal study finding but instead as an editorial in a journal not normally read by most doctors.* (Castelli clearly found it hard to believe that this finding could be true, and he insisted in an interview that the problem must have been one of imprecise collection of the dietary data, but the methodology Mann used was meticulous by the standards of the field, so Castelli's explanation doesn't seem likely.)

Despite his other successes, being on the unpopular side of the cholesterol debate made a bitter man of George Mann. As he approached retirement in the late 1970s, a tone of torment crept into his papers. An article he wrote in 1977 began: "A generation of research on the diet-heart question has ended in disarray," and he called the diet-heart hypothesis a "misguided and fruitless preoccupation."

I last spoke to Mann when he was ninety years old (he died in 2012). Although his memory was not perfect, he seemed to have total recall for the deprivations he perceives himself to have suffered for having opposed Keys. "It was pretty devastating to my career," he said. Finding journals that would accept his scientific articles, for instance, grew increasingly difficult, and after he spoke out against the diet-heart hypothesis, he says he was virtually barred from prominent AHA publications such as *Circulation*.

---

*The *Archives of Internal Medicine* is a respected journal, but Castelli, who was in charge of the largest study on heart disease risk factors in the country, could have probably placed his article anywhere, including a journal more commonly read by doctors, such as *The New England Journal of Medicine*.

Mann also believes that Keys's sizable influence at NIH led to the cancellation of Mann's longtime research grant. "One day," recalls Mann, "the woman who was the study section secretary asked me to step out in the hall. 'Your opposition to Keys is going to cost you your grant,' she said. And she was right."

How could one man's ideas rule the field in such a way? Mann explains, "You have to understand what a forceful and persuasive person Keys was. He could talk to you for an hour and you would utterly believe everything he said."

The Diet-Heart Hypothesis Comes to Rule

These stories about Mann being marginalized by the AHA and NIH illustrate a larger reality about how the diet-heart hypothesis solidified into nutritional dogma among a universe of experts. Keys was clearly the most influential proponent of the diet-heart hypothesis, but it would be naïve to think that a form of scientific bullying on the part of a few men could steamroll over an entire field of intelligent and objective academic researchers. Instead, what happened was that after the diet-heart hypothesis became adopted by the AHA and NIH, Keys's bias was institutionalized. These two organizations set the agenda for the field and controlled most of the research dollars, and scientists who didn't want to end up like Mann had to go along with the AHA-NIH agenda.

The AHA and NIH were parallel, entwined forces from the start. In 1948, when the AHA was launched as a national, volunteer-run organization, one of its first tasks was to establish a "heart lobby" in Washington, DC, to convince President Eisenhower to set up the National Heart Institute—which he did, also in 1948. NHI morphed over the years into the National Heart, Lung, and Blood Institute (NHLBI) that exists today. And every step of the way, this new institute moved in concert with its close sibling, the AHA. In 1950, for instance, the two jointly held the first national conference on heart disease, in Washington, DC. In 1959, they jointly reported "to the nation" on "A Decade of Progress against Cardiovascular Disease." In 1964, the two agencies together held a second national conference on heart disease in Washington. In 1965, the AHA president worked closely with Congress to establish the Regional Medical Programs Service as part of the NHI, which, through a contract with the AHA, went through an elaborate process to set up standards for cardiovascular care across the country. And so on. The NHLBI and the AHA celebrated their thirtieth anniversaries together in 1978.

In all this time, the NHLBI and AHA have regularly issued joint reports as well as co-hosted conferences and task forces. These, along with the activities of top cardiology societies, have together constituted the official history of heart disease research. Put another way, any event from the early 1950s on that was *not* convened by the AHA, the NHLBI, or one of these few societies has had virtually no impact on the writing of that history.

The nucleus of control steering these groups was a tiny group of experts with overlapping responsibilities. The number of those in this nutrition elite was small enough for them all to be on a first-name basis with each other and they came to control pretty much every large clinical trial on diet and disease. These were the nutrition "aristocrats," to use a term coined by Thomas J. Moore, a journalist who wrote an explosive critique of the cholesterol hypothesis in 1989.* They came from the academic faculties of medical schools, teaching hospitals, and research establishments, mainly along the Eastern Seaboard but also in Chicago. (As air travel grew less expensive, experts from California and Texas were able to join.) The group of nearly all men worked closely with the AHA and the NHLBI. Members of this academic haut monde were appointed to official committees and expert panels; they co-authored influential articles, sat on the editorial boards of major scientific journals, and peer-reviewed each other's papers. They attended and dominated the major professional conferences.

In all these contexts, the same names continually come up. For example, AHA founder Paul Dudley White was also appointed by President

---

*Moore's original work appeared as a cover story in the *Atlantic* in 1989 and sold more copies than any other issue in the magazine's history. Later that year, he published a book on the subject. Also in 1989, Moore's reporting prompted Congress to hold hearings on the question of whether the NIH's programs were needlessly recommending that millions of Americans take cholesterol-lowering drugs. (Moore, "The Cholesterol Myth," 1989; Moore, *Heart Failure*, 1989; Anon, Associated Press, 1989.)

Harry S. Truman to be the first director of the National Heart Advisory Council, which guided all NHI activities with respect to cardiovascular disease. White then established a number of joint AHA-NHI scientific committees, including the community service and education committee, which he himself chaired before passing the mantle to Keys. AHA presidents "almost routinely" directed the NIH Advisory Council or served as members, noted the AHA's official history. AHA leaders also dominated the professional medical societies. White helped found the International Society for Cardiology, and he, together with Keys, co-chaired its research committee. And in 1961, the AHA and the NHI jointly began planning the huge National Diet Heart Study, the biggest-ever endeavor to test the diet-heart hypothesis, for which the executive committee read like a *Who's Who* of nutrition science, including, of course, both Keys and Stamler.

The AHA and NHLBI together also administered the vast majority of grants for all cardiovascular research. By the mid-1990s, the NHLBI's annual budget had reached $1.5 billion, with most of those funds going to heart disease research; the AHA, meanwhile, was devoting about $100 million a year toward original research. These two pots of money dominated the field. The NIH or AHA financed virtually all the American-led studies we will discuss in this book. The only other significant source of research funding came from the food and drug industries, which researchers tried to avoid for the obvious reason of avoiding any conflict of interest or even the appearance of one. As George Mann wrote in 1991, when he hosted a small meeting of researchers with alternative views, "This was a daunting task, because we cannot obtain federal funding, and we must not accept food industry funding lest we be seen as speaking for a vested interest."

Ultimately, for every million more dollars spent by the AHA and NIH trying to prove the diet-heart hypothesis, the harder it became for those groups to reverse course or entertain other ideas. Although studies on the diet-heart hypothesis had a surprisingly high failure rate, these results had to be rationalized, minimized, and distorted, since the hypothesis itself had become a matter of institutional credibility.*

---

*Today, this interlocking system operates in much the same way, with the exception that open skeptics such as Pete Ahrens and Michael Oliver, who in the 1970s and

The dissenting voices were fading. An "almost embarrassingly high number of researchers boarded the 'cholesterol bandwagon,' " lamented the editors of the *Journal of the American Medical Association* in 1967, referring to the narrow, "fervent embrace of cholesterol" to the "exclusion" of other biochemical processes that might cause heart disease. In the pages of sympathetic scientific journals, Ahrens and Mann, plus their handful of like-minded colleagues, continually sent up futile cries against the relentless march of the diet-heart hypothesis, but they were powerless in the face of the elite. As George Mann wrote at the end of his career in 1978, a "heart Mafia" had "supported the dogma" and hoarded research funds. "For a generation, research on heart disease has been more political than scientific," he declared.

---

early eighties were included on expert panels, since they had been involved in the field since its birth, are now even less well tolerated. Since those men retired, no member of the nutrition elite has published a comprehensive critique of the diet-heart hypothesis.

4

The Flawed Science of Saturated versus Polyunsaturated Fats

Although Keys behaved as if the Seven Countries study had proven his diet-heart hypothesis, he was always careful in his published papers to include the caveat that his study could only demonstrate an association; "causal relationships are not claimed." This was a necessary statement reflecting the limitations inherent to epidemiology.

To establish cause and effect with any reliability, investigators must almost always undertake a type of research called a clinical trial.

Clinical nutrition trials are controlled experiments, where people are actually fed a specified diet over a period of time instead of simply being questioned about what they are already eating. In the best (most "well-controlled") trials, researchers prepare or provide food to study participants to control exactly what they eat. Sometimes subjects are invited to dine in a special cafeteria, or sometimes the researchers will go so far as to deliver meals to their subjects' homes—although these kinds of measures can be quite expensive. In less well-controlled trials, subjects are simply counseled about what to eat and perhaps given a diet book to take home.

Ideally, people on a special diet are compared to a similar group of "controls" who do not change their diet, so the effect of the intervention can be isolated. If a large-enough study population is divided randomly into these two groups, they can theoretically be assumed to be the same in every relevant way. They should have the same age distribution, the same tendency to smoke or exercise, and be the same in a thousand other ways that researchers might never think to measure. The *one* difference between the two groups in a clinical trial should be the intervention, be it a drug or diet. Starting with two identical groups allows any differences that emerge between them to be reasonably attributed to the intervention.

That is the great strength of clinical trials: unlike epidemiological studies, where researchers must try to think of and then measure all the many things that might be contributing to a disease, a clinical trial, by virtue of its very design, holds all these factors constant, regardless of whether the researchers have thought to account for them.

These types of clinical trials on the diet-heart hypothesis started in the late 1950s and they're important to lay out, so that a reader can see for him- or herself the scientific origins of why we think saturated fat is bad for us, as well as some of the surprising side effects of the diet that Keys proposed. These were not low-fat trials—the idea of avoiding *all* types of fat only became common decades later. What obsessed researchers during these midcentury years was Keys's idea that a diet low in *saturated* fat and cholesterol could prevent heart disease. Therefore, the total fat content of these foundational trials was still quite high by today's standards; only the type of fat varied.

An early and celebrated trial was called the Anti-Coronary Club, launched by Norman Jolliffe, director of the New York City Health Department, in 1957. Jolliffe was a well-regarded authority in his day, the author of a popular diet book called *Reduce and Stay Reduced on the Prudent Diet*, which even President Eisenhower had used. Jolliffe had also read Keys's work, and decided to test these ideas over a sustained period. He signed up eleven hundred men to his Anti-Coronary Club and instructed them to reduce their consumption of red meat, such as beef, lamb, or pork, to no more than four times a week (which would be considered a lot by today's standards!) while consuming as much fish and poultry as they liked. Eggs and dairy were limited. The men also drank at least two tablespoons of polyunsaturated vegetable oil a day. Overall, the diet was about 30 percent fat, but the ratio of polyunsaturated fats (vegetable oils, mostly) to saturated fats was four times greater than what Americans regularly ate. Jolliffe also recruited a control group to eat normal American fare, with an estimated 40 percent fat, although he failed to record the diet of the controls.

"Diet Linked to Cut in Heart Attacks," reported the *New York Times* in 1962, when the coronary trial results started to come out: they showed that men who stayed on the diet saw a drop in both cholesterol and blood pressure and lost weight. Their risk for heart disease appeared to be slamming into reverse, an outcome that looked like a reassuring condemnation of saturated fats. But then, a decade into the trial, investigators began to find "somewhat unusual" results: twenty-six members of the diet club had died during the trial, compared to only six men from the controls. Eight members of the club had died of heart attacks, but not one of the controls. In the discussion section of the final report, the authors (who no longer included Jolliffe, because he had died of a heart attack in 1961) emphasized the improved risk factors among the men in the diet club but ignored what those risk factors had blatantly failed to predict: their higher death rate. That result was buried in the study report. The authors avoided the very question that mattered most: Would someone live longer on a "prudent" diet? The answer from the Anti-Coronary Club was clearly no.

Far from an anomaly, this sort of finding comes up again and again, and is an extremely uncomfortable fact for the promoters of the diet-heart hypothesis: people who eat less fat, particularly less saturated fat, appear not to extend their lives by doing so. Even though their cholesterol inevitably goes down, their risk of death does not. It is an unpleasant result that has plagued the field ever since Keys first noticed it in his Seven Countries study, and the result has been confirmed by other studies—whose authors have also, on the whole, decided that this is a detail best ignored.

The Anti-Coronary Club trial, despite its scientific weaknesses, became one of the foundational studies for the idea that a diet low in saturated fat will protect against heart disease. I will mention just a few more of these studies, which are continually cited by scientists as the bedrock proof for that hypothesis. Once, when I was talking to a specialist who had chaired the prestigious AHA nutrition committee for three years, she listed the citations for these studies off the top of her head, like a preacher rattling off Bible verses: "*Lancet* 1965, pages 501 to 504, *Circulation* by Dayton, 1969, volume 60, supplement 2, page 111. . . ." I couldn't keep up.

Everyone in the field knows these studies, and they have been cited in practically every paper on diet and atherosclerosis for decades, yet every one of these experiments appears upon examination to be riddled with shortcomings and contradictions similar to those in the Anti-Coronary Club trial. Only recently have investigators begun to reexamine these studies, the actual details of which are a bit shocking, like discovering a foundation made of sand.

The first study mentioned by that AHA specialist is the Los Angeles Veterans Trial. It was conducted by UCLA professor of medicine Seymour Dayton on nearly 850 elderly men living in a local Veterans Administration (VA) home in the 1960s. For six years, Dayton fed half the men a diet in which corn, soybean, safflower, and cottonseed oils replaced the saturated fats in butter, milk, ice cream, and cheese. The other half of the men acted as controls and ate regular foods. The first group saw their cholesterol levels drop almost 13 percent more than did the controls. More impressively, only forty-eight men on the diet died from heart disease during the study, compared to seventy on the regular diet.

This would appear to be extremely good news, except that the total rates of deaths from all causes for the two groups were the same. Worryingly, thirty-one men on the vegetable oil diet died of cancer, compared to only seventeen of the controls.

Dayton was clearly concerned about this cancer finding and wrote about it at length. Indeed, the unknown consequences of a diet high in vegetable oils were the reason for undertaking the study in the first place: "Was it not possible," he asked, "that a diet high in unsaturated fat . . . might have noxious effects when consumed over a period of many years? Such diets are, after all, rarities." This was an odd new reality: vegetable oils had been introduced into the food supply only in the 1920s, yet suddenly the oils were being recommended as a cure-all. In fact, the upward curve of vegetable oil consumption happened to coincide *perfectly* with the rising tide of heart disease in the first half of the twentieth century, but researchers and doctors at the time barely discussed this coincidence. It was just an association, of course, and there were so many other changes occurring in American life during that time (including car ownership and refined carbohydrates, as we've seen).

Because researchers in the field were focused on the role of saturated fat in heart disease, Dayton's study received a largely enthusiastic reception in the United States when it came out in 1969. The bottom line for most experts was simply that a prudent diet had reduced the risk of heart attacks. A number of European scientists were more skeptical, and the editors of Britain's oldest and most prestigious medical journal, *The Lancet*, wrote a withering critique. They cited such problems as the rate of heavy smoking being twice as high among the controls as it was in the experimental group* and that people on the special diet ate only about half their food in the hospital (nothing was known about the food they ate outside). Moreover, as even Dayton admitted, only half the men in the experimental group stayed on the diet successfully during the six years of the study. The results were also skewed because there was a tendency for men who got well to leave the VA center and be lost to the trial. Dayton defended his study in a letter to *The Lancet*, standing squarely by his conclusion that a "prudent diet" could lower heart disease risk. And "LA Veterans" has since frequently been cited as evidence for that point, even as the original controversy surrounding the trial has been forgotten.

A third famous clinical trial that is cited again and again is the Finnish Mental Hospital study. I first heard about this study from a top nutrition expert who assured me that it was really "the best possible proof" that saturated fat is unhealthy.

In 1958, researchers seeking to compare a traditional diet high in animal fats to a new one high in polyunsaturated fats selected two mental hospitals near Helsinki. One they called Hospital K and the other, Hospital N. For the first six years of the trial, inmates at Hospital N were fed a diet very high in vegetable fat. Ordinary milk was replaced with an emulsion of soybean oil in skim milk, and butter was replaced by a special margarine high

---

*Dayton wrote a reply in *The Lancet*, in which he analyzes the smoking data and, based on a number of assumptions, asserts that it had "no net effect whatsoever" on the outcome of the trial (Dayton and Pearce 1970).

in polyunsaturated fats. The vegetable oil content of the special diet was six times higher than in a normal diet. Meanwhile, inmates of Hospital K ate their regular fare. Then the hospitals swapped, and for the next six years, Hospital K inmates got the special diet while Hospital N returned to their normal one.

In the special-diet group, serum cholesterol went down by 12 percent to 18 percent, and "heart disease was halved." This is how the study is remembered and is the conclusion that the study directors, Matti Miettinen and Osmo Turpeinen, themselves drew. In a population of middle-aged men, they said, a diet low in saturated fats "exerted a substantial preventive effect upon coronary heart disease."

But a closer look reveals a different picture. Heart disease incidence (which the investigators defined as deaths plus heart attacks) *did* go down dramatically for the men at Hospital N: there were sixteen such cases among men on the normal diet compared to only four on the special diet. But the difference found in Hospital K was not significant. Nor was any difference observed among the women. The biggest problem with the study, however, was that, like the subjects in the LA Veterans Trial, its population was a moving target. With admissions and discharges over the years, the composition of the groups changed by half. A shifting population means that an inmate in the group who died of a heart attack might have been admitted three days earlier and the death would have had nothing to do with his diet; and, vice versa, a patient who was released might have died soon thereafter but would not have been recorded in the study.

This and other design problems were so great that two high-level NIH officials together with a professor at George Washington University felt moved to criticize the study in a letter to *The Lancet* asserting that the authors' conclusions were too statistically weak to be used as any kind of evidence for the diet-heart hypothesis. Miettinen and Turpeinen acknowledged that their study design was "not ideal," including the fact that the study population was far from stable, but asserted in their defense that a perfect trial would be "so elaborate and costly . . . [that it] may perhaps never be performed." Their imperfect trial, meanwhile, would have to stand: "we do not see any reason to change or modify our conclusions," they wrote. The research community accepted this "good-enough" reasoning, and the Finnish Mental Hospital study earned a spot as one of the linchpins of evidence for the diet-heart hypothesis.

The fourth frequently cited diet trial "proving" the diet-heart hypothesis was known as the Oslo study, conducted in the early 1960s.

Paul Leren, a medical doctor in Oslo, Norway, selected 412 middle-aged men who had suffered a first heart attack (rates of heart disease among men in Oslo had skyrocketed from 1945 to 1961) and divided his subjects into two groups. One group followed a traditional Norwegian diet, which Leren describes as high in cheese, milk, meat, and bread as well as vegetables and fruit in season—altogether, 40 percent fat. The second group undertook a "cholesterol-lowering" diet featuring lots of fish and soybean oil but very little meat and no whole milk or cream. In all, the diets contained about the same amount of fat, but in the "cholesterol-lowering" diet most of the fat was polyunsaturated.

Leren chose to study men who had already had a heart attack, in part because such men tend to be highly motivated to stick to a doctor-prescribed diet. This was especially valuable since, as Leren acknowledged, the special high-vegetable-oil diet was received "not with enthusiasm," and some of the men felt weakened and nauseated by it. The other advantage of working with such a population and why post-heart-attack men are so often chosen for these types of trials is that these men are more likely to have another heart attack soon, and so researchers will have enough "events" to generate statistically significant results.

The experiment lasted five years, and in 1966, Leren published his findings. Like all these other large trials, his diet had successfully lowered the men's serum cholesterol, in this case by about 13 percent more than the controls. Fatal heart attacks were definitely down in the dieting group: ten versus twenty-three among the controls, which was an impressive result. However, a major wrench in the experiment, and one that has gone unnoticed because until recently no one was looking for it, was that in addition to saturated animal fats, the control group was eating a great deal of hard margarine and hydrogenated fish oils, then staples of the Norwegian diet, amounting to nearly half a cup of trans fats per day. This was many times more than the average American was eating when the Food and Drug Administration deemed trans fats dangerous enough to put them on food labels. The experimental diet, which sought to maximize polyunsaturated soybean oil, did not contain trans fats, and this was a significant difference that might easily have affected the outcome. Also, the experimental group, following a public health campaign of the time, cut out tobacco use by 45 percent more than the control group, a large difference that the investigators could not explain but which alone could have accounted for most of the difference in heart attack numbers. Despite these issues, however, the Oslo experiment is remembered only for the success of its cholesterol-lowering diet.

Reading these studies in the literature, one is reminded of a game of telephone. Maybe the first person in line says: "Fewer heart attacks, but remember several important caveats." Yet twenty years later, the message is simply remembered as "Fewer heart attacks!"*

Deeply flawed though they were, the Anti-Coronary Club trial, the VA Hospital study, the Finnish Mental Hospital study, and the Oslo experiment are the clinical trials most frequently cited in support of the diet-heart hypothesis. In the same way that any number of zeros can never add up to one, these studies, even taken together, cannot really amount to a convincing pile of evidence, but they have nevertheless endured over time.

What these trials *do* show are the enduring, enormous challenges of studying the link between nutrition and heart disease in a rigorous, definitive way. As many scientists have lamented, it's close to impossible to feed a study population and keep all the variables constant over enough years to yield a statistically significant number of "hard end points" (e.g., heart attacks). This is why these early trials were valuable: they were, on the whole, conducted on institutionalized populations who were, at least in theory, relatively easy to control. Ethical guidelines now rightly prohibit such experiments. Yet, as we've seen, even these hospital populations were hard to keep constant. And in one of the most ironic complications, investigators of these early studies couldn't prevent members of the control group from

---

*A formal description of this problem was written in 1973 by Texas A&M's Raymond Reiser: "It is this practice of referring to secondary or tertiary sources, each taking the last on faith, which has led to the matter-of-fact acceptance of a phenomenon that may not exist" (Reiser 1973, 524).

hearing the emerging public health recommendations against animal fats and smoking—which would inevitably change their behavior, too. The control group thus ended up looking like the experimental group. The difference of intervention was lost.

Another pitfall of these diet trials is that neither the study investigators nor the participants could really be "blind" to the intervention. An ideal trial is designed to prevent either party from knowing whether a participant is assigned to the treatment or the control group. The hope is to avoid the preferential treatment that an experimenter might feel inclined to give to the intervention group (a form of bias called the "performance effect") or, equally, the participant's often-unconscious positive response to knowing that he or she is receiving an intervention (known as the "placebo effect"). The latter is the reason why drug studies usually hand out placebos to the control group: so that everyone has the same experience of taking a pill.

Realistically, though, a diet that includes butter, cream, and meat does not look or taste like a diet without them, so a truly blind diet experiment is difficult. And unlike an experiment on exercise, where you can compare exercisers to nonexercisers, the same cannot be done for eaters and noneaters. Instead, foods must be selectively eliminated. Whenever one thing is removed from the diet—saturated fat, say—something else must replace it. What should that be? Soybean oil? Carbohydrates? Fruits and vegetables? Diet experiments are really always measuring two things at once: the absence of one nutrient and the addition of another. Sorting out the impact of one versus the other requires multiarm trials, and these are often prohibitively expensive.

The biggest attempt to create a truly blind trial, in which subjects would switch to a vegetable-oil-based diet without knowing it, was conducted by the National Heart, Lung, and Blood Institute with Jerry Stamler as one of the principal investigators. NHLBI was aware of the ongoing problems with the diet trials. It was clear that only an enormous, well-controlled clinical trial could definitively establish the link between saturated fat and heart disease. Such a trial would need to enroll a hundred thousand Americans in order to get statistically significant results and

NINA TEICHOLZ

would need a follow-up period of forty-five years. To see if such a giant undertaking was even possible, NHLBI first conducted a feasibility study in 1962. This in itself was a giant effort involving multistep studies on nearly twelve hundred subjects in five different cities, including Baltimore, Boston, Chicago, the Minnesota Twin Cities, and Oakland, as well as a mental hospital in Minnesota.

Coincidentally, the oversight for these studies fell to those most invested in their outcome: Keys and Stamler. Stamler remembers walking the streets in New York City "all night long" with Keys, debating how they might set up the study so people could be "blinded" to the food they ate. Eventually, they came up with a solution that satisfied them: the food company Swift & Co. would make custom margarines with varying levels of fatty acids that both groups would eat; butter would therefore be a non-issue. Even so, the undertaking remained daunting, because other special foods also had to be made for all diet groups, in order to assure that the taste, texture, and cooking experience for all participants would be the same. Hamburger patties and hot dogs were therefore made in two versions: one high in vegetable oil and one made with tallow or lard. Milk and cheese for the intervention group came "filled" with soybean oil. (No one could figure out how to make a simulacrum of an egg, however, so everyone just got two normal eggs a week.) "A housewife would order once a week from a special store that had been set up for the study and was sent the proper foods assigned to her group," says Stamler. Neither the participants nor the study administrators knew who was getting which diet, in an attempt to "double-blind" the study, which was a milestone in diet-heart research. No one had ever managed to do this before, and according to various confirmation tests performed by the investigators, their methods were largely successful: "No one noticed who was getting which types of food! It was all done so well," Stamler asserted.

In retrospect, it is perplexing why scientists did not question the assumption that entirely newfangled foodstuffs could restore a population to good health. How could it be that a healthy diet would depend upon these just-invented foods, such as milk "filled" with soybean oil?

It's true that vegetable oils had been shown to lower total cholesterol successfully, and this effect held great appeal to a research community obsessed with cholesterol. Yet cholesterol-lowering was just one of the many effects of these oils on biological processes, not all of which seemed to be so beneficial.* In fact, no human population had been documented surviving long-term on oils as a major source of fat until 1976, when researchers studied the Israelis, who at the time consumed "the highest reported" quantity of vegetable oils in the world. Their rates of heart disease turned out to be relatively high, however, contradicting the belief that vegetable oils were protective.

When I asked Stamler about the novelty of vegetable oils he said that he and Keys had been concerned about the absence of any historical record for human consumption of these oils, but that ultimately it wasn't considered an impediment to promoting a "prudent" diet.

How Vegetable Oils Became King of the Kitchen

That Americans came to see vegetable oil as the healthiest-possible kind of fat was one of the more astonishing changes in our attitudes about diet in the twentieth century. The change in consumption itself was astronomical: the oils went from being completely unknown before 1910 to representing somewhere around 7 percent or 8 percent of all calories consumed by Americans by 1999, according to two scholarly estimates.

These fats came into the US food supply in two ways: in bottles of salad and cooking oil with brands like Wesson and Mazola; and, more commonly, as hardened oils, used in margarine, Crisco, cookies, crackers, muffins, breads, chips, microwave popcorn, TV dinners, coffee whiteners, mayonnaise, and frozen foods. These solid oils also came to be used in many of the foods sold in cafeterias, restaurants, amusement parks, and sports stadia: anything baked or fried in these settings over the past forty years has typically been made with hardened oils.

The health consequences of these oils, hardened or not, remain largely

---

*NIH researcher Christopher Ramsden went back to some of the early clinical trials to try to tease out the effect of vegetable oils and concluded that they were associated with higher death rates—although the effects he found were small, and since the trials had been so poorly controlled, open to question (Ramsden et al. 2013).

unknown. When consumed as liquid oils, they lower cholesterol in the body, which is the reason health experts have given since the early 1960s for advising us to eat them in ever-increasing amounts (the AHA currently recommends that Americans consume 5 percent to 10 percent of all calories in the form of polyunsaturated oil), but these oils have also had worrisome side effects—like cancer, potentially. When heated, they were shown already by the early 1960s in more than a few experiments to significantly shorten rats' lives. And in their hardened form, they contain trans-fatty acids, which the FDA has deemed enough of a health danger to include on food labels.

Consumption of Fats in the United States, 1909-1999

*Note: Pre-1936 shortening is comprised mainly of lard while afterward, partially hydrogenated oils came to be the major ingredient.

Source: Tanya L. Blasbalg et al., "Changes in Consumption of Omega-3 and Omega-6 Fatty Acids in the United States During the 20th Century," *American Journal of Clinical Nutrition* 93, no. 5 (May 2011): Figures 1B and 1C, 954.

Since 1900, Americans have switched from eating animal fats to vegetable oils.

As the accompanying graph shows, the only fats that could be found in any American kitchen up until about 1910 were those that came exclusively from animals: lard (the fat from pigs), suet (the fat from around an animal's kidneys), tallow (a harder fat from sheep and cattle), butter, and cream. Some cottonseed and sesame oils were produced locally on farms in the South (the slaves brought sesame seeds from Africa), but none was produced nationally or in large quantities; and efforts to make olive oil foundered upon an inability to successfully cultivate olive trees (although no less a man than Thomas Jefferson tried). The fats used by housewives in the United States and also in most of Northern Europe were therefore those from animals. Cooking with oil was a largely unfamiliar idea.

Oils weren't even considered edible. They didn't belong in the kitchen. They were used to make soaps, candles, waxes, cosmetics, varnishes, linoleum, resins, lubricants, and fuels—all of which were increasingly needed for burgeoning urban populations as well as the machinery of industrialization in the nineteenth century. Whale oil was the primary material for all these purposes starting in 1820; a boom in that oil's production enriched two generations of New Englanders living on the coast, but the industry had collapsed by 1860.

The development of cottonseed oil from Southern cotton plantations helped fill the void. Americans still didn't consider oil acceptable for cooking or baking, but that didn't stop some companies from mixing the oil with beef fat to make a "compound lard." Swift & Co., for instance, introduced a product called Cottonsuet in 1893. Unbeknownst to consumers, manufacturers had also been sneaking cottonseed oil into butter from the 1860s on as a way of reducing costs. Indeed, here was the enduring and compelling logic of vegetable oils: they were cheaper than animal fats. Starting in the early 1930s, when the mechanized process of hulling and pressing cottonseeds came to be widely used, this and then other oils pressed from seeds and beans were simply less expensive than raising and slaughtering animals.

Although we know them as "vegetable oils," they're actually pressed mainly from seeds: cottonseeds, rapeseeds, safflower seeds, sunflower seeds, sesame seeds, and corn, as well as from soybeans. We've seen how these oils started to become popular for culinary use when the AHA endorsed them for "heart health" in 1961. Having the backing of the country's highest medical authority on heart disease gave them an enormous boost. "The rush to get aboard the polyunsaturated bandwagon has become a stampede," gushed the trade publication *Food Processing* in that same year. New products containing "higher and higher amounts of polyunsaturated oils" included salad dressings, mayonnaise, and margarine. Even breads and rolls were promoted for containing these new oils. Mazola was just one of the manufacturers enthusiastically advertising the potential health benefits of its oils. "Polyunsaturates are the *plus* in Mazola," said a magazine ad in 1967. And by 1975, Mazola was practically pushing its oil as a medical product.

"Take This Ad to Your Doctor," Mazola, 1975

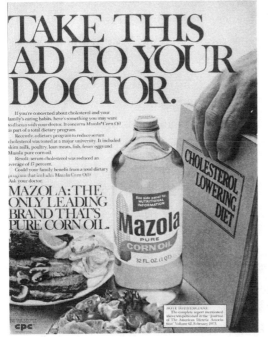

Vegetable oils were marketed in the 1970s for their polyunsaturated-fat content and ability to lower cholesterol, following the advice of the American Heart Association.

While Keys and others firmly believed that polyunsaturated oils would help prevent heart disease due to their cholesterol-lowering properties, it's also true that the AHA received millions of dollars in support from the food companies that manufactured those oils. Remember that the AHA's very launch as a nationally influential group in 1948 depended upon Procter & Gamble's "Truth or Consequences" radio show. Campbell Moses, AHA medical director in the late 1960s, even posed with a bottle of Crisco Oil in an AHA educational film. And remarkably, when Jerry Stamler reissued his 1963 book, *Your Heart Has Nine Lives*, it was published as a "professional" red leather edition by the Corn Products Company and distributed free of charge to thousands of doctors. Inside, Stamler thanks both that company and the Wesson Fund for Medical Research for "significant" research support. "Scientists in public health *must* make alliances with industry," he told me, unabashedly, when I asked him about the connection. "It's tough."

Stamler is correct; nutrition studies are expensive and funding sources limited (although less so in his day), and researchers have long solicited food companies to fill the financing gap. Yet one could reasonably argue that the connections forged by Stamler, Keys, and others in those early days had an exceptionally outsized influence on the course of the American diet. Replacing saturated fat with vegetable oils, after all, became the backbone of the "prudent diet," which endures to the present day.

As we've seen, Americans started following this advice religiously in the early 1960s, yet one of the unpleasant realities of these oils was that they were often too greasy for cooking and baking and turned rancid easily. This explains why very few human civilizations have a history of using an oil as its principal source of cooking fat. For thousands of years the Greeks have used olive oil, but its fatty acids are monounsaturated (with only one double bond) and are therefore more stable. By contrast, the oils pressed from cottonseeds, corn, soybeans, peanuts, linseeds, and rapeseeds* are polyunsaturated (with multiple double bonds). Each double bond provides an additional opportunity for the fatty acid to react with the air (that extra "handshake," as described earlier), so the oils oxidize—and go bad quickly. They are especially unstable when heated and cannot travel long distances, whereas olive oil is relatively safe at high temperatures and, as so many ancient Greek jars can attest, traveled the length of an empire.†

---

*The oils from linseed and rapeseed, in a genetically modified form, are blended to make "canola" oil. The "can" in canola is named for its origin, in Canada.
†The Inuit of the north Pacific coast devised a way to thicken the oil of the oolichan fish by fermenting and boiling it to create a "grease" that could travel over long distances and be used year-round (Phinney, Wortman, and Bibus 2008).

Greasy, rancid-turning oil was not as useful as a long-lasting solid fat, such as butter, tallow, or lard. But if oil could be turned into a solid, the conversion would solve these problems magically, like spinning straw into gold. That is why the ability to harden polyunsaturated oils, through a process called hydrogenation, was such an enormously important discovery. Converting oil into a hard fat transformed it from a relatively useless culinary commodity into one of the most important and serviceable ingredients that the food industry has ever known. Hydrogenated oils were far more useful than the liquid form had ever been. Employed in manufacturing tens of thousands of food products and in making over-the-counter meals across the country, hydrogenated oils would change the landscape of food processing in America for decades to come.

The hydrogenation of oil was invented by a chemist in Hanover, Germany, and was adopted in the United States by Procter & Gamble, which filed two patents for the process in 1908. The original idea at the company had been to employ this new substance to make soap, but the white or yellowish creamy product, which looked so much like lard, also suggested a food use. P&G announced its results in 1911: a new, nonlard shortening called Krispo! Well, almost. That name had to be scuttled over trademark problems, so another name, Cryst, was used until someone noted its rather obvious religious connotations. Finally P&G settled on the name Crisco, derived from its chief ingredient, *crys*tallized *co*ttonseed oil.

Because hydrogenated oil contains trans-fatty acids, Crisco was the product that introduced these fats into the American food supply.* Only *part* of a hydrogenated oil is comprised of trans fats, however, which is why the name on the ingredient list is usually *partially* hydrogenated oil. Manufacturers control the process carefully to get the exact amount of hydrogenation they want. The more of the oil that is hydrogenated, the harder it is—and the more trans fats it contains. Highly hydrogenated oils are ideal

---

*"Trans" refers to the type of double bond between two carbon atoms on a fatty acid chain. A double bond in the *trans* form will make a zigzag-shaped molecule, which allows adjacent fatty acids to lie neatly against each other and create a fat that is solid at room temperature. (The other type of double bond is called "cis" and produces U-shaped twists in the fatty acid chain; these molecules cannot lie closely together and therefore form oils.)

for making chocolate coatings on candies and hard cake icings. A lightly hydrogenated oil is used in fluid products such as sauces or dressings, while an oil in-between is used for creamy fillings and baked goods—and for a product such as Crisco.*

Of course, American housewives didn't jump into a whole new way of cooking overnight. P&G ran a massive advertising campaign to draw them into using this new kind of shortening. In *The Story of Crisco* (1913), the first of several cookbooks that P&G published entirely on this new product, much of the language is devoted to portraying Crisco as a "*new*" and "*better*" fat that would appeal to a housewife's longing to be up to date. While Crisco may be "a shock to the older generation born in an age less progressive than our own," it says, a modern woman is "glad" to give up butter and lard just as her "Grandmother" was happy to forgo the "fatiguing spinning wheel." The cookbook also claimed that Crisco was easier to digest than butter or lard, and that it was produced in "sparkling bright rooms" where "white enamel covers metal surfaces." (This last point was meant to set Crisco apart from pig lard and recent scandals over its squalid production conditions.) And unlike lard, Crisco didn't smoke up the house when used in frying: "Kitchen odors are out of place in the parlor," it advised.†

Crisco's sales multiplied forty times in merely four years following its introduction, luring other brands into the market with names such as Polar White, White Ribbon, and Flakewhite. During World War I, the government required that bakers use all-vegetable shortening so that lard could be exported to European allies, and this provided an enormous boost to the

_____

*Trans-fatty acids comprise up to 70 percent of the most highly hydrogenated oils, while a lightly hydrogenated oil has 10 to 20 percent trans-fatty acids.

†P&G further recognized Crisco's special appeal for kosher dietary needs. The cookbook quotes Rabbi Margolies of New York as saying, "The Hebrew Race had been waiting 4,000 years for Crisco." Crisco "conformed to the strict dietary laws of the Jews. It is known in the Hebrew language as a 'parava,' a neutral fat." "Unlike dairy fats, Crisco can be used with both 'milchig' and 'fleichig' (milk and flesh) food," said the rabbi. Special packages of Crisco bearing the seals of Rabbi Margolies and Rabbi Lifsitz of Cincinnati were sold to the Jewish trade, and American Jews would consume more of these vegetable-based fats than others in the United States due to the convenience in keeping kosher (P&G 1913, 10).

industry. Once commercial bakers discovered how to use vegetable shortening, they stayed with it.

By the early 1940s, one and a half billion pounds of this shortening were being produced in sixty-five plants around the country, and vegetable shortening became the eighth-ranking food item by sales, with the Crisco brand always in the lead. "And so the nation's cookbook has been hauled out and revised. Upon thousands of pages the words 'lard' and 'butter' have been crossed out and the word 'Crisco' written in their place," celebrated *The Story of Crisco*.

Meanwhile, there was another pioneering food item delivering hydrogenated oils to Americans: margarine.* Compared to Crisco, margarine had a far more mixed reception. For one, it didn't arrive in a class of its own, like Crisco. And it was intended not just for cooking but for direct consumption. Margarine replaced butter, a symbol of America's pure and hallowed heartland, and was therefore far more suspect. As the first ersatz food to be widely manufactured, it raised a near-metaphysical question about the essential nature of food. What should a person make of a butter substitute? Artificial food products were not the norm in the early twentieth century. There were no imitation crab cakes, meatless "sausages," or coffee "whiteners." Now we're fairly blasé about the coconut oil that might be masquerading as cheese, but back then food was still pretty much as it had been for generations. Thus, margarine "and its kindred abominations" were considered a "mechanical mixture" created by "the ingenuity of depraved human genius," as Minnesota governor Lucius Frederick Hubbard declaimed in the 1880s. It was common to call margarine manufacturers "swindlers" and their trade "counterfeiting."†

On the other hand, margarine was cheaper than butter, and that was

---

*Margarine was originally made with lard and some brands were made from coconut oil, but by the 1950s, margarine was comprised primarily of partially hydrogenated vegetable oils.

†There is a famous passage illustrating this in Mark Twain's *Life on the Mississippi*: " 'Now as to this article,' said [the salesman], '. . . look at it—smell of it—taste it. . . . Butter, ain't it? Not by a thundering sight—it's oleomargarine! You can't tell it from butter; by George! . . . You are going to see the day, pretty soon, when you can't find an ounce of butter to bless your self with. . . . Why we are turning out oleomargarine now by the thousands of tons. And we can sell it so dirt-cheap that the whole

its main appeal for housewives, who slowly began to embrace it. The dairy industry reacted fiercely, lobbying for an unparalleled number of taxes and other restrictions on margarine. From 1917 to 1928, bills attempting to protect the dairy industry from margarine were introduced in every session of Congress, although most died in committee. The federal government passed four major pieces of margarine legislation, the last of which, in 1931, almost entirely prohibited the sale of all yellow-colored margarines (white margarines that did not imitate butter were considered more acceptable). State governments also passed their own laws, with varying degrees of restrictions on margarine sales.

In a nod to how ludicrous the legislation became, a *Gourmet* magazine cartoon showed an elegantly dressed woman standing before her seated guests at a dinner party, announcing, "In accordance with Title 6, Section 8 Chapter 8 of the laws of this state, I wish to announce that I am serving oleomargarine." And newspapers commonly recounted stories of housewives carpooling across state borders to buy margarine where laws weren't so strict.

Responding to consumer demand for the product, the federal government finally dropped all its taxes and restrictions on margarine in 1950, and a decade later, AHA endorsed margarine as part of its "prudent diet." Now, ironically, the spread, which had been so villainized, turned golden almost overnight. In 1961, for instance, Mazola margarine advertised itself as being the choice "For people concerned about saturated fats in the diet." A few years later, Fleischmann's margarine claimed to be the "lowest in saturated fat." Margarine's reputation was thus rehabilitated as a key part of a healthy, cholesterol-lowering diet.

Decades later, margarine underwent another ironic conversion, this time into a scary trans-fat-containing health threat. (The early margarines contained far more trans fats—up to 50 percent of the total fat content—than did later versions.) But in the meantime, the food industry ensured that margarine, Crisco, and all their other products containing hydrogenated oils were considered safe and healthy. From the early 1960s, consum-

---

country has got to take it. . . . Butter don't stand any show . . . and from this out, butter goes to the wall' " (Twain [1883] 2011, 278–288).

ers were advised to replace butter with margarine or Crisco and always to choose vegetable fats over animal fats as part of a healthy, prudent diet.

NIH Invests $250 Million Attempting to Show Healthfulness of Oils

The National Diet Heart Study that Stamler and Keys were helping to run was a rigorous effort to test the feasibility of a full-sized study of the "prudent diet." Seen now through the prism of industrial history, however, it seems entirely plausible that the endeavor, to which Swift & Co. devoted one of its employees full-time and developed high-polyunsaturated margarines and fake hamburgers, could reasonably be viewed in part as an industry-driven effort to broaden the market for its commodity oil.* Companies contributing to the study included nearly every major food corporation in the country, including the vegetable oil giant Anderson, Clayton & Company, Carnation, The Corn Products Company, Frito-Lay, General Mills, H.J. Heinz, the Pacific Vegetable Oil Corporation, Pillsbury, and Quaker Oats, among others.

A "feasibility" study doesn't produce results; it's meant simply to test out the practicalities of a certain kind of experiment before ramping up to the full-scale version. And on these terms, it was clearly unsuccessful. Keys, Stamler, and their team found that fully a quarter of the men had dropped out during the first year because they found it too hard to eat all their meals at home and because their wives were "uncooperative or disinterested." The third principal reason the men gave was simply that they didn't like the special diets; they missed their regular foods.

Whether the NIH should go on to invest in a larger study after this pilot effort was a question that administrators circled around repeatedly in a series of review committees throughout the 1960s. It was obviously a frustrating situation because, for the sake of the science, a full-scale clinical trial was urgently needed. Doctors following AHA guidelines had been

---

*The foods that made up the experimental diet of the LA Veterans trial, including filled milk, imitation ice cream, and filled cheese, were also donated by industry (Editors, "Diet and Atherosclerosis" 1969, 940), as were the foods in the Oslo study (Leren 1966, 88).

recommending a diet low in animal fats and cholesterol for nearly a decade already, based on weak epidemiological associations and some loosely controlled trials which had not reduced overall mortality.

Ultimately, however, in 1971, the NIH decided against conducting a definitive test of the diet-heart hypothesis. It was just too impractical and uncertain. To make all those margarines and other special foods to sell in special stores for so many people over so many years could cost upwards of a billion dollars. And since participants could barely be persuaded to stick with the diet anyway, the whole endeavor seemed futile. The NIH thus decided as a fallback to spend $250 million on two smaller trials, which would nevertheless be among the largest, most expensive diet trials in the history of diet-heart research.

One of these was the Multiple Risk Factor Intervention Trial, known as MRFIT (pronounced Mr. Fit), which ran from 1973 to 1982. Stamler had the prestigious job of directing it. After his lackluster efforts to get people to adhere to the ersatz foods he had invented for the National Diet Heart Study, Stamler thought that perhaps a better intervention would be to focus less on diet and more on controlling other factors, such as smoking, weight loss, and blood pressure. MRFIT therefore used the "everything but the kitchen sink" approach to fighting heart disease. It was one of the biggest and most demanding medical experiments ever performed on a group of human beings, involving twenty-eight medical centers nationwide at a cost of $115 million.

Stamler's teams measured the cholesterol of 361,000 middle-aged American men and found twelve thousand whose cholesterol was above 290 mg/dL—so high that they were considered to be at imminent risk of heart attack.* Most of the twelve thousand were obese, had high blood pressure, and smoked, so they had plenty of risks to modify. Half of them then received "multiple" interventions: counseling to quit smoking, medication to lower high blood pressure, if necessary, and advice on how to fol-

---

*This group was likely to include a disproportionate number of men with a rare (1 in 500) genetic disorder that causes exceptionally high cholesterol (genetic screenings were not performed on subjects). These men's physiological responses cannot be generalized to the rest of the population, but many diet-heart studies selected these men in order to increase the likelihood of generating more "events" (heart attacks), and the whole field of research was distorted as a result.

low a low-fat, low-cholesterol diet. They drank skim milk, used margarine instead of butter, limited eggs to two or fewer per week, and avoided meat and desserts; the target for saturated fat was 8 percent to 10 percent of calories. The other half were told to eat and live however they liked. Stamler followed all twelve thousand men for seven years.*

The results, announced in September 1982, were a disaster for the diet-heart hypothesis. Although men in the intervention group had been spectacularly successful in changing their diets, quitting smoking, and reducing their blood pressure, they died at slightly higher rates than the controls. The MRFIT investigators acknowledged this and floated various possible explanations. One was that the control group had also, independently, reduced rates of smoking and sought medication to control blood pressure, so by the end of the study the differences between the two groups were not as great as expected. Another possible explanation was that the diuretics used to treat high blood pressure were toxic (this idea was disproved). A final idea was that perhaps people would need to start such interventions earlier in life or keep them up over a longer period of time to see results.

MRFIT triggered widespread comment and criticism in the research community, but after much hand-wringing, its failure did not generate a change of course or even a serious reevaluation of the direction of heart disease research. And that was true even after MRFIT's follow-up findings delivered more bad news: at the sixteen-year follow-up to the study in 1997, the treatment group was found to have higher rates of lung cancer even though 21 percent of them had quit smoking, compared to only 6 percent of the controls.

When I asked Stamler about this apparent paradox, he took it straight on. "I don't know! That could be a chance finding. . . . It's just one of those findings. Troublesome. Unexpected. Not explained. Not rationalized!" (Stamler meets even the most timid challenge to his ideas with enthusiasm, delivered through an earthy Chicago accent. One colleague described him in his nineties as "frail but on fire.")

---

*Stamler has said the only problem with the study is that it didn't include women (Stamler interview). Men used to contract heart disease at rates far higher than women, but by the mid-1980s these rates had equalized. Women as a separate category for the study of diet and disease will be discussed in the next chapter.

Low Cholesterol and Cancer

One of the things that Stamler told me at the beginning of my visit with him was that he remembered certain things very well, "and other things I don't remember at all." What that meant, I discovered, is that Stamler recalled the smallest detail of the evidence in favor of the diet-heart hypothesis and little of the evidence against it. Regarding cancer, for instance, he probably should have remembered that his MRFIT findings were far from unusual. By 1981, nearly a dozen sizable studies on humans had found a link between lowering cholesterol and cancer, principally for colon cancer.

In the Framingham study, men with cholesterol levels below 190 mg/dL were three times more likely to get colon cancer than men with cholesterol greater than 220 mg/dL. In fact, ever since corn oil had been shown to double the rate of tumor growth in rats in 1968, there had been a baseline level of concern about vegetable oils and cancer. (Other studies from this time led to the supposition that corn oil might cause cirrhosis of the liver.) And there were other problems. People who had successfully lowered their cholesterol in trials of diet or drugs turned out to have higher rates of gallstones.* Strokes were also a concern. In Japan, for instance, a country of interest to heart disease researchers due to the relatively low rates of heart disease found in rural areas, NIH investigators found that Japanese people with cholesterol levels below 180 mg/dL suffered strokes at rates two to three times higher than those with higher cholesterol.

The NHLBI became so concerned about the cancer findings that it hosted three workshops in 1981, 1982, and 1983. The evidence on the topic was reviewed and rereviewed by an extremely prominent group of scientists, including Keys and Stamler. One suggestion was that low cholesterol might be an early *symptom* of cancer, rather than a cause. It was a plausible bit of logic. In the end, however, although the assembled

---

*Autopsies of subjects on the LA Veterans Trial, which used a diet high in polyunsaturated fats, revealed that people on the diet were more than twice as likely to have gallstones as those in a control group (Sturdevant, Pearce, and Dayton 1973). Excessive rates of gallstones were also observed among participants in a cholesterol-lowering clofibrate trial (Committee of Principal Investigators 1978).

researchers could find no convincing explanation for the cancer findings, they concluded that they did "not present a public health challenge" and did not "contradict" the more urgent, "commonsense" public health message for everyone to lower their cholesterol.

On the whole, said Manning Feinleib, an associate director at the NHLBI who attended the meetings as a rapporteur, the committee seemed to consider the downside of cancer to be less important than the upside of reducing heart disease. I spoke to him in 2009, and he was clearly dismayed that the issue of low cholesterol and cancer had still not been settled. "Oh boy, it's been more than twenty-five years, and they have still not shed more light on what's going on, and why not? That's even more puzzling."

In 1990, the NHLBI held yet another meeting on the problem of "significantly increased" death rates from cancer and other noncardiovascular causes for people with low cholesterol. The lower the cholesterol, the worse it looked for cancer deaths, and damningly, it looked especially bad for healthy men who were actively trying to reduce their cholesterol through diet or drugs. But there was no follow-up to these meetings, and the results did not change the enthusiasm for the "prudent diet." The effects of low cholesterol are still not well understood.

When I mentioned all this to Stamler, he didn't remember any part of this cancer-cholesterol debate. In this way, he is a microcosm of a larger phenomenon that allowed the diet-heart hypothesis to move forward: inconvenient results were consistently ignored; here again, "selection bias" was at work.

An Extreme Case of Selection Bias

There has been a lot of selective reporting and ignoring of the methodological problems over the years. But probably the most astonishing example of selection bias was the near-complete suppression of the Minnesota Coronary Survey, which was an outgrowth of the National Diet Heart Study. Also funded by NIH, the Minnesota Coronary Survey is the largest-ever clinical trial of the diet-heart hypothesis and therefore certainly belongs on the list along with Oslo, the Finnish Mental Hospital Study, and the LA Veterans Trial, but it is rarely included, undoubtedly because it didn't turn out the way nutrition experts had hoped.

Starting in 1968, the biochemist Ivan Frantz fed nine thousand men and women in six Minnesota state mental hospitals and one nursing home either "traditional American foods," with 18 percent saturated fat, or a diet containing soft margarine, a whole-egg substitute, low-fat beef, and dairy products "filled" with vegetable oil. This diet cut the amount of saturated fat in half. (Both diets had a total of 38 percent fat overall.) Researchers reported "nearly 100% participation," and since the population was hospitalized, it was more controlled than most—although, like the Finnish hospital study, there was a good deal of turnover in the hospital (the average length of stay was only about a year).

After four-and-a-half years, however, the researchers were unable to find any differences between the treatment and control groups for cardiovascular events, cardiovascular deaths, or total mortality. Cancer was higher in the low-saturated-fat group, although the report does not say if that difference was statistically significant. The diet low in saturated fat had failed to show any advantage at all. Frantz, who worked in Keys's university department, did not publish the study for sixteen years, until after he retired, and then he placed his results in the journal *Arteriosclerosis, Thrombosis, and Vascular Biology*, which is unlikely to be read by anyone outside the field of cardiology. When asked why he did not publish the results earlier, Frantz replied that he didn't think he'd done anything wrong in the study. "We were just disappointed in the way it came out," he said. In other words, the study was selectively ignored by its own director. It was another inconvenient data point that needed to be dismissed.

The Evidence against Saturated Fat: Epidemiological Studies

Of the vast quantities of imperfect data that were interpreted to support the diet-heart hypothesis, much came not from clinical trials but from large epidemiological undertakings, of the kind that Keys had pioneered with his Seven Countries study. These are studies where the diets of populations are not changed in any way: they are simply observed over time, and at the end, investigators try to link health outcomes such as disease and death back to their subjects' dietary patterns. Researchers had done these kinds of studies earlier—on the Italians in Roseto, the Irish, the Indians, and others—but those efforts had all been much smaller. The new studies followed thousands of people over many years, and their results made a highly influential contribution to the growing body of scientific papers that were used by experts to support the diet-heart hypothesis.

Stamler inherited one of the earliest of these studies, involving two thousand men who worked at the Western Electric Company near Chicago. The men were medically evaluated and their diets measured from 1957 onward. In the paper's abstract, which is often the only part of scientific papers that busy doctors and scientists ever read, Stamler wrote that his results supported cholesterol-lowering through diet. But the results, after twenty years of study, actually showed that diet affected blood cholesterol only a tiny bit and that the "amount of saturated fatty acids in the diet was not significantly associated with risk of death from CHD [coronary heart disease]," as the authors wrote. It seems clear that Stamler could not countenance such results. In the discussion section of the paper, he and his colleagues dismiss their own data outright and immediately move on to talk about other studies that *did* have the "correct" outcome.

When I asked Stamler about that, he said, "What we showed was that saturated fat had no *independent* effect on end points."

"So, in the end, saturated fat in the diet didn't matter, right?" I asked.

"It had no INDEPENDENT effect," Stamler yelled, meaning that on its own, it didn't matter. The Western Electric Study has nevertheless been regularly cited in support of the diet-heart hypothesis.

Another study in Israel followed ten thousand male civil service and government employees for five years and found no correlation between heart attacks and anything they ate. (The best way to avoid a heart attack, according to the study, was to worship God, since the more men identified themselves as being religious, the lower was their risk of having a heart attack.)*

---

*At the twenty-three-year follow-up of this study, researchers found a very weak relationship between saturated fat and myocardial infarctions, which the authors themselves dismissed as unimportant (Goldbourt 1993). Nevertheless, the Israeli Civil Service Study, as it's called, is routinely cited by prominent scientists demonstrating a

The other large epidemiological study during this period dealt with the Japanese, who have long been a source of fascination because they had very low rates of heart disease and lived on what appeared to be a near-vegetarian diet.

A study called NiHonSan tried to tease out the influences of genes and diet by comparing Japanese men living in Hiroshima and Nagasaki to their fellow citizens who had emigrated to either Honolulu or the San Francisco Bay Area. The middle-aged men were healthy in 1965, when their diet was first assessed, and were followed for five years. It turned out that the men who moved to California developed heart disease (as judged by abnormal electrocardiograph tests) twice as often as those in Hawaii or Japan. Saturated fat seemed to provide a reasonable explanation, since the Japanese in San Francisco ate roughly five times more saturated fat than did their counterparts in Japan. (The possible radiation exposure of these men to the atomic bombs dropped on their cities at the end of World War II was not factored into the analysis.)

The NiHonSan results have been widely trumpeted. The problems with the conclusions, however, ranged from the obvious to the obscure. First, the study authors circumvented their data on mortality, which did *not* support the diet-heart hypothesis, by selecting definite plus "possible" cardiovascular disease as their end points. ("Possible" heart disease includes vaguely defined symptoms such as chest pain.) This expansion of the definition to include uncertain diagnoses introduced a significant degree of error into the risk calculations yet it allowed the study leaders to show results consistent with the diet-heart hypothesis: a stepwise progression between heart disease and saturated fat consumption rising from Japan to Hawaii to California.

Looking only at the "definite CHD," however, the men in Honolulu, who ate just about as much saturated fat as the Californians, suffered *lower* rates of heart disease than their fellow Japanese back in Japan (34.7 v. 25.4 per 1,000). Serum cholesterol levels didn't line up so neatly, either. In fact, none of the risk factors that researchers knew—serum cholesterol, hyper-

---

"positive relationship" between saturated fat intake and coronary heart disease risk (Griel and Kris-Etherton 2006, 258).

tension, or blood pressure—could explain the differences in heart disease that they observed. Nor could they explain how men in Japan avoided coronary disease when nearly all of them smoked.

These inconsistencies indicated to me that maybe there might be something generally awry about this data. I wondered, for instance, what the authors meant when they wrote that diet information had been collected from only a "*sub*-sample of the cohort in San Francisco [italics added]." So I dug up the paper on NiHonSan's diet methodology, published two years earlier. It seems that the team in the San Francisco Bay Area had completely fallen down on the job. Not only did they get diet information from only 267 men, compared to the 2,275 interviewed in Japan and a whopping 7,963 in Honolulu, but they had done these interviews only one time and in only one way (a twenty-four-hour recall questionnaire), whereas the other two teams had assessed diet on two different occasions, several years apart, and in four different ways; this was clearly not the "same method" that the authors claimed. Yet these issues were never mentioned, and I wouldn't have known about them if I hadn't decided to look them up myself.

In any case, although the Japanese men in California did eat more saturated fat, they also met with any number of other factors found in wealthier Western societies, such as more stress, less physical activity, more industrial pollution, and more packaged and refined foods. Any of these factors could have provoked heart disease. That the authors blamed only saturated fat and took pains to obscure the questionable nature of their data almost certainly reflects the general bias in favor of the fat hypothesis for heart disease by 1970.*

And were the Japanese back in the homeland actually healthier? True, they suffered less from ischemic heart disease, but compared to Americans, they had much higher rates of stroke—which dropped when Japanese men migrated to the United States. Other studies have shown a higher incidence

---

*At the six-year follow-up to the study, the authors reported that the association of heart disease with saturated-fat consumption had disappeared and that lower rates of coronary mortality were associated only with less alcohol, higher carbohydrate consumption, and a lower-calorie diet overall (Yano et al. 1978).

of stroke in populations with diets low in meat, dairy, and eggs, compared to those eating more of those foods. Men in Japan were also found to have higher rates of fatal cerebral hemorrhages, which were associated with their low blood cholesterol and have been, by contrast, quite uncommon in the United States. Keys and his colleagues attempted to dismiss these findings when they emerged in the late 1970s. However, high rates of stroke and cerebral hemorrhage, associated with low cholesterol, have endured until today in Japan, and researchers have been unable to explain whether a low-cholesterol diet might be causing these health problems.

Also, although the Japanese have recently been eating far more meat, eggs, and dairy than they used to since the end of World War II, rates of heart disease have dropped to levels seen by Keys in the 1950s. This means that although the story of diet and disease in Japan is complex, we can pretty well say that based on this trend alone, a diet low in saturated fat was not the factor that spared the Japanese from heart disease in the postwar years.

After the publication of NiHonSan and the trial on the Israeli civil servants, *The Lancet* took stock of the evidence in 1974. "So far, despite all the effort and money that has been spent," wrote the editors, "the evidence that eliminating risk factors will eliminate heart disease adds up to little more than zero."

"One thing is clear," they continued about the two recently published epidemiological studies, "statistical association must not be immediately equated with cause and effect." It was an obvious point but one worth re-peating in a community of nutritional experts who were tempted to stretch the epidemiological evidence in favor of the diet-heart hypothesis.

The Lancet editors were consistently outspoken about adopting the diet-heart hypothesis too soon, and for many years, the debate in England was more lively and open than it was in the United States. In England, skepticism and even hostility toward the diet-heart hypothesis were wide-spread. The passionate embrace of the diet-heart hypothesis by American scientists was something that their British colleagues found perplexing. "There was a very big emotional component into the interpretation in those days," said the influential British cardiologist Michael Oliver. "It was quite extraordinary to me. I could never understand this huge emotion towards lowering cholesterol." His colleague in the United Kingdom, Gerald Shaper, the researcher who studied the Samburu tribe in Kenya, also found the American diet-heart proponents incomprehensible: "People like Jerry Stamler and Ancel Keys raised the blood pressure of British cardiologists to a level which was not believable. It was something strange; it was not rational, it was not scientific."

The Lancet editors sometimes mocked the American obsession. Why would Americans put up with the sacrifices of a low-fat diet? They were appalled that "some believers long past their prime were to be seen in public parks in shorts and singlets,* exercising in their free time, later returning home to a meal of indescribable caloric severity [when] there is no proof that such activity offsets coronary disease."

The Lancet also sounded a note of alarm that would soon be picked up by others: "The cure should not be worse than the disease," wrote the editors, echoing the medical dictum, "First, do no harm." Perhaps reducing fat in the diet might lead to some unintended consequence, such as a lack of "essential" fatty acids in the diet (these are fats that the body itself cannot make). In fact, Seymour Dayton was concerned about the extremely low levels of arachidonic acid, an essential fatty acid present mainly in animal foods, among his prudent dieters. Another possible consequence of cutting back on fat was the seemingly inevitable increase in carbohydrate consumption that would result, for the simple reason that there are only three kinds of macronutrients: protein, fat, and carbohydrates. Reducing animal foods (mainly protein and fat) shifts consumption toward the only type of macronutrient remaining: carbohydrate. In practical terms, a breakfast without eggs and bacon (fat and protein) becomes one of cereal or fruit (carbohydrates). Dinner without meat is often pasta, rice, or potatoes. Experts now lament that this dietary change came to pass in the latter half of the twentieth century, with disturbing results for health. *The Lancet's* fear was therefore clearly justified.

In the United States, Pete Ahrens, who was still the prudent diet's most

---

*A "singlet" is the English word for a tank top.

prominent critic, continued to publish his central point of caution: the diet-heart hypothesis "is still a *hypothesis* . . . I sincerely believe we should *not* . . . make broadscale recommendations on diets and drugs to the general public now." *

By the late 1970s, however, the number of scientific studies had grown to such "unmanageable proportions," as one Columbia University pathologist put it, that it was overwhelming. Depending on how one interpreted the data and how one weighed all the caveats, the dots could be connected to point in different directions. The ambiguities inherent to nutrition studies opened the door for their interpretation to be influenced by bias— which hardened into a kind of faith. There were simply "believers" and "nonbelievers," according to cholesterol expert Daniel Steinberg. A number of interpretations of the data were possible and equally compelling from a scientific perspective, but there was only one for "believers," while "disbelievers" became heretics outside the establishment.

Thus, the normal defenses of modern science had been flattened by a perfect storm of forces gathered in postwar America. In its impressionable infancy and compelled by an urgent drive to cure heart disease, nutrition science had bowed to charismatic leaders. A hypothesis had taken center stage; money poured in to test it, and the nutrition community embraced the idea. Soon there was very little room for debate. The United States had embarked upon a giant nutritional experiment to cut out meat, dairy, and dietary fat altogether, shifting calorie-consumption over to grains, fruits, and vegetables. Saturated animal fats would be replaced by polyunsaturated vegetable oils. It was a new, untested diet—just an idea, presented to Americans as the truth. Many years later, science started to show that this diet was not very healthy after all, but it was too late by then, since it had been national policy for decades already.

---

*By "drugs" Ahrens meant the first generation of cholesterol-lowering drugs, clofibrate and niacin, which in three large trials failed to show that lowering cholesterol made any difference in reducing heart attacks among middle-aged men after five years ("Trial of Clofibrate in the Treatment of Ischaemic Heart Disease" 1971).

5

The Low-Fat Diet Goes
to Washington

The low-cholesterol diet became national policy not only because the American Heart Association and nutritionists enthusiastically endorsed it as a solution to heart disease but even more importantly because the vast power of the US government swung behind it. Starting in the late 1970s, Congress intervened in the question of what Americans ought to eat, and this involvement by government propelled the low-fat diet down a new path, taking it out of the realm of science and into the world of politics and government. For the previous fifteen years, the research community, having endorsed an idea about diet and heart disease before it had been properly tested, had pretty much failed on its own terms. Whatever chance these experts might have had for self-correction was lost, however, when the federal government got involved. With its massive bureaucracies and obedient chains of command, Washington is the very opposite of the kind of place where skepticism—so essential to good science—can survive. When Congress adopted the diet-heart hypothesis, the idea gained ascendancy as an all-ruling, unassailable dogma, and from this point on, there has been virtually no turning back.

It all started in 1977, when the Senate Select Committee on Nutrition and Human Needs turned toward the question of diet and disease in America. With a sizable budget of nearly half a million dollars, the committee had previously dealt with issues of hunger, or *under*nutrition. Now the group turned to the new question of *over*nutrition: whether eating too much of certain foods might lead to disease. After all, what middle-aged male senator would not support an investigation into heart disease, the number one cause of death among middle-aged male senators?

So in July of that year, the committee, led by Senator George McGovern, held two days of hearings entitled "Diet Related to Killer Diseases."* The committee staff was comprised of lawyers and former journalists who knew little more than interested laymen on the subject of fat and cholesterol and nearly nothing about the scientific controversy that had been simmering on this topic for years. McGovern himself came to the subject with a potential bias, since he had recently attended a weeklong clinic at the center founded by lifestyle guru and low-fat devotee Nathan Pritikin.

After the hearings, committee staffer Nick Mottern spearheaded the research and writing of the report. He was a conscientious progressive, a former labor reporter for the small weekly newsletter *Consumer News* in Washington, DC, and a crusader against corporate influence. Mottern had no background in nutrition or health, however. He was therefore woefully ill-equipped to examine the subtleties of, say, study sample size or confounding issues in epidemiology. He didn't have the experience to know that when interpreting science, it's always wise to seek a variety of opinions. Instead, he relied almost exclusively on Mark Hegsted, a professor of nutrition at the Harvard School of Public Health and diet-heart stalwart. (Keys would have been a likely candidate for this role, but he had retired in 1972.) With Hegsted as his guide, Mottern recommended a diet in line with the one the AHA had been recommending, with overall fat reduced from 40 percent to 30 percent of calories, saturated fat capped at 10 percent of calories, and an increase in carbohydrates to between 55 percent and 60 percent of calories. (Mottern introduced the term "complex carbo-

---

*The story of the committee's work on this topic was first revealed in a 2001 article in *Science* magazine (Taubes 2001).

NINA TEICHOLZ

hydrates" to the nutrition lexicon, referring to whole grains, as compared to refined carbohydrates like sugar.)*

The committee ultimately adopted this view of a healthy diet, which dovetailed with Mottern's own skeptical views of the meat, dairy, and egg industries. Mottern found them objectionable for environmental and ethical reasons (He would later run a vegetarian restaurant in upstate New York for several years). And he believed the meat industry to be wholly corrupt, having been exposed to it up close—since McGovern represented South Dakota, a big cattle-raising state, and members of the National Cattlemen's Association often came striding through the office to meet with the senator. Mottern himself received calls from cattlemen trying to interfere with his report.

This influence by lobbyists rankled Mottern's idealism. Perhaps because he worked on Capital Hill, he viewed the fat and cholesterol issue to be as much a political contest between competing food interests as a scientific debate about nutrition and disease. In his eyes, the controversy pitched the virtuous, AHA-endorsed low-fat diet against the debased meat and egg industries, whose "cover-up" on the fat issue was, in his mind, like Big Tobacco's efforts to obscure negative health data on smoking. "Nick really wanted to find an enemy and make it a matter of good guy versus bad guy," recalled Marshall Matz, general counsel of the committee. For Mottern, the choice was clear. Impressed by researchers such as Jerry Stamler, who testified on behalf of the AHA, Mottern thought that "these scientists were willing to stand up to a lot of industry money and pressure," as he told me. "I admired them."

The reality was that, for all their obvious self-interest, the egg, meat, and dairy groups were hardly the most hard-core lobbies among the food interests. The real heavyweights were the big food manufacturers, such as General Foods, Quaker Oats, Heinz, the National Biscuit Company, and the Corn Products Refining Corporation. In 1941 these companies had set up the Nutrition Foundation, a group that worked to influence opinion

---

*Mottern's report also advised a reduction in sugar consumption (this was the fifth of six recommendations), but this goal fell by the wayside as researchers became more focused on fat and cholesterol.

with far more subtle techniques than striding through senators' offices. The foundation steered the course of science at its very source by developing relationships with academic researchers, funding important scientific conferences, and funneling many millions of dollars directly into research (even before the NIH began funding nutrition research). The foundation, along with food companies working individually, was therefore able to influence scientific opinion as it was being formed.*

The promotion of carbohydrate-based foods, such as cereals, breads, crackers, and chips, was exactly the kind of dietary advice large food companies favored, since those were the products they sold. Recommending polyunsaturated oils over saturated fats also served them well because these oils were a major ingredient of their cookies and crackers and were the principal ingredient in their margarines and shortenings. The pro-carbohydrate, anti-animal-fat orientation of Mottern's emerging report thus suited food manufacturers just perfectly. By contrast, that report did nothing for the egg, meat, and dairy interests, despite their high-profile reputation as bogeymen about Washington. So as hard as they might have tried, their lobbying efforts clearly hadn't been so successful.

A Bias against Meat

The disdain that Mottern felt for the cattle lobby reflected a bias against red meat that was already strong by the late 1970s when he was writing his report. This view of red meat as impure and unhealthy is now so ingrained in our beliefs that it's hard to imagine otherwise, but readers of this book will now be aware that a dose of skepticism for conventional wisdom is always merited. What *is* the scientific evidence against red meat? The question of exactly what data might be underpinning anti-meat health claims is important to know, especially as the drumbeat of seemingly bad news about red meat appears to intensify with each passing year.

In the 1950s and sixties, Ancel Keys and his colleagues didn't single out red meat as any worse than other foods high in saturated fat and choles-

---

*Many large food companies also had their own research institutes, such as the Corn Products Institute and the Wesson Fund for Medical Research.

terol; red meat, cheese, cream, and eggs were equally condemned for their ability to raise total cholesterol and hence potentially cause heart disease. Red meat, however, has long held a place of distrust in Western culture: it has been associated with greed as well as the power to incite sensuality and virility, which are generally considered to be impediments to a spiritual life.* And killing animals for their meat poses an ethical dilemma, more with respect to large animals such as cows, perhaps because they seem more sentient to us, than birds, like chickens. These moral qualms have heightened over the past century, fueled by the especially inhumane and corrupt practices of industrialized meat production. Also, as Americans became aware of world poverty and population pressures, red meat came to be seen as wasteful. The landmark 1971 book *Diet for a Small Planet* by Frances Moore Lappé made the case that the livestock raised to satisfy Americans' lust for meat represented a monumental waste of protein that could instead be feeding malnourished people in poor countries. Beef eating was particularly inefficient, she wrote, since cattle consumed 21 pounds of vegetables to produce one pound of meat.

These and other arguments against eating red meat dovetailed with Ancel Keys's advice about cutting back on saturated fat and made his recommended diet seem that much more intuitive to a nation of responsible consumers. The result has been that since the 1970s, a bias against red meat has settled in, even in the scientific research community, and this bias can be seen in the way that experiments are performed and interpreted.

---

*Pythagorus was a vegetarian partly for these reasons. The Reverend William Cowherd, who was one of the founders of the Vegetarian Society in Britain in the early nineteenth century, preached that "partaking of flesh" was partly responsible for the fall of man, and that meat's ability to inflame passions prevented the reception of the soul into "heavenly love and wisdom." These ideas were adopted in the United States by nineteenth-century Protestant reformers such as Reverend Sylvester Graham. However, it's worth pointing out that in both ancient Greek texts and the Bible, meat is portrayed as the food of the Gods. For instance, in the first book of Moses, Cain brings vegetables as an offering, while Abel brings "the firstlings of his flock and of the fat thereof." And "the Lord had respect unto Abel and to his offering: But unto Cain and to his offering he had not respect" (Genesis 4:4) (Spencer 2000, 38–69, on Pythagorus; Spencer 2000, 243, on Cowherd).

One of the more stark examples of prejudice in the field is the most famous study of vegetarians ever performed, involving 34,000 Seventh-day Adventist men and women who were followed by researchers throughout the 1960s and seventies. The Seventh-day Adventist Church prescribes a vegetarian diet that allows eggs and dairy but little meat or fish, and in 1978, investigators reported that the Seventh-day Adventist men on this diet had lower rates of all kinds of cancer (except prostate cancer, which was higher) than non-Adventist men, as well as fewer deaths from heart disease. Women, by contrast, saw no benefit* and an increased risk for endometrial cancer—in one of many examples of a contrary result on women that has gone unpublicized.

This study is widely cited as the bedrock evidence that a vegetarian diet is superior to one with meat. Yet again, it's easy to see many problems with the study that make the findings less than reliable. For example, one cohort of the Seventh-day Adventist subjects were compared to a control group living at the opposite end of the country, in Connecticut, where environmental factors could not be assumed to be similar (indeed, coronary mortality was 38 percent higher on the East Coast than in the West, and this variance alone could have explained the different rates of heart disease observed). More important, however, was the fact that the Adventist men following the church's vegetarian teachings were also very likely to be following other Seventh-day Adventist advice as well. They would probably have refrained from smoking and participated in the church's social and religious community. They were also known to be better educated than the control group. All these variables are associated with better health and therefore make it impossible to say how much diet alone affected outcomes. (Moreover, the diet itself was assessed only once in twenty years, and then only for those subjects who chose to return a questionnaire, which creates a distortion, because people who participate tend to be healthier than those who can't or don't.)† Even the study director acknowledged these prob-

---

*Elderly women in the study did see slightly lower rates of heart disease, however.
†This "healthy volunteer bias" was acknowledged by the study leaders, who tried to account for it (Fraser, Sabate, and Beeson 1993, 533).

lems.* Finally, one glaring bias not mentioned in any of the papers on the study is that Loma Linda University, home of the Seventh-day Adventist study, is an institution run for and by Seventh-day Adventists.

The Seventh-day Adventist study, despite its obvious flaws, was one of the foundational pieces of evidence used as "proof" for the belief that red meat is unhealthy. More recent studies cited to solidify this idea contain similar flaws. On March 12, 2012, for instance, there was a profusion of especially scary headlines, including one in the *New York Times*: "Risks: More Red Meat, More Mortality." This story referred to a research finding that just three additional ounces of red meat a day were associated with a 12 percent greater risk of dying overall, including a 16 percent greater risk of cardiovascular death and a 10 percent greater risk of cancer death. The study's announcement echoed around the world, with news reports in virtually every country.

The data for that report came from the so-called Nurses' Health Study II, which has followed more than 116,000 nurses for more than twenty years and is among the longest and largest epidemiological studies ever undertaken. For the red meat analysis, researchers at the Harvard School of Public Health, which directs the study, combined the nurses' data with a similar, smaller data set on male physicians from another epidemiological study they oversee. In the questionnaires answered by these doctors and nurses, the investigators discovered an association between eating red meat and reduced mortality. However, an association, as we know, can be merely coincidental—it does not demonstrate cause and effect, and this association, it turned out, was tiny.

The actual numbers underlying the 12 percent finding (percentages often look more dramatic when they are calculated from small numbers)

---

*Gary Fraser, the epidemiologist at Loma Linda University who has recently led the study (which is ongoing), wrote that these "possible confounding variables" made it difficult to zero in on what, exactly, might be protecting health. He objected, even, to the way that nutrition experts such as William Castelli, then director of the Framingham Study, were exaggerating his study's results. Castelli claimed that Seventh-day Adventists experienced only "one seventh" the risk of heart attacks of other Americans, but the difference was really only "modest," corrected Fraser (Fraser 1988; Fraser, Sabaté, and Beeson 1993, 533).

show that the increase in the risk of dying was only one person per hundred over the twenty-one years of the study. Moreover, the risk did not rise in lockstep with meat eating (meaning that eating a certain amount more red meat didn't translate smoothly to a certain amount of increased risk, which is that "dose-response" relationship that epidemiologists consider crucial for establishing the reliability of an association). Indeed, the risk associated with red meat eating in the Harvard study dropped steadily as meat consumption grew, and then only worsened in the group of biggest meat eaters—an odd finding that suggested there might be no real association after all.

But what about that group of biggest meat eaters? Could they not be seen as a cautionary tale? Many other observational studies have shown an association between eating a great deal of red meat and negative health outcomes. Possibly a high consumption of red meat triggers an effect only seen at a very high threshold? Or, more likely, maybe this effect is seen because people consuming a lot of red meat today are living less healthy lifestyles overall for reasons that have nothing to do with meat. In choosing to eat a lot of red meat, most of these people have consistently ignored the linchpin of dietary advice from doctors, nurses, and health officials for decades. It's quite likely, therefore, that these people are failing to prioritize their health in other ways: they probably don't visit their doctors regularly, don't take medications, don't exercise frequently, attend cultural events, or embed themselves in meaningful ways in their communities—all factors that have been shown to be associated with good health. It is therefore not surprising that in the Harvard study, the top meat eaters were also found to be less physically active, more obese, and more likely to smoke.

By the same token, it is also true that people eating a lot of fruits and vegetables over the past few decades are healthier in ways that have nothing to do with diet. People who make a conscientious effort to follow doctor's orders, whether to take a pill or exercise more regularly, have long been found by researchers to be healthier than people who don't. This effect, called the "compliance" or "adherer" effect, was discovered during the Coronary Drug Project in the 1970s, when researchers found that the men who took the intervention drug most faithfully cut their heart disease risk by half. But surprisingly, men taking the placebo most faithfully *also* cut their risk by half. The objective value of the intervention mattered less than the willingness to follow the doctor's orders. It turns out that people who dutifully follow advice are somehow quite different from the sort of people who don't; maybe they take better care of themselves in general. Maybe they're richer. But whatever the reason, statisticians generally agree that this compliance effect is quite large.

Therefore, any associations found between meat eating and disease, in order to be meaningful, must be big enough to overcome this compliance effect as well as other confounding variables. Yet, like the small association that Harvard researchers found in their 2012 study, the associations seen between red meat consumption and heart disease have generally been minimal, a scientific detail that study leaders tend not to emphasize and that the mainstream media have also, on the whole, overlooked.

The same kind of soft evidence pervades the other major health problem assumed to be related to red meat: cancer. According to a 2007 report by the World Cancer Research Fund and the American Institute for Cancer Research, a 500-page document that is the most authoritative review of diet and cancer conducted to date, red meat causes colorectal cancer. Yet, again, the reported difference between those who ate the most red meat and those who ate the least was minuscule—only 1.29 (this number, called a "relative risk," was even lower for processed meat, only 1.09). This is far from the "convincing evidence" that the 2007 report labeled it, since the National Cancer Institute itself recommends interpreting any relative risk below 2 "with caution." Experts lambasted the report's red meat findings for this and other reasons. As one critic pointed out, "If anything, the available evidence could only support a link with so-called HCA carcinogens, generated when red meat is cooked or fried."* And as we'll see later, this apparent carcinogenic effect could very well have less to do with the meat itself and more to do with the oil in which it is fried.

---

*Konrad Biesalski, a nutrition expert at the University Hohenheim in Stuttgart, also noted the counterintuitive reality that many of the nutrients implicated in protecting against cancer, such as vitamin A, folic acid, selenium, and zinc, for which we have been told to eat more fruits and vegetables, are not only more abundant in meat but are also more "bioavailable," meaning that they are more easily absorbed by humans into the bloodstream when eaten in meat rather than in vegetables (Biesalski 2002).

How Americans Used to Eat

Yet despite this shaky and often contradictory evidence, the idea that red meat is a principal dietary culprit has thoroughly pervaded our national conversation for decades. We have been led to believe that we've strayed from a more perfect, less meat-filled past. Most prominently, when Senator McGovern announced his Senate committee's report, called *Dietary Goals*, at a press conference in 1977, he expressed a gloomy outlook about where the American diet was heading. "Our diets have changed radically within the past fifty years," he explained, "with great and often harmful effects on our health." Hegsted, standing at his side, criticized the current American diet as being excessively "rich in meat" and other sources of saturated fat and cholesterol, which were "linked to heart disease, certain forms of cancer, diabetes and obesity." These were the "killer diseases," said McGovern. The solution, he declared, was for Americans to return to the healthier, plant-based diet they once ate.

The *New York Times* health columnist Jane Brody perfectly encapsulated this idea when she wrote, "Within this century, the diet of the average American has undergone a radical shift away from plant-based foods such as grains, beans and peas, nuts, potatoes, and other vegetables and fruits and toward foods derived from animals—meat, fish, poultry, eggs and dairy products." It is a view that has been echoed in literally hundreds of official reports.

The justification for this idea, that our ancestors lived mainly on fruits, vegetables, and grains, comes mainly from the USDA "food disappearance data." The "disappearance" of food is an approximation of supply; most of it is probably being eaten, but much is wasted, too. Experts therefore acknowledge that the disappearance numbers are merely rough estimates of consumption. The data from the early 1900s, which is what Brody, McGovern, and others used, are known to be especially poor. Among other things, these data accounted only for the meat, dairy, and other fresh foods shipped across state lines in those early years, so anything produced and eaten locally, such as meat from a cow or eggs from chickens, would not have been included. And since farmers made up more than a quarter of all workers during these years, local foods must have amounted to quite a lot.

Experts agree that this early availability data are not adequate for serious use, yet they cite the numbers anyway, because no other data are available. And for the years before 1900, there are no "scientific" data at all.

In the absence of scientific data, history can provide a picture of food consumption in the late-eighteenth- to nineteenth-century in America. Although circumstantial, historical evidence can also be rigorous and, in this case, is certainly more far-reaching than the inchoate data from the USDA. Academic nutrition experts rarely consult historical texts, considering them to occupy a separate academic silo with little to offer the study of diet and health. Yet history can teach us a great deal about how humans used to eat in the thousands of years before heart disease, diabetes, and obesity became common. Of course we don't remember now, but these diseases did not always rage as they do today. And looking at the food patterns of our relatively healthy early American ancestors, it's quite clear that they ate far more red meat and far fewer vegetables than we have commonly assumed.

Early Americans settlers were "indifferent" farmers, according to many accounts. They were fairly lazy in their efforts at both animal husbandry and agriculture, with "the grain fields, the meadows, the forests, the cattle, etc, treated with equal carelessness," as one eighteenth-century Swedish visitor described. And there was little point in farming since meat was so readily available.

The endless bounty of America in its early years is truly astonishing. Settlers recorded the extraordinary abundance of wild turkeys, ducks, grouse, pheasant, and more. Migrating flocks of birds would darken the skies for *days*. The tasty Eskimo curlew was apparently so fat that it would burst upon falling to the earth, covering the ground with a sort of fatty meat paste. (New Englanders called this now-extinct species the "doughbird.")

In the woods, there were bears (prized for their fat), raccoons, bobolinks, opossums, hares, and virtual thickets of deer—so much that the colonists didn't even bother hunting elk, moose, or bison, since hauling and conserving so much meat was considered too great an effort.*

---

*The availability of game in early America stands in sharp contrast to the more heavily settled lands of Europe, where peasants continually craved more meat than they could obtain (Montanari 1996).

A European traveler describing his visit to a Southern plantation noted that the food included beef, veal, mutton, venison, turkeys, and geese, but he does not mention a single vegetable. Infants were fed beef even before their teeth had grown in. The English novelist Anthony Trollope reported, during a trip to the United States in 1861, that Americans ate twice as much beef as did Englishmen. Charles Dickens, when he visited, wrote that "no breakfast was breakfast" without a T-bone steak. Apparently, starting a day on puffed wheat and low-fat milk—our "Breakfast of Champions!"— would not have been considered adequate even for a servant.

Indeed, for the first 250 years of American history, even the poor in the United States could afford meat or fish for every meal. The fact that the workers had so much access to meat was precisely why observers regarded the diet of the New World to be superior to that of the Old. "I hold a family to be in a desperate way when the mother can see the bottom of the pork barrel," says a frontier housewife in James Fenimore Cooper's novel *The Chainbearer.*

Like the primitive tribes mentioned in Chapter 1, Americans also relished the viscera of the animal, according to the cookbooks of the time. They ate the heart, kidneys, tripe, calf sweetbreads (brains), pig's liver, turtle lungs, the heads and feet of lamb and pigs, and lamb tongue. Beef tongue, too, was "highly esteemed."

And not just meat but saturated fats of every kind were consumed in great quantities. Americans in the nineteenth century ate four to five times more butter than we do today, and at least six times more lard.*

In the book *Putting Meat on the American Table*, researcher Roger Horowitz scours the literature for data on how much meat Americans actually ate. A survey of eight thousand urban Americans in 1909 showed that the poorest among them ate 136 pounds a year, and the wealthiest more than 200 pounds. A food budget published in the *New York Tribune*

---

*Butter consumption was between 13 and 20 pounds per person annually in the nineteenth century, compared to less than 4 pounds per person in 2000. Lard consumption was 12 to 13 pounds per person in the nineteenth century, compared to less than 2 pounds today. (Lard consumption hit a high of nearly 15 pounds per person from about 1920 to 1940.) (Nineteenth-century numbers are from Cummings 1940, 258; current numbers are from the USDA.)

in 1851 allots two pounds of meat per day for a family of five. Even slaves at the turn of the eighteenth century were allocated an average of 150 pounds of meat a year. As Horowitz concludes, "These sources do give us some confidence in suggesting an average annual consumption of 150–200 pounds of meat per person in the nineteenth century."

About 175 pounds of meat per person per year! Compare that to the roughly 100 pounds of meat per year that an average adult American eats today. And of that 100 pounds of meat, about half is poultry—chicken and turkey—whereas until the mid-twentieth century, chicken was considered a luxury meat, on the menu only for special occasions (chickens were valued mainly for their eggs). Subtracting out the poultry factor, we are left with the conclusion that per capita consumption of red meat today is about 50 pounds per person—or only a third to a quarter of what it was a couple of centuries ago.

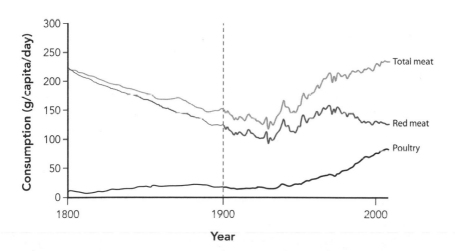

Meat Consumption in the United States, 1800-2007:
Total, Red Meat and Poultry

Source: Roger Horowitz, *Putting Meat on the American Table* (Baltimore, MD: Johns Hopkins University Press, 2000):11–17; Adapted from Carrie R. Daniel et al., "Trends in Meat Consumption in the USA," *Public Health Nutrition* 14, no. 4 (2011): Figure 2, 578.

Americans in the eighteenth and nineteenth centuries ate three to four times more red meat than they do today.

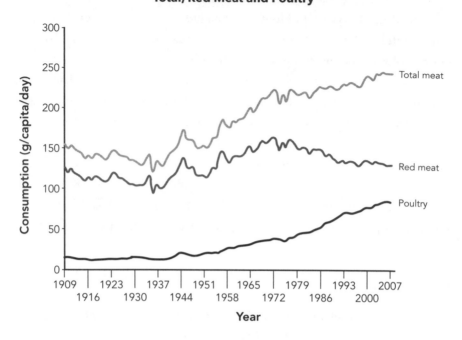

Meat Consumption in the United States, 1909-2007:
Total, Red Meat and Poultry

Source: US Department of Agriculture, Economic Research Service; Adapted from Carrie R. Daniel et al., "Trends in Meat Consumption in the USA," *Public Health Nutrition* 14, no. 4 (2011): Figure 2, 578.

Americans now consume more meat than a century ago, but that is due to eating more poultry, not red meat.

Yet this drop in red meat consumption is the exact opposite of the picture we get from public authorities. A recent USDA report says that our consumption of meat is at a "record high," and this impression is repeated in the media. It implies that our health problems are associated with this rise in meat consumption, but these analyses are misleading because they lump together red meat and chicken into one category to show the growth of meat eating overall, when it's just the chicken consumption that has gone up astronomically since the 1970s. The wider-lens picture is clearly that we eat far less red meat today than did our forefathers.

Meanwhile, also contrary to our common impression, early Americans appeared to eat few vegetables. Leafy greens had short growing seasons and were ultimately considered not worth the effort. They "appeared to yield so little nutriment in proportion to labor spent in cultivation," wrote one eighteenth-century observer, that "farmers preferred more hearty foods." Indeed, a pioneering 1888 report for the US government written by the country's top nutrition professor at the time concluded that Americans living wisely and economically would be best to "avoid leafy vegetables," because they provided so little nutritional content. In New England, few farmers even had many fruit trees, because preserving fruits required equal amounts of sugar to fruit, which was far too costly. Apples were an exception, and even these, stored in barrels, lasted several months at most.

It seems obvious, when one stops to think, that before large supermarket chains started importing kiwis from Australia and avocados from Israel, a regular supply of fruits and vegetables could hardly have been possible in America outside the growing season. In New England, that season runs from June through October or maybe, in a lucky year, November. Before refrigerated trucks and ships allowed the transport of fresh produce all over the world, most people could therefore eat fresh fruit and vegetables for less than half the year; farther north, winter lasted even longer. Even in the warmer months, fruit and salad were avoided, for fear of cholera. (Only with the Civil War did the canning industry flourish, and then only for a handful of vegetables, the most common of which were sweet corn, tomatoes, and peas.)

Thus it would be "incorrect to describe Americans as great eaters of either [fruits or vegetables]," wrote the historians Waverly Root and Richard de Rochemont. Although a vegetarian movement did establish itself in the United States by 1870, the general mistrust of these fresh foods, which spoiled so easily and could carry disease, did not dissipate until after World War I, with the advent of the home refrigerator.

So by these accounts, for the first two hundred and fifty years of American history, the entire nation would have earned a failing grade according to our modern mainstream nutritional advice.

During all this time, however, heart disease was almost certainly rare. Reliable data from death certificates is not available, but other sources of information make a persuasive case against the widespread appearance of the disease before the early 1920s. Austin Flint, the most authoritative expert on heart disease in the United States, scoured the country for reports of heart abnormalities in the mid-1800s, yet reported that he had seen very few cases, despite running a busy practice in New York City. Nor did William Osler, one of the founding professors of Johns Hopkins Hospital, report any cases of heart disease during the 1870s and eighties when working at Montreal General Hospital. The first clinical description of coronary thrombosis came in 1912, and an authoritative textbook in 1915, *Diseases of the Arteries including Angina Pectoris*, makes no mention at all of coronary thrombosis. On the eve of World War I, the young Paul Dudley White, who later became President Eisenhower's doctor, wrote that of his seven hundred male patients at Massachusetts General Hospital, only four reported chest pain, "even though there were plenty of them over 60 years of age then."* About one fifth of the US population was over fifty years old in 1900. This number would seem to refute the familiar argument that people formerly didn't live long enough for heart disease to emerge as an observable problem. Simply put, there were some ten million Americans of a prime age for having a heart attack at the turn of the twentieth century, but heart attacks appeared not to have been a common problem.

Was it possible that heart disease existed but was somehow overlooked? The medical historian Leon Michaels compared the record on chest pain with that of two other medical conditions, gout and migraine, which are also painful and episodic and therefore should have been observed by doctors to an equal degree. Michaels catalogs the detailed descriptions of migraines dating all the way back to antiquity; gout, too, was the subject of lengthy notes by doctors and patients alike. Yet chest pain is not mentioned. Michaels therefore finds it "particularly unlikely" that angina pectoris, with its severe, terrifying pain continuing episodically for many years, could have gone unnoticed by the medical community, "if indeed it had been anything but exceedingly rare before the mid-eighteenth century."†

---

*In Britain, the Scottish doctor Walter Yellowlees hunted down every last case of heart disease he could find and came to the conclusion that in prewar Britain the condition was "a very rare disease." The first case of an infarction in the Edinburgh Royal Infirmary was recorded in 1928 (Yellowlees 1982; Gilchrist 1972).

†Michaels recounts that William Heberden, one of the "most learned physicians of the day," presented the first properly recorded cases of chest pain to the Royal Col-

So it seems fair to say that at the height of the meat-and-butter-gorging eighteenth and nineteenth centuries, heart disease did not rage as it did by the 1930s.*

Ironically—or perhaps tellingly—the heart disease "epidemic" began after a period of exceptionally *reduced* meat eating. The publication of *The Jungle*, Upton Sinclair's fictionalized exposé of the meatpacking industry, caused meat sales in the United States to fall by half in 1906, and they did not revive for another twenty years. In other words, meat eating went down just before coronary disease took off. Fat intake did rise during those years, from 1909 to 1961, when heart attacks surged, but this 12 percent increase in fat consumption was not due to a rise in animal fat. It was instead owing to an increase in the supply of vegetable oils, which had recently been invented.

Nevertheless, the idea that Americans once ate little meat and "mostly plants"—espoused by McGovern and a multitude of experts—continues to endure. And Americans have for decades now been instructed to go back to this earlier, "healthier" diet that seems, upon examination, never to have existed.

"We Cannot Afford to Wait"

In the late 1970s in America, the idea that a plant-based diet might be the best for health as well as the most historically authentic was just entering the popular consciousness. Active efforts to demonize saturated fat had been underway for more than fifteen years by that time, and we've seen how the McGovern committee's staff were in short order persuaded by these ideas. Even so, the draft report that Mottern wrote for the McGovern committee sparked an uproar—predictably—from the meat, dairy,

---

lege of Physicians of London on July 21, 1768. The afflicted "are seized, while they are walking . . . a painful and most disagreeable sensation in the breast, which seems as if it would take their life away if it were to increase or to continue." These attacks would continue for months, or even years, until the final blow came. Heberden called the condition angina pectoris (severe pain of the breast) (Michaels 2001, 9).
*The dramatic takeoff in the number of reported cases in the early twentieth century may have also been due to improved diagnostic techniques (Taubes 2007, 6–8).

and egg producers. They sent representatives to McGovern's office and insisted that he hold additional hearings. Under pressure from these lobbies, McGovern's staff carved out an exception for *lean* meats, which Americans could be advised to eat. Thus, *Dietary Goals* recommended that Americans increase poultry and fish while cutting back on red meat, butterfat, eggs, and whole milk. In the language of macronutrients, this meant advising Americans to reduce total fat, saturated fat, dietary cholesterol, sugar, and salt while increasing carbohydrate consumption to between 55 percent and 60 percent of daily calories.

While Mottern would have liked the final report to advise against meat altogether, some of the senators on the committee were not so unequivocally confident about their ability to weigh in on matters of nutritional science. The ranking minority member, Charles H. Percy from Illinois, wrote in the final *Dietary Goals* report that he and two other senators had "serious reservations" about the "divergence of scientific opinion on whether dietary change can help the heart." They described the "polarity" of views among well-known scientists such as Jerry Stamler and Pete Ahrens and noted that leaders in government, including no less than the head of the NHLBI as well as the undersecretary of health, Theodore Cooper, had urged restraint before making recommendations to the general public.

Yet this hesitation turned out to be too little too late to stop the momentum that Mottern's report had set in motion. *Dietary Goals* revived the same argument that Keys and Stamler had used before: that *now* was the time to take action on an urgent public health problem. "We cannot afford to await the ultimate proof before correcting trends we believe to be detrimental," said the Senate report.

So it was that *Dietary Goals*, compiled by one interested layperson, Mottern, without any formal review, became arguably the most influential document in the history of diet and disease. Following publication of *Dietary Goals* by the highest elective body in the land, an entire government and then a nation swiveled into gear behind its dietary advice. "It has stood the test of time, and I feel very proud of it, as does McGovern," Marshall Matz, general counsel of the McGovern committee, told me thirty years later.

Proof of the report's substantiality, according to Matz, is that its basic recommendations—to reduce saturated fat and overall fat while increasing carbohydrates—have endured down to today. But such logic is circular. What if the US Congress had said exactly the opposite: to eat meat and eggs and nothing else? Perhaps that advice, supported by the power of the federal government, would have lived on equally well. In the decades since the publication of *Dietary Goals*, Americans have seen the obesity and diabetes epidemics explode—a hint, perhaps, that something is wrong with our diet. Based on these facts, the government might have deemed it appropriate to reconsider these goals, but it has nevertheless stayed the course because governments are governments, the least nimble of institutions, and unable easily to change direction.

No Looking Back: Washington's Wheels Begin to Turn

Once the US Congress had thrown its official heft behind a set of dietary recommendations, bureaucratic wheels all over Washington, DC, began slowly, inexorably, to turn. Diet and disease had long been ignored by various government agencies, but no longer.

Congress designated the USDA as the lead agency on nutrition, and coincidentally, Mark Hegsted turned up there in the post of the agency's new nutrition division director as well. He therefore effectively moved from being the scientific architect of the *Dietary Goals* to being their chief administrator. At the USDA, he worked with assistant secretary Carol Foreman, a vigorous consumer advocate who, like Mottern, saw her role as protecting unsuspecting Americans from the overconsumption of fatty foods ostensibly being foisted upon them by the corrupt egg and meat producers.

It was Hegsted's and Foreman's role to figure out how to implement the *Dietary Goals*. And this task required at the very least some imagination, because by September 1978, the only thing USDA staffers had published on the subject was a suggested menu of thirteen slices of bread each day in order to meet the report's recommended amount of carbohydrates. Could no one even come up with some palatable menu suggestions, asked a dietician quoted in the *Washington Post*.

Well, no, because although Congress had decided upon the components of a healthy diet, scientists were still quarreling over the basic evidence supporting those choices. Hegsted tried to put together an authoritative report on the matter at the USDA, but his effort fell apart amid bureaucratic infighting. Meanwhile, the esteemed American Society for Nutrition, which was also concerned about the need for a stronger scientific consensus before moving ahead with advice for the entire American population, had set up a formal task force to take another look at the diet and disease data and evaluate their strength. Hegsted decided to let his USDA recommendation be guided by the work of that task force. After all, the USDA's efforts could only be made more credible by having expert support, since it remained true that *no* group of nutrition scientists other than the AHA nutrition committee (dominated by Keys and Stamler) had ever formally been convened to review the evidence on diet and disease to date. Hegsted knew that he was "taking a big chance . . . since Pete Ahrens of Rockefeller University was co-chairing the committee and was known to oppose general dietary recommendations." Yet despite that risk, Hegsted agreed to abide by the panel's decision.

Ahrens chose a nine-member task force representing the full range of scientific views on the diet-heart hypothesis. The panel deliberated for several months over each link in the chain of the diet-heart hypothesis, from eating saturated fat, to total cholesterol, to heart disease. The results, however, were not exactly welcome news to diet-heart supporters like Hegsted or Keys. For instance, one issue the panel agreed upon was that the evidence condemning saturated fat was not persuasive. Moreover, the most they could say about fat generally was that it could be linked to heart disease only indirectly. The core problem was, as it had always been, the near-absence of clinical trial data on the low-fat diet, leaving only epidemiological studies. These studies, as we know, could show association but not prove causation. They had been enough for the Hegsted camp but not for the Ahrens camp.

The final report from the Ahrens task force in 1979 made it clear that the majority of its members remained highly skeptical of the idea that reducing fat or saturated fat could deter coronary disease. The group hadn't explicitly said that the dietary goals would do harm, however, and so Hegsted chose to take this as a green light. Using the same tenuous logic as did Keys in assuming that he was right until proven wrong, Hegsted asked rhetorically: "The question . . . is not why should we change our diet, but why not? What are the risks associated with eating less meat, less fat, less cholesterol?" The view in ascendance among nutrition experts was that Americans should "hedge their bets" against heart disease by reducing dietary fat until more evidence emerged. Hegsted imagined that "important benefits could be expected," and he could not imagine the costs. Ahrens's committee countered that the principle of "doing no harm" demanded harder proof before proceeding with a change in the American diet, but Hegsted was not persuaded by this argument. And ultimately, the USDA was accountable not to academic scientists but to the US Congress, which had ruled definitively in favor of a new low-fat regime.

Thus, in February 1980, despite the lack of an endorsement from Ahrens's committee, Hegsted went ahead with the publication of the *Dietary Guidelines for Americans*, the first set ever issued to the American public.* Eventually, these guidelines became the basis for the USDA food pyramid (which has morphed into the USDA's "My Plate" in recent years). Despite having grown from the work of a single congressional staffer and his single academic advisor and despite the lack of endorsement from nutrition experts, these are the now most broadly recognizable food guidelines in the United States, familiar to all schoolchildren and highly influential in determining school lunches and nutrition education across the country.

War Among Experts over Evidence

Aside from Ahrens's panel, there was one other group of nutrition experts who did not buy Hegsted's argument about the science being good enough to justify these guidelines. This was the National Academy of Sciences, a private society created by Congress in 1863 to be a resource for advice on scientific matters. Its Food and Nutrition Board has been the most respected expert group in Washington, DC, on matters of nutrition since it

---

*They are distinct from *Dietary Goals*, which the McGovern committee had published and which set the policy from which Hegsted's *Dietary Guidelines* flowed. *Dietary Guidelines for Americans* has been issued by the USDA jointly with the US Department of Health and Human Services every five years since 1980.

was established in 1940, and it sets the Recommended Dietary Allowances (RDAs) of nutrients every few years. The board had actually been solicited by the USDA to write up a review of the *Dietary Goals*, but the contract was never signed. Someone canceled it, quite likely, as the magazine *Science* reported, because USDA officials had caught wind of the board's lack of sympathy for the Senate's new low-fat diet.

Unwilling to be silenced, the academy used its own funds to prepare a review. An academy panel went through the now-familiar process of reviewing those same studies that everyone else had been looking at. Its conclusion on the available diet-heart evidence, published in a report called *Toward Healthful Diets*, was that the studies had "generally unimpressive results."

One of the more forceful points made by the academy was that Americans had been doing fairly well on their diet to date. The traditional diet was abundant in essential vitamins and high-quality proteins and was, as Gil Leveille, head of the Food and Nutrition Board, described it in 1978, "better than ever before and is one of the best, if not *the* best in the world." The average height of the American male—a fairly reliable indicator of life-long nutrition—had been fast rising throughout the first half of the twentieth century. Compared to countries with comparable statistics, Americans were among the tallest people on earth.*

So now there was a giant tug-of-war in Washington over the future of US nutrition. On one side were the USDA and the DHHS, mammoth branches of government backed up by the McGovern report, and also the US Surgeon General, who had responded to *Dietary Goals* by weighing in with his own like-minded report in 1979. Opposing all of these offices in the federal government, on the other side, was the lone and increasingly beleaguered Food and Nutrition Board of the National Academy of Sciences. It alone backed the view that a fat-reduced diet should not be recommended to all Americans.

---

*The steadily increasing height of the American male came to a halt for men born in the year 1970 and onward. Declining nutrition is one of a number of reasons that experts hypothesize might be the cause.

The media had a heyday—after all, fat and cholesterol were extremely hot topics, and, as Hegsted said gleefully, "the government and the academy were at odds!"

There were prominent stories in the *New York Times* and the *Washington Post*, and both papers saw fit to editorialize on the subject. Members of the board appeared on television talk shows, and the *MacNeil/Lehrer Report* ran a full segment on the subject. Even *People* magazine published an item, with a photo of the academy board chairman, Alfred E. Harper, at home, looking on affectionately as his wife scrambled up a batch of eggs.

Generally, the media coverage was fiercely in favor of the government's low-fat recommendations. The *New York Times* accused the academy's report of being "one-sided" and failing to represent "more than a single view." What the *Times* misunderstood was that the scientific disagreement was not about two dueling hypotheses, each with its own tangle of supporting arguments. There was only one hypothesis on the stand, and scientists were simply voting up or down on the evidence behind it. Was it enough? Or not?

The *New York Times* essentially took a poll: "at least 18 other health organizations and the Federal Government supported a reduction in fat and cholesterol," wrote the editors, with only the academy and the American Medical Association on the other side. The diet's potential costs—an increased heart disease risk from the carbohydrates, an increased risk of cancer from polyunsaturated oils, or a lack of adequate nutrition for children—were not part of the discussion. The *Times* concluded, "The Federal Government still thinks a prudent person should eat less fat and cholesterol. Unless the academy can authoritatively demonstrate Government error, a prudent person will do just that."

Here, then, was the new reality: a political decision had yielded a new scientific truth. Contrary to the normal scientific method, which requires that a hypothesis be tested before it can be considered viable, in this case politics short-circuited the process, and an untested hypothesis was elevated as the reigning doctrine, presumed to be right until proven wrong.

For the academy's report, the death knell was surely sounded on June 1, 1980, when the *New York Times* ran a front-page story about two board members and their ties to industry: Robert E. Olson, a biochemist at St. Louis University School of Medicine, had consulted for the egg and dairy industries, and Chairman Harper for the meat industry. These accusations were true. But again, corporate food interests were attempting to influence both sides of the debate. At the same time that two board members had been found to have ties to the meat, dairy, and egg industries, two other members of the academy's board were food company *employees*, one with the spice maker McCormick and Company, and another with the Hershey Foods Corp. And from the start, the board had been funded by the Nutrition Foundation, whose members included General Foods, Quaker Oats, Heinz Co., and Corn Products Refining Co., among other major food corporations.

Even despite this powerful lobby, the board had stood firm against the new low-cholesterol, low-fat diet recommendations. "Our attitude at the time," said Chairman Harper unapologetically in an interview when he was eighty-four years old, "was that if you had a competent person who was an adviser to a food company, there was no reason why they shouldn't serve on the board."

The press and public knew little of these widespread entanglements on all sides of the debate. They only picked up the impression that meat packers and egg farmers were corrupt, a view fostered by the press coverage. The health dangers of saturated fats had already come to be taken so much for granted by this point that pro-animal-food voices were presumed to have ulterior motives. Critics called *Toward Healthful Diets* "conspiratorial" and "slipshod," and US Representative Fred Richmond of New York stated openly that lobbyists for the food industry "must have been at work here."

The furor over the report startled academy scientists unaccustomed to this public gnashing of teeth. Philip Handler, head of the academy, told a friend that *Toward Healthful Diets* received more attention than had all the academy's numerous other erudite publications in recent years. "We were naïve about the politics," he said, and quipped, "you lose some, you lose some."

In the summer of 1980, the House and the Senate each held hearings on the report, and the academy's reputation was raked over the coals.

"Without too much doubt, the [House] committee's intention was to crucify Handler," judged *Science* magazine. Indeed, wrote the *Washington Post* editorial board, the report had "soiled" the board's and the academy's reputations for giving "careful scientific advice." The report had been a rigorous and fair-minded effort and contained far more expert analysis than did Mottern's, but publicity is powerful, and the widespread disparaging view of the board's work on the *Toward Healthful Diets* report has unfortunately endured until today. Because the academy is one of the few scientific groups that provides checks and balances against the work of other authoritative bodies on the subject of nutrition and disease (the others being the NIH, the USDA, and the AHA), the collapse of the academy's skeptical report on this issue was a significant event, for it left no formal scientific group to weigh in as the opposition.

The LRC Trial Puts an End to Debate

The last word on the debate over the diet-heart hypothesis came from the NHLBI in the early 1980s. Remember that two trials had been planned a decade earlier, when the institute decided against spending a billion dollars on a single, definitive full-scale trial of the prudent diet. One of these two smaller trials was MRFIT, the experiment run by Stamler using the "kitchen sink" model that had such a disappointing outcome. The other trial was the $150 million Lipid Research Clinic Coronary Primary Prevention Trial (LRC), the largest-ever experiment to test the idea that lowering one's cholesterol could protect against heart disease. MRFIT was a huge disappointment for the diet-heart hypothesis, so everyone was waiting for the LRC results, hoping they'd be better.

LRC was led by Basil Rifkind, chief of NHLBI's Lipid Metabolism Branch, together with Daniel Steinberg, a cholesterol specialist at the University of California, San Diego. They screened nearly half a million middle-aged men and found 3,800 with levels of cholesterol high enough (265 mg/dL or above) to be considered likely to have a heart attack soon; these men were divided into two groups. Both received counseling to eat a cholesterol-lowering diet, with fewer eggs, leaner meat, and lower-fat dairy than the national average. The treatment group was also given a cholesterol-lowering drug called cholestyramine, while the controls received a placebo.

It's important to understand that this trial did not test diet. Both groups in the study were advised to eat the same low-fat fare. Therefore, diet was not a variable tested in the trial; only the drug cholestyramine was tested in this design. The reason for not testing different diets, the investigators explained to critics, was that the NHLBI could not, in good conscience, deprive any high-risk man of a cholesterol-lowering diet—even though one of the trial's original goals was to test whether such a diet could protect against heart disease in the first place. It was a Kafkaesque circle of reasoning. Keys's hypothesis had evidently managed to sail over the normal hurdles of scientific proof such that the mere act of testing the diet was now considered unethical.

Despite this omission of diet as a variable in the trial, the LRC results, when they came out in 1984, were nevertheless hailed as a triumph for the diet-heart hypothesis. Part of that hypothesis dealt with the importance of lowering total cholesterol to prevent plaque buildup, and the drug *did* cause cholesterol to drop more in the treatment group compared to the controls. The treatment group also had slightly fewer heart attacks, and fewer of those that did occur were fatal.*

As we have come to expect, however, these results seem promising only until we look a little more closely at the data. The difference in heart attacks, for instance, was relatively small and turned out not to be statistically significant according to the statistical test that the authors had originally chosen to use. At the end of the study, investigators took the unorthodox and controversial step of retroactively selecting a more lenient test by which

---

*The group taking the drug saw cholesterol drop by an average of 13 percent, compared to only 4 percent in the control group. Even so, the result was considered a failure for the drug, since investigators had expected a more than fourfold difference in serum cholesterol between the two groups. Explanations given by study leaders for the lack of better results included the difficulty of adherence (the drug had many unpleasant side effects) and the fact that the liver compensates for the depletion of cholesterol by ramping up its own production (homeostasis at work).

their results *could* be called statistically significant.* They also decided to report their data on LDL-cholesterol as percentage changes, which skewed the results and obscured the relatively small changes in absolute numbers. Even with this statistical sleight of hand, however, there was still the problem that while the treatment had reduced coronary deaths, it had not, curiously enough, improved total mortality hardly at all; sixty-eight men in the treatment group had died from all causes compared to seventy-one of the controls, a mere 0.2 percent difference.

All-cause mortality was always the pitfall of cholesterol-lowering trials. Bizarrely but consistently, men whose cholesterol had gone down were found to die at significantly higher rates from suicides, accidents, and homicides. Rifkind thought the results were a fluke, yet this strange finding had shown up before in trials that reduced saturated fat, such as the Helsinki Heart Study. In fact, a metanalysis of six cholesterol-lowering trials found that the chance of dying from suicide or violence was twice as high in the treatment groups as it was in the control groups, and the authors posited that the diet might cause depression. (Researchers have subsequently suggested that cholesterol depletion in the brain may lead to impaired functioning of seratonin receptors.) Other cholesterol-lowering studies where diet had been the only intervention consistently found higher rates of cancer and gallstones in the experimental group, which is why the NHLBI itself had held that series of workshops on the problem only a few years earlier. In addition, populations found to have very low cholesterol, such as the Japanese, suffer from higher rates of strokes and cerebral hemorrhage compared to groups whose average cholesterol is higher.

A number of biostatisticians felt strongly that the LRC leaders should account for the trial's "fluke" findings. "Any statistician would turn in his badge if he couldn't find an excuse for such an outcome," said Paul Meier,

---

*In their protocol, LRC investigators stated that they would use a "two-tailed" test for significance, which recognizes that a treatment can go in two directions with either beneficial or detrimental effects. At the end of the study, however, investigators switched over to use a less-restrictive, one-tailed test, which assumes that the treatment can have only a beneficial effect. This looser statistical standard has been a source of controversy surrounding the LRC (Kronmal 1985).

one of the most influential biostatisticians of his generation. Nor could NHLBI administrator Salim Yusuf dismiss the LRC findings so easily. "I can't fully explain it and it worries the hell out of me," he told *Science* at the time.

Yet Rifkind and Steinberg did not attempt to account for these problems; they announced that the trial had been a resounding success in showing the health benefits of reducing cholesterol. Moreover, they did not merely conclude that cholysteramine prevented heart attacks; they came to the further conclusion that cholesterol-lowering changes in the *diet* must also reduce heart attacks—even though diet itself had not been tested. The assumption that reducing cholesterol with a drug must equal reducing cholesterol with diet represented a leap of faith and it was a questionable one. It led the biostatistician Richard A. Kronmal to write in the *Journal of the American Medical Association* that while it was tempting to assume that a low-fat, prudent diet would result in a reduction in heart attacks similar to what the drug had produced, the results of the trial "do not provide evidence to support this conclusion." Kronmal was concerned that Rifkind and colleagues had pushed the data to such an extent that it seemed more like "advocacy than science." The biostatistician Paul Meier commented that to call the results "conclusive" would constitute "a substantial misuse of the term."

Despite these criticisms, however, Rifkind told *Time* magazine, "It is now indisputable that lowering cholesterol with diet and drugs can actually cut the risk of developing heart disease and having a heart attack." Steinberg triumphantly declared LRC to be the "keystone in the arch" of the diet-heart hypothesis. Rifkind and Steinberg also assumed that their findings, based on extremely high-risk middle-aged men, "could and should be extended to other age groups and women," as well as low-risk men, based on the commonly held assumption that the fight against heart disease could never start too soon.

Their study results were hailed as definitive in part because experts so badly wanted them to be. The NHLBI had spent $250 million on two trials, each among the most expensive studies in the history of nutrition. This investment by the government virtually demanded that the trials lead to conclusive recommendations. Decades had gone by with supporters of the diet-heart hypothesis waiting for a "definitive" trial, and this pent-up demand put pressure on experts to overlook the study's problematic numbers and alarming side effects. According to the optimistic view of LRC taken by its lead investigators, the public could now be advised to lower their cholesterol by cutting back on saturated fat, or by taking a drug, or both.

LRC was therefore far from just the latest study on the stack. This trial, that did not even test diet at all, turned out to be one of the most influential studies of all time because its findings were subsequently used by the NHLBI to set up an entire bureaucracy devoted solely to lowering the serum cholesterol of every "high risk" person in America. Part of this effort involved telling people to cut back on dietary fat, especially saturated fat. And the effort came to encompass every man, woman, and child in the nation.

The Consensus Conference

If a large portion of middle-aged American adults are now cutting back on meat and taking statin pills, it is due almost entirely to the step that the NHLBI took next. Dispensing drugs and dietary advice to the entire US population is a huge responsibility, and the NHLBI decided it needed to create a scientific consensus, or at least the appearance of one, before moving forward. Also, the agency needed to define the exact cholesterol thresholds above which it could tell doctors to prescribe a low-fat diet or a statin. So once again, in 1984, NHLBI convened an expert group in Washington, DC, with a public meeting component attended by more than six hundred doctors and researchers. Their job—in an unrealistic two-and-a-half days—was to grapple with and debate the entire, massive stack of scientific literature on diet and disease, and then to come to a consensus about the recommended cholesterol targets for men and women of all ages.

The conference was described by various attendees as having preordained results from the start, and it's hard not to conclude otherwise. The sheer number of people testifying in favor of cholesterol lowering was larger than the number of spaces allotted to challengers, and powerful diet-heart supporters controlled all the key posts: Basil Rifkind chaired the planning committee, Daniel Steinberg chaired the conference itself, and both men testified.

The conference "consensus" statement, which Steinberg read out on the last morning of the event, was not a measured assessment of the complicated role that diet might play in a little-understood disease. Instead, there was "no doubt," he stated, that reducing cholesterol through a low-fat, low-saturated-fat diet would "afford significant protection against coronary heart disease" for every American over the age of two. Heart disease would now be the most important factor driving dietary choices for the entire nation.

After the conference, in March 1984, *Time* magazine ran an illustration on its cover of a face on a dinner plate, comprised of two fried-egg eyes over a bacon-strip frown. "Hold the Eggs and Butter!" stated the headline, and the story began: "Cholesterol is proved deadly, and our diet may never be the same."

NIH Consensus Conference: *Time*, March 26, 1984

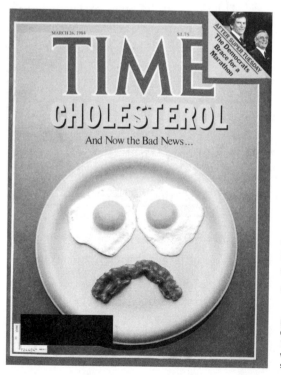

An NIH "Consensus" Conference in 1984 enshrined the idea that saturated fat causes heart disease.

From *TIME* Magazine, March 26, 1984 © 1984, Time Inc. Used under license. *TIME* and Time Inc. are not affiliated with, and do not endorse products or services of, Licensee.

As we've seen, LRC had nothing to say about diet, and even its conclusions on cholesterol were only weakly supported by the data, but Rifkind had already demonstrated that he believed this extrapolation was fair. He told *Time* that the results "strongly indicate that the more you lower cholesterol and fat in your diet, the more you reduce the risk of heart disease."

Gina Kolata, then a reporter for *Science* magazine, wrote a skeptical piece about the quality of the evidence supporting the conference's conclusions. The studies "do not show that *lowering* cholesterol makes a difference," she wrote, and she quoted a broad range of critics who worried that the data were not nearly strong enough to recommend a low-fat diet for all men, women, and children. Steinberg attempted to dismiss the criticisms by calling her article a case of the media's appetite for "dissent [which] is always more newsworthy than consensus," but the *Time* cover story in support of Steinberg's stated conclusions was clearly an example of the opposite, and on the whole, the media supported the new cholesterol guidelines.

The consensus conference spawned an entirely new administration at the NIH, called the National Cholesterol Education Program (NCEP), whose job it remains to advise doctors about how to define and treat their "at-risk" patients, as well as to educate Americans themselves about the apparent advantages of lowering their cholesterol. In the following years, the NCEP's expert panels became infiltrated by researchers supported by pharmaceutical money, and cholesterol targets were ratcheted ever lower, thereby bringing greater and greater numbers of Americans into the category that qualified for statins. And the low-fat diet, even though it had never been properly tested in a clinical trial to ascertain whether it could prevent heart disease, became the standard, recommended diet of the land.

For longtime critics of the diet-heart hypothesis such as Pete Ahrens, the consensus conference was also significant because it marked the last time they could speak openly. After this conference, Ahrens and his colleagues were forced to fold their case. Although members of the nutrition elite had, over the previous two decades, been allowed to be part of the debate, in the years following the consensus conference, this was no longer true. To be a member of the elite now meant, ipso facto, supporting the low-fat diet. So effectively did the NHLBI-AHA alliance silence its antagonists, in fact, that among the tens of thousands of researchers in the worlds of medicine and nutrition over the next fifteen years, only a few dozen would publish research even gingerly challenging the diet-heart hypothesis. And even then, they worried about putting their careers on the line. They saw Ahrens, who had risen to the very top of his field and yet found himself having a hard time getting grants, because there was "a price to pay for going up against the establishment, and he was well aware of that," as one of his former students told me.

No doubt this is why Ahrens, in looking back on the conference, which came to be his swan song, spoke with an uncharacteristic lack of reserve. "I think the public is being hosed by the NIH and the American Heart Association," he declared. "They desire to do something good. They're hoping to God that this is the right thing to do. But they are not acting on the basis of scientific evidence, but on the basis of a plausible but untested idea." Plausible or even probable, however, that untested idea had now been launched.

6

How Women and Children Fare on a Low-Fat Diet

It's hard to overstate what a radical departure from the government's stand on nutrition the *Dietary Guidelines for Americans* represented when it came out in 1980. Since 1956, the USDA had been advising people to seek out nutritious foods by eating a "well-balanced" diet of the basic food groups—first five of them, then seven, then four. The four food groups were milk, meat, fruits & vegetables, and cereals & grains. Americans had been encouraged to eat some foods from each group every day. The USDA has always suffered from a conflict of interest, since its entire mission is to promote American food commodities, and the agency has long been heavily influenced by those very industries. In any case, now its message was shifting from one of ensuring that people got enough servings of nutritional foods to one of restricting them—and the irony was that, in most instances, these were the very same foods! Meat, butter, eggs, and whole milk, all long associated with prosperity, went from being salubrious to dangerous.

Because Americans were questioning accepted norms in the 1970s, with public-interest advocates turning up ugly truths about consumer items, from cigarettes to pesticides that had long been assumed safe, the questioning of such basic foodstuffs as meat, milk, and eggs seems understandable as part of that skepticism. Advice to ditch traditional foods came at a moment when the public lacked confidence in once-sacrosanct beliefs, and this explains in part why the *Dietary Guidelines* found a willing public when it recommended replacing these foods with more vegetables, fruits, and grains.

In the wake of the *Dietary Guidelines*, the low-fat, low-cholesterol diet spread far and wide in the 1980s, expanding from the original class of high-risk, middle-aged men to encompass all Americans, women and children alike. It became the diet of the entire nation. Setting strict cholesterol targets, the new NCEP guidelines were not only directed at more people, but they also extended their dietary reach. The proposed regime no longer required cutting back just on saturated fat and cholesterol but on fat overall. The rationale was based on that powerfully intuitive, straightforward logic, as Jerry Stamler expressed in 1972, that fat was "excessive in calories . . . so that obesity develops." This seemingly obvious but nonetheless unproven assumption was that fat made you fat. It was, again, that unfortunate homonym.

This idea about the cause of obesity had always been lurking in the background of the diet-heart conversation, but it did not become a formal dietary recommendation until 1970, when the AHA, ever on the forefront of ratcheting back fat, first published a guideline setting a 35 percent limit on fat as a portion of total calories. By contrast, just two years earlier, the AHA committee had warned *against* reducing fat due to a concern that this would lead to an increase in carbohydrates. The committee was especially concerned about refined carbohydrates and counseled against the "excessive use of sugar, including candy, soft drinks, and other sweets."

However, when the AHA nutrition committee changed its leadership for the 1970 set of guidelines, with the influential Jerry Stamler once again onboard, that warning was lost. And for the next twenty-five years until 1995, AHA pamphlets told Americans to control their fat intake by increasing refined-carbohydrate consumption. Choose "snacks from other food groups such as . . . low-fat cookies, low-fat crackers, . . . unsalted pretzels, hard candy, gum drops, sugar, syrup, honey, jam, jelly, marmalade," stated a 1995 AHA publication. In short, to avoid fat, people should eat sugar, the AHA advised.

Later, many nutrition experts lamented the so-called "SnackWell's phenomenon," referring to the fact that people seeking to be health-conscious by reducing fat would plow their way through bags of nonfat or low-fat cookies full of refined carbohydrates instead. "We could not have foreseen this—it was *industry* that made these high carb–concentrated calories," Stamler told me, in a view that has been widely aired. Yet the AHA itself had clearly steered Americans—and the food industry—toward exactly that solution. The AHA even rode the profit wave of refined carbohydrates from the 1990s onward by charging a hefty fee for the privilege of putting the AHA's "Heart Healthy" check mark on products, with the label ending up on some dubious candidates, such as Kellogg's Frosted Flakes, Fruity Marshmallow Krispies, and low-fat Pop-Tarts. Eventually, the AHA was chastened into removing its endorsement from those blatantly unhealthy products, yet in 2012, the check mark still appeared on boxes of Honey Nut Cheerios and Quaker Life Cereal Maple and Brown Sugar, which might have healthier-sounding names but are both higher in sugar and carbohydrates than Kellogg's Frosted Flakes. Given the AHA's role in promoting high-sugar foods, it therefore seems disingenuous to blame the food industry for the shift from fat to refined carbohydrates.

The AHA's emphasis on reducing total fat *did* encounter a degree of high-level official criticism in its day. Indeed, Donald S. Fredrickson, a top NIH official who later went on to lead that government agency, wrote an article taking the AHA guidelines to task: "Do we know enough," he asked, "to advise everyone to eat a diet which will provide more than half of the calories as carbohydrates?" There was something about the AHA report "to be pitied" he wrote, condescendingly, referring to the lack of scientific evidence for the low-fat diet.

It's important to realize that in 1970, when the AHA started telling Americans to cut back on total fat, this regime had not been tested in clinical trials. All those famous big, early trials had been on the "low-cholesterol," or "prudent" diet—high in vegetable oils and low in saturated fats—but when it came to reducing fat *overall*, as the AHA was now advising, the evidence was nonexistent. In fact, the data underpinning the low-fat diet amounted to only a couple of tiny studies, one from Hungary and one from Britain, in which fat was severely reduced to an unrealistic 1.5 ounces a day to see if such a diet could reduce heart disease. And these two studies had contradictory results. Trials aimed at testing the 35 percent fat limit that was already being recommended had simply not been performed.

This lack of evidence had clearly not impeded the AHA from issuing its low-fat guidelines, however, and the group now went a step further. It called for a vast overhaul of the country's food production systems: development of new strains of leaner livestock, low-fat dairy products and low-fat bakery goods, the promotion of margarine, the virtual elimination of egg yolks, and revisions of school lunches and food stamps, as well as meals for both the Armed Forces and veterans' facilities. As we know, most of these changes have since come to pass. Not only have government food programs switched over to low-fat products, but pretty much every food company in the country has reformulated its products, from Tyson's skinless chicken breasts to low-fat soups, spreads, yogurts, and cookies. You name it, and there's a low-fat version of it. In some cases, it's not even possible to buy the full-fat version of a food product anymore. For instance, the major American yogurt manufacturers to this day sell only low- or nonfat yogurts. (In 2013, the only full-fat yogurts on the national market came from Greece.) In the mid-1990s, at the height of the consumer craze to get rid of all dietary fat, fully one quarter of all new food products coming on the market were labeled as "low-fat." *

Throughout the 1980s and nineties, magazines and newspapers overflowed with articles on how to cut fat and live happily without meat. Jane Brody, the health columnist for the *New York Times* and the most influential promoter of the low-fat diet in the press, wrote, "If there's one nutrient that has the decks stacked against it, it's fat," and in 1990, she published her seven-hundred-page message to the public: *The Good Food Book: Living the High-Carbohydrate Way.*

_____

*Since 1990, the FDA has regulated these kinds of health claims on food packages, which also include claims such as "high fiber" and "low cholesterol."

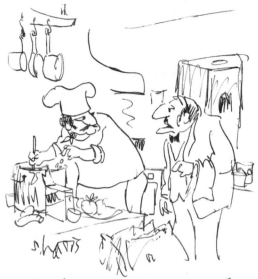

"TABLE 4 SENDS ITS COMPLIMENTS. TABLE 7 WANTS TO KNOW IF YOU'RE TRYING TO KILL THEM WITH ALL THOSE SATURATED FATS AND CHOLESTEROL."

Dean Ornish and the Near-Vegetarian Diet

As anyone who grew up during the 1980s can remember, the low-fat craze reached its height during that decade, as the diet evolved toward its nonfat pole. Leading the way in this direction was the self-educated Nathan Pritikin, who, in struggling with his own high cholesterol, found the low-fat diet as a solution. He then popularized the regime through his best-selling books and the Pritikin Longevity Center in San Diego. Pritikin's condemnation of fat grew over the years, and by the early 1980s, he had eliminated almost all fat from his diet. This nonfat, vegan fare is what he liked to call "mankind's original meal plan."* Pritikin advocated that fully 80 percent

---

*Some of the scientific literature on the Paleolithic human diet has reinforced the idea that our prehistoric diet was formerly comprised of mostly plants, although Loren Cordain, author of *The Paleo Diet*, the founding book of this field, argues that early humans, "whenever and wherever it was ecologically possible," ate 45 percent to 65 percent of their calories as animal foods. This idea coincides with the work of Richard Wrangham, an anthropologist at Harvard University, who argues that the evolution of *Homo sapiens* only became possible when early humans shifted their diet to one of predominantly meat, for the reason that meat and especially viscera like

of daily calories be eaten as carbohydrates—a kind of AHA low-fat diet for extremists.

The 1970s and eighties were generally a sustained era of famous diet doctors. The doctor who was squarely in Pritikin's camp yet who ultimately proved to be far more powerful—indeed, arguably the most enduringly influential diet doctor of the past thirty years—was Dean Ornish. (At the other end of the spectrum during these years, there was Robert C. Atkins, discussed in Chapter 10.)

Ornish has been promoting the near-vegetarian diet since the 1980s. Exiled from his diet are red meat, liver, butter, cream, and egg yolks. These are in what he calls "Group Five," the lowest, most forbidden, rung of his diet "ladder," below Group Four foods, which include "doughnuts, fried pastries, cakes, cookies, and pies." If you seriously aim to reverse heart disease, counsels Ornish, then you must eat mostly fruits, vegetables, and grains; in all, nearly three quarters of calories should come from carbohydrates. High-fat diets, by contrast, he claims, make people "tired, depressed, lethargic and impotent."

However, it turns out that people have a hard time adhering to the Ornish diet even when their meals are provided for them, as Frank Sacks, a professor at the Harvard School of Public Health, found when he conducted a study on the Ornish program in the early 1990s. "We pulled out all the stops. We had a superb staff," he said, but the study subjects "could not stick with it." Ornish agrees that his diet can take work, but, he argues, "It's hard to do a lot of things in life that are worth doing. It's hard to exercise every day but I don't think most people would say it's not worth doing. It's hard to quit smoking. It's hard to raise a family."

Although Ornish is an internist with no research training, he became

---

kidney and liver are far more nutrient-dense than plant food (Wrangham argues that the ability to cook meat was especially crucial, since this process increases the availability of nutrients for digestion). By contrast, chimpanzees who subsist mainly on plant food must spend much of their day in the act of eating in order to acquire enough nutrients for survival, and their large mouths are an indication of the volume of plant food they needed to ingest, compared to the smaller mouth size of humans surviving on meat, according to Wrangham (Cordain et al. 2000; Wrangham 2009; Werdelin 2013, 34–39).

NINA TEICHOLZ

famous because in the 1990s, he was one of the first people ever to publish evidence apparently demonstrating the benefits of a diet low in fat. Ornish's studies have been among the most highly cited papers in nutrition history, and he claims that his program, which involves not just diet, but also aerobic exercise, yoga, and meditation, is the only one ever to demonstrate an actual *reversal* of heart disease. His studies are therefore worth looking at more closely.

The 1990 study upon which Ornish's spectacular claims are based involved twenty-one San Francisco residents who participated in Ornish's diet-and-exercise program for a year. According to a medical imaging process called angiography, which uses X-rays to take a two-dimensional picture of blood vessels, the subjects in the intervention program saw their arteries widen. Meanwhile, nineteen members of a control group, without any diet or exercise intervention over the same period of time, saw their arteries contract.* Reducing arterial blockage was a key finding, because never before had anyone been able to demonstrate that heart disease could be reversed.†

"Healer of Hearts!" announced a *Newsweek* cover story in 1998 when Ornish published an article in the *Journal of the American Medical Association* (JAMA). The article portrayed Ornish as the opposite of a cynic, spontaneously hugging people and striving to approach his work from a "spirit of service" rather than an "ego-driven" effort. And in a world where cardiologists are pushing patients toward invasive surgery or a lifelong dependence on statin drugs, Ornish has been virtually alone in the cardiology world in suggesting, alongside nutritionists, that diet and exercise are enough to keep people healthy.

---

*Ornish started with 28 patients in the experimental group, but one died while exercising, and follow-up data for the others could not be obtained (Ornish et al. 1990, 130).

†Five years later, with only twenty subjects left on the program, Ornish reported in two articles that the results were on track: the arteries of his experimental patients had widened by 3 percent since day one of the experiment, whereas those of the controls had narrowed by nearly 12 percent. Imaging with positron-emission tomography (PET) scans revealed that blood flow to the heart had improved by some 10 percent to 15 percent among the diet-and-exercise group (Gould et al. 1995; Ornish et al. 1998; Ornish et al. 1990).

Yet Ornish's study, like so many in nutrition research, is troublesome. Twenty-one patients is not a lot, nor did all of them make it through the full five years of follow-up.* And importantly, Ornish's study has never been successfully replicated by independent researchers, the hallmark of credibility in "hard" sciences.

Curious about the findings, I called Kay Lance Gould, director of cardiology at the University of Texas, who helped Ornish launch his research career and was a co-author with Ornish on the JAMA papers. (Altogether, they published three JAMA papers, which is an unusually high number for one small trial.) On the phone, I could almost hear Gould's incredulity over how Ornish had promoted their study results. "Most people do a study and get one paper. Dean does one study and gets a bunch of papers. It's a miracle. There's a certain skill in marketing a small little piece of data. He's really a genius at PR."

Gould is also perfectly up-front about the fallibility of the angiographic evidence that supposedly demonstrated widening of the subjects' arteries. These images have not been shown to be the bedrock evidence that Ornish routinely asserts, nor do they necessarily translate into the good news that he implies. While an artery getting wider seems intuitively like a good sign, the gradual narrowing of arteries has not been reliably correlated with coronary mortality.† And widening arteries by the insertion of a stent (a mesh

---

*Another study, looking at the need for repeat heart surgery among subjects on the Ornish program, failed to produce statistically significant results (Ornish 1998).
†Cardiologists have been debating the reliability of such angiographic evidence since the late 1950s. The narrowing of the arteries is caused by an accumulation of lesions on the arterial walls, called "atherosclerosis," and this buildup of plaque has long been thought to indicate heart attack risk. However, George Mann was one of the first researchers to make observations that did not support this idea: despite "extensive" lesions in the arteries of the fifty Masai men he autopsied, equal to "that of old U.S. men," electrocardiogram evidence revealed almost no evidence of heart attacks. He postulated that atherosclerosis was a natural part of the aging process and that only certain kinds of unstable plaques broke off, creating the blockages that cause heart attacks. This theory has been widely embraced. One of the problems with angiography is that its images cannot reveal the differences between normal plaque and the dangerous, unstable kind. Its reliability is also hampered by the fact that the

tube that expands the arterial walls) has not been shown to extend life. Major scientific journals were publishing articles on this issue in the mid-1980s when Ornish undertook his experiments.

When I asked Ornish about this point, he wavered. "Why do you want to know?" he asked, so I explained. "Well, it's not the best evidence," he admitted. Yet two days later, in another conversation, he was back to claiming that his studies had "actually reversed heart disease," including "quantitative arteriography" as a central part of the proof of that assertion. When I challenged him again, there was silence. Then: "You're absolutely right . . . I'm totally in agreement." (Ornish would repeat this claim again—most recently in an opinion piece in the *New York Times* in 2012, defending the near-vegetarian diet.)

In our conversation, Ornish moved on to his next assertion that "we also found improvements in blood flow. . . . [which] is the bottom line in coronary heart disease. We showed 300 percent improvement in blood flow," he said. Yet Gould, who had interpreted that data for the study, had told me that this number was around 10 percent to 15 percent. I reported this to Ornish. "Well, I'm not going to quibble about that," he said.

But even accepting Ornish's claim of heart disease "reversal," the question remains: Was it the very low-fat diet that made the difference? Or the smoking cessation, the drop in refined carbs, the aerobic exercise, the group psychosocial support, the stretching, the yoga, the meditation, or the other interventions to reduce stress? All these were part of his program. Possibly the fat reduction was irrelevant. How could even Ornish know, let alone anyone else?

Vegetarian diets generally have not been shown to help people live longer. The 2007 report by the World Cancer Research Fund and the American Institute for Cancer Research, discussed in the last chapter, found that "in no case" was the evidence for the consumption of fruits and vegetables in the prevention of cancer "judged to be convincing." And despite the fact that vegetarians tend to be "compliers" who follow doctors' orders and are

---

technique is difficult and the results therefore quite variable (Jones 2000; Mann et al. 1972).

generally more aware of their health, meaning that they should live longer than other people, many studies have found this not to be true. Indeed, in the largest observational study on vegetarians, which followed 63,550 middle-aged men and women in Europe for a decade, overall mortality for vegetarians and nonvegetarians turned out to be the same.*

Since we now live in a time when the vegetarian (or near-vegetarian) diet is so heavily favored by health authorities as well as the popular press, these researcher findings are probably a surprise, but they would not have been to nutrition experts in the 1920s. Remember those Masai warriors in Kenya who ate little other than milk, blood, and meat? Decades before George Mann arrived in Kenya, the British government commissioned scientists in 1926 to compare the Masai to a neighboring tribe, the Akikuyu. They had lived side by side for many generations, in "very similar" conditions, according to the researchers. However, whereas the Masai ate mainly animal foods, the Akikuyu subsisted on a near-vegetarian diet that was very low in fat, with the "great bulk" of their food consisting of "cereals, tubers, plantains, legumes, and green leaves."

Investigators spent several years in detailed examination of 6,349 Akikuyu and 1,546 Masai adults, and in the end, found that the health of the two groups differed dramatically, though not in ways one might expect. The vegetarian Akikuyu men were found to be far more likely to suffer from bone deformities, dental caries, anemia, lung disease, ulcers, and blood disorders; the Masai were more likely to contract rheumatoid arthritis. The Masai men were on average 5 inches taller than the Akikuyu and

---

*This result came out a few years before the Harvard Nurses' Health Study findings on red meat and disease, but it did not, unsurprisingly, get the same number of headlines. Nor has it received the same level of publicity as the China Study, the subject of at least eight books and cookbooks since 1990, by the nutritional biochemist T. Colin Campbell, who argues in favor of a vegan diet. These books are based on one epidemiological study, with a number of significant methodological problems, that was never published in a peer-reviewed issue of a scientific journal. Campbell's two papers were instead published as part of conference proceedings in journal "supplements," which are subject to little or no peer review (Campbell and Junshi 1994; Campbell, Parpia, and Chen 1998; Masterjohn 2005, on the "significant methodological problems").

23 pounds heavier, and much of that extra weight was apparently muscle, since the Masai had narrower waists and broader shoulders and possessed far more muscular strength than the Akikuyu, who were generally less fit and had little capacity for manual labor.*

The modern-day Ornish version of this very low-fat, near-vegetarian diet was not scientifically examined by experts until 1998, when Tufts University nutrition professor Alice Lichtenstein and a colleague reviewed the very low-fat diet for the AHA. The limited available evidence for the diet, including Ornish's studies, showed that drastically lowering fat to 10 percent or less seemed only to exacerbate the problems associated with a 30 percent–fat diet. The bad kind of cholesterol dropped (which was good), but so did the good cholesterol (which was bad), and triglycerides went up (also bad), sometimes by as much as 70 percent (very bad). Lichtenstein concluded that very low-fat diets "are not beneficial and may be harmful."

Ornish's impact has nevertheless been profound and enduring.† Unlike Atkins, whose high-fat recommendations were dismissed by the AHA and NIH as dangerous to health, Ornish's extremely low-fat, near-vegetarian "lifestyle" program is one of only two diet-and-exercise regimes that Medicare covers, as do some forty private insurance companies to varying degrees, including the giants Mutual of Omaha and Blue Shield of California. For them, the simple logic is that months of diet, yoga, meditation, and exercise, if they can prevent a heart attack, represent a bargain compared to $40,000 for bypass surgery.

---

*Muscular strength of the hands was assessed with a dynamometer, which measures mechanical force. With this test, the Masai were found to be 50 percent stronger than the Akikuyu. Another sign of physical weakness among the Akikuyu men was that 65 percent were "immediately rejected on medical grounds" when turning up for army reserve service in 1917. The women of the two tribes, by contrast, had more similar diets and did not have such dramatic differences in health (Orr and Gilks 1931, 9 and 17 "immediately rejected").

†Ornish was close to the Clintons and revamped their White House kitchen to make way for soy burgers and dessert sauces derived from pulped bananas (Bill Clinton is now a vegan). And Ornish is still in the debate, with a prominent opinion piece in the *New York Times* in 2012, arguing for the near-vegetarian diet (Squires July 24, 2001; Ornish September 22, 2012).

Starting out Life in a Position of Defense

While mainstream nutrition experts continued to have doubts about Ornish's extreme diet, they were confident that the standard AHA-recommended low-fat diet, plus all the new cholesterol benchmarks and guidelines set forth by the NCEP, would be a boon for every American in the enduring fight against heart disease. This belief was fostered by the Senate as part of its 1977 *Dietary Goals* report. One of its headlines read, "Benefits Would Be Shared by All," meaning not just middle-aged men, but women and children, too. No studies had been done on whether a low-fat diet was better—or even safe—for infants, children, adolescents, pregnant or lactating women, or the elderly, yet the diet-heart hypothesis had taken hold to such a degree in the expert community that it was just considered a commonsense measure of prevention against heart disease for everyone at any stage of life over the age of two to start on this regime.

The compelling rationale for including children in the dietary recommendations was that in the 1920s, German scientists performing autopsies on children had found some of their arteries to contain fatty streaks and lesions, which are early signs of atherosclerosis. It was assumed that if left unchecked, these streaks and lesions would inevitably lead to the fatal disease. The question of how to halt this progression early in life became a source of extreme worry and concern in the diet and disease research community.

Indeed, in the late 1960s, the NHLBI had been putting children as young as four years old on cholesterol-lowering diets and also giving them cholestyramine, the same drug that would be used in the LRC trial. Convinced that cholesterol was a crucial part of the heart disease puzzle, the NHLBI went so far as to propose universal umbilical cord blood screening in order to start treatment as early as possible, even at birth. In 1970, mass screening of cord blood at "no more than" five dollars per baby was given serious consideration. Such was the preoccupation with heart disease that researchers believed healthy children ought to start out life in a position of defense.*

---

*Starting in 1970, Fleischmann's, the margarine company, ran ads that asked, "Should an eight-year-old worry about cholesterol?" Due to the lack of evidence for any connection between childhood diet and adult heart disease, however, the Federal

Quite a few experts challenged this line of thinking as it was being developed. "What evidence do we have that an egg yolk a day spells jeopardy for *all* Americans?" asked Donald S. Fredrickson, a top NHLBI official, in the *British Medical Journal* in 1971. "What of sucklings and older infants? . . . Are we convinced of the safety of a diet containing 10 percent of polyunsaturates to the extent that we want to insist on this in baby's formula?" He went on to point out that the specific problem of middle-aged men "is not to be solved by general dietary advice" to the entire population. The National Academy of Sciences, in its *Toward Healthful Diets* report, agreed, objecting that it was "scientifically unsound" for the government to include children in its low-fat recommendations. "The nutritional needs of the young, growing infant are distinctly different from those of the inactive octogenarian," stated the academy, but because that report was so lambasted by Congress and the press, this cautionary note became lost in the controversy.

The arguments about including children continued vociferously at the NIH Consensus Development Conference in 1984. Researchers and doctors were concerned that no trial had ever been conducted on children to test a diet low in fat or low in saturated fat. "There is absolutely *no* evidence that it's safe for children to be on a cholesterol-lowering diet," Thomas C. Chalmers, former president of the Mount Sinai Medical Center, told *Science*. "I think they [the NIH leaders] made an *unconscionable* exaggeration of all the data." The government was not impeded by this absence of evidence in issuing its dietary recommendations for children, however, and other expert groups adopted this point of view as well.

The only professionals holding out against this generalized advice for all children were those entrusted with child health: the pediatricians. Even as experts at the NHLBI and the AHA pressed the American Academy of Pediatrics (AAP) to prescribe the low-fat diet to all children, the AAP refused. In an editorial published in the AAP journal, *Pediatrics,* in 1986, the group's nutrition committee said that any change toward a more restrictive diet in the first two decades of life should "await demonstration that such

---

Trade Commission in 1973 ordered the company to stop the advertisements (FTC 1973).

dietary restrictions are needed." The editorial emphasized the differences in the nutritional needs of growing children, especially during the growth spurt of adolescence, compared to those of middle-aged men with high cholesterol. "The proposed changes would affect consumption of foods currently providing high quality protein, iron, calcium, and other minerals essential for growth," stated the authors.

The AAP had long considered high-quality proteins to come from meat, dairy products, and eggs, which would be restricted under the low-cholesterol, low-fat diet. "Dairy products provide 60 percent of dietary calcium; and meat is the best source of available iron," the academy wrote. The AAP feared that rates of iron deficiency, which had not been a problem among children for decades in the United States, might rise if children started cutting back on meat.

Not so many years earlier, meat, dairy, and eggs had been considered the best foods to promote growth. The expert who chaired the National Academy of Science's controversial report had alluded to this point when he said the country should not abandon a diet that produced Americans who were healthy and tall. This belief was based on research conducted before the field of nutrition became absorbed by the study of heart disease. Nutrition experts in the 1920s and thirties were less interested in athero-sclerosis, which was still emerging, and focused instead on what constituted an optimal diet for growth and reproduction. These stages have always been critical to any animal's success, which, in a Darwinian sense, meant growing from youth to adulthood, with the capacity to produce healthy offspring.

One of the more important early nutrition researchers looking at these questions was Elmer V. McCollum, an influential biochemist at Johns Hopkins University. He performed endless feeding studies on rats and pigs because they, like humans, are omnivores and are therefore considered instructive for human nutritional needs. His book *The Newer Knowledge of Nutrition* (1921) is populated with pictures of scrawny, scruffy-furred rats raised on poor nutrition, compared to large, lustrously furred ones raised on better nutrition. He found that animals on a vegetarian diet had an especially difficult time reproducing and rearing their young. In one experi-ment, McCollum describes the fate of a rat on this kind of diet:

They grew fairly well for a time but became stunted when they reached a weight of about 60 percent of normal adult size. They lived 555 days, whereas omnivores had an average span of life of 1,020 days. The vegetarians grew to be approximately half as large, and lived half as long as did their fellows which received animal food.

Experimenting with various kinds of oats, grains, alfalfa leaves, legumes, maize, and seeds, the ingredients of the mostly carbohydrate, near-vegetarian diet, McCollum found that he could improve the animals' growth—which "made it evident that there is nothing in vegetarianism per se" that made it unable to sustain life; however, it was by far the more difficult route and required the careful selection and combining of grains and legumes "in the right proportions."

McCollum found it easier to keep rats healthy by feeding them milk, eggs, butter, organ meats, and green leafy vegetables. He came to call these foods "protective" because they supported healthy growth and reproduction for the omnivorous animal.

In the 1920s, when nutrition investigators started identifying some of the specific vitamins in "protective" foods, the focus of research turned away from these whole foods and toward the vitamins instead. An entire era of vitamin-based research took off. Ultimately, the idea of separating vitamins from their native foods would prove to have some unfortunate consequences, since Americans mistakenly came to believe that they could meet their nutritional needs simply by taking a supplement or eating fortified foods such as breakfast cereal. Yet a number of essential vitamins, including calcium and the fat-soluble vitamins A, D, K, and E, cannot be fully absorbed if eaten unaccompanied by fat. Without the saturated fat in milk, for example, calcium forms insoluble "soaps" in the intestine instead. And the vitamins in fortified cereal can only be well absorbed if consumed with milk that has not been stripped of its fat content; the same is true of the vitamins in a salad with a fat-free dressing. That is why mothers in the early twentieth century dispensed cod-liver oil to their children as a dose of protection against sickness; the fat is what made the spoonful of vitamins go down.

In the late 1940s, following more than two decades of vitamin-focused research, the field of nutrition shifted its orientation once again, turning toward heart disease as the country's leaders trained its resources on the ailment that most afflicted their ranks. Over the next decades, cardiovascular and cholesterol experts came to dominate the nutrition conversation, and childhood growth and development were neither their expertise nor their main concern. Thus the line of research on protective foods forged by McCollum and others was overrun, and the focus on child nutrition gave way to a preoccupation with heart disease and the low-fat diet.

The AAP, which had long embraced McCollum's views, did its best to resist the tidal wave of pressure from the health and medical establishments to get in line with the low-fat diet. But, as had happened with so many other groups, including the National Academy of Sciences when it tried to take a stand against the country's new dietary advice, the pediatricians were losing the battle for public opinion. Experts had been telling Americans to reduce cholesterol and fat for so many years that parents had long since absorbed the message. Bombarded by low-fat advice, parents had swapped out whole milk for the reduced-fat variety and were restricting their children's consumption of eggs. Between 1970 and 1997, consumption of whole milk dropped from 214 to 73 pounds per person, while low-fat and skim milk consumption together increased from 14 to 124 pounds. These were worrying trends for a former generation of pediatricians schooled in the idea that growing children needed fat and animal foods to ensure good health.

"I have seen figures that 25 percent of the infants in this country under the age of 2 are on reduced fat milk," Lloyd Filer, a professor of pediatrics at the University of Iowa, is quoted as saying in the *New York Times* in 1988. Children on such diets had been turning up in hospitals showing "failure to thrive," he said, and when restored to higher-fat diets, "they gained weight and began to grow."

Yet the concerns of pediatricians continued to be drowned out by advocacy from expert groups, the government, and the media for a diet low in fat. By 1995, a survey of about a thousand mothers found that 88 percent of them believed that a low-fat diet was "important" or "very important" for their infants, and 83 percent responded that they sometimes or always avoided giving fatty foods to their children.

Clearly, these mothers didn't realize that the scientific evidence for their dietary choices was virtually nonexistent. Indeed, the argument for including children in the official guidelines had never been based in science at all. The foundation instead had always primarily been that entirely speculative notion that the fatty streaks observed during autopsies in the arteries of young people would develop into full-blown atherosclerosis later in life.

A second theory for including children in the low-fat diet recommendations came from Mark Hegsted, the Harvard professor and USDA administrator. He used an infectious-disease model of prevention, which suggests that treating a healthy population would benefit society at large. Vaccinating a population against measles is an obvious example of this model in action, and Hegsted extended it to heart disease. His analogy was this: if an entire population could lower its cholesterol levels by a certain percent, some number of people would avoid having a heart attack. Hegsted even developed a mathematical formula that he claimed could predict the exact number of lives that would be spared. Those saved would mainly be middle-aged and elderly men, but it was simply assumed that the rest of the population would join in the project.

Yet it seems obvious that atherosclerosis is not like the measles. A healthy family might give up steak for dinner in the hopes of prolonging the life of the at-risk father, but eating steak is not contagious. Children might eat one thing, and the father another. Thus Hegsted's model might have made sense on a practical level, since the whole family sits down to one meal together, but the public health logic was clearly tenuous. From the point of view of a baby's biological needs, for instance, it would be logically equivalent to advise all family members at dinner to consume only breast milk, since this is the healthiest option for the infants at the table. However, Hegsted and his colleagues did not seem to consider how ridiculous it was for the whole family to eat according to the dietary needs of a single one of its members.

In 1989, Fima Lifshitz, a professor of pediatrics at Cornell University, described in a paper a number of cases where a father or mother had received a diagnosis of heart disease, thereby triggering a dietary shift in the family home, including drastic reductions in dietary fat. It was exactly the kind of family diet changeover that Hegsted had recommended, but some parents had clearly gone overboard. The "overzealous application of a low-fat, low-cholesterol diet" was leading to "nutritional dwarfing," insufficient weight gain, and delayed puberty, Lifshitz found, and the worst vitamin deficiencies occurred on the lowest-fat diets, even when protein intake was adequate.

Hegsted's theoretical model nevertheless prevailed among leaders at the AHA, the NHLBI, and universities around the country, where the nutritional needs of children were debated. Even so, NHLBI in the 1980s finally decided that it needed to establish a scientific foundation for its guidelines for children. It therefore funded a trial called the Dietary Intervention Study in Children (DISC). Starting in 1987, three hundred seven- to ten-year-old children were counseled, along with their parents, to eat a diet in which saturated fat was limited to 8 percent of calories and total fat to 28 percent, and this group was compared to an equal-sized group of controls. Investigators found that those put on the diet low in fat (and animal fat) grew just as well as the children eating normally during the three years of the experiment, and the authors emphasized this point.

Yet it was problematic for the study that the boys and girls in the trial did not represent a normal sample. For their study population, the DISC leaders had selected children who had unusually high levels of LDL-cholesterol (in the 80th to 98th percentile). In other words, these children could very well have had familial hypercholesterolemia, the genetic condition that causes heart disease through a metabolic defect, which is entirely different from the way that cholesterol is altered by diet. These at-risk children were chosen because they were thought to need help more urgently in fighting the early onset of a life-threatening disease, yet their unusually high cholesterol levels meant that the results could not be generalized to the larger population of normal children.

Beyond this problem, another giant complication in the study's ability to support the low-fat diet for children was that subjects on the DISC intervention diet ended up consuming less than two thirds of the RDAs for calcium, zinc, and vitamin E. They also got less magnesium, phosphorus, vitamin B12, thiamin, niacin, and riboflavin than did children in the control group. This result was not surprising, actually, since this type of vitamin deficiency had also been observed, along with faltering growth,

in a few other small studies of children on vegetarian or low-fat diets.*†
Indeed, these preliminary findings had been among the principal concerns
originally driving the DISC study. In the Bogalusa Heart Study on children
aged eight to ten, for instance, those children eating less than 30 percent of
calories as fat were found to have a significantly higher chance of failing to
meet the RDAs for vitamins B1, B12, and E, as well as thiamin, riboflavin,
and niacin, compared to the group eating more than 40 percent fat.

Moreover, the children on the DISC intervention diet saw virtually no
improvement in total cholesterol, LDL-cholesterol, or triglycerides compared to the control group. Therefore, even setting aside the skewed study
population, the results clearly suggested that the low-fat diet presented no
particular benefits and one clear cost to children, since the diet appeared to
pose a nutritional risk according to the targets set by the RDAs.

When these studies came out in the mid-1990s, however, the bias
toward a low-fat diet was already so intense that a reader can almost see
the study leaders straining, in their published report, to support the established, NIH-endorsed dietary recommendations. In the case of DISC,
moreover, the NIH had not only helped conduct the study but had funded
it. The study's authors concluded that "lower fat intakes . . . are safe for
growth and are nutritionally adequate." On the lookout for psychological
problems, since earlier studies of the cholesterol-lowering diet had found
higher rates of suicide and violent deaths, DISC researchers reported no
evidence of any emotional impairment. The diet's nutritional deficiencies
were hardly mentioned.

---

*The finding has been seen among adults, too. Even the USDA, which recommends
getting a majority of calories from fruits, vegetables, and grains, acknowledged in its
latest *Dietary Guidelines* that more research was needed on the "potential limitations
of [a] plant-based diet for key nutrients, especially in children and the elderly" (Dietary Guidelines Advisory Committee 2010, 277).

†Slightly stunted growth was consistently found among children eating vegetarian
diets. Children were also found to experience growth spurts when incorporating
more animal foods in their diets. Growth faltering was particularly pronounced
among children on a vegan diet, which cuts out all animal foods (Kaplan and
Toshima 1992, 33–52).

Flawed as it was, DISC is one of only two controlled clinical trials anywhere in the Western world ever conducted on children to look at the nutritional adequacy of the low-fat diet. Other studies, such as the Bogalusa Heart Study, were epidemiological surveys rather than trials, and the few other actual experiments on children that had been conducted were either very small or based on abnormal study populations. The second large trial, conducted in Finland, was the Special Turku Coronary Risk Factor Intervention Project (STRIP). The limitation of this low-fat experiment was that it intervened in the diet of children only up to the age of three.

STRIP was a loosely controlled experiment, starting in 1990, on 1,062 Finnish babies as young as seven months. Breast milk was replaced with nonfat milk after one year of age, and parents were instructed, through counseling sessions every few months, on how to eliminate saturated fat by using lean meat products, low-fat cheese, and nondairy ice cream. The children were also given multivitamin supplements, and when they reached the age of three, they returned to their normal higher-animal-fat diets. The researchers observed no difference in the children's growth, both in terms of height and weight, either during the study or during follow-up exams of the children until the age of fourteen. However, the intervention children ended up with significantly lower levels of HDL-cholesterol, which was a bad sign for heart disease risk. And although investigators found no vitamin deficiencies, the supplements they provided may have masked this problem. It is also significant that 20 percent of the families in both groups left before the end of the study.

DISC and STRIP are often cited as justification for the low-fat dietary recommendations for all children, yet these studies clearly do not come close to establishing the sort of evidence base that one would want, in order to warrant altering the food habits of an entire nation of children. Taken together, the studies had tested a low-fat diet on only eight hundred children, three hundred of whom couldn't be called representative due to their singularly high LDL-cholesterol. The rest were under the age of three. Additionally, the children weren't followed to adulthood, so reproductive consequences could not be studied. Based on such a small, irregular sample, it seemed unconscionable to counsel millions of normal American children of all ages to change their diets.

Yet perhaps inevitably, the AAP's resistance to the low-fat diet slowly eroded. By the late 1990s, a universe of experts had believed in the diet for so long that alternative viewpoints could not realistically hold out. Criticism of the diet-heart hypothesis, which had been lively until the 1984 Consensus Conference, was afterward virtually silenced in the United States. In the nutrition community worldwide, criticism was reduced to a trickle, coming mainly from a handful of researchers in Europe and Australia. And this monolithic adoption of the low-fat dogma finally made inroads into the AAP. A new generation of leaders took the helm there, and they now argued, as Hegsted had before them, that even though only scant evidence existed in favor of the low-fat regime for children, the diet should be assumed right until proven wrong. After all, they reasoned, the diet had not, in these two short trials, shown too much harm. Thus, in 1998, the AAP officially adopted the standard advice and recommended a diet with 10 percent of calories as saturated fat and 20 percent to 30 percent for fat overall for all children over the age of two.

No Harm for Children?

Sitting on the AAP nutrition committee at the time was Marc Jacobson, then a professor of pediatrics and epidemiology at Albert Einstein College of Medicine. In an interview, I asked him about the possible shortfalls in vitamins and minerals that had turned up among children on a low-fat diet in these trials. He replied that while these deficits were problematic, they were not as important as growth as a measure for good health.

Still, the children in the higher-fat groups grew just as well and did not have any problems getting adequate amounts of vitamins and minerals. So why did the AAP not opt for that kind of diet instead? It seems to be a hard position to defend the low-fat diet as the default choice when children were doing just as well or even better on their normal diets, and without the need for vitamin supplements.

Jacobson emphasized the original argument: that the fight against plaque formation in the arteries should start as early as possible.

As it turns out, though, research over the years has yielded no solid evidence for the claim that lowering serum cholesterol in children has an impact on their future risk for heart disease. As studies have accumulated, they have revealed that most of these fatty streaks do not become dangerous, fibrous plaques and more importantly, that a child's diet is completely unrelated to the appearance of these streaks in the first place. Instead, for babies, it is the lipid profile of the mother that seems to be the main determinant.

Nor, as the DISC study found, could lowering dietary fat of any kind lead to meaningful improvements in blood cholesterol measures. And even if eating fat did raise LDL-cholesterol in children, the implications for adulthood are hazy. Only about half of children with high total cholesterol turn into adults with high total cholesterol (this holds true for LDL-cholesterol, too). In fact, the whole chain of apparent causation, from diet to cholesterol to heart disease, in children now looks very questionable. The justification for including children in the original low-fat recommendations therefore appears to break down.

When the authoritative Cochrane Collaboration, an international group that commissions experts to perform objective reviews of science, finally weighed in on the evidence in 2001, it concluded that avoiding fat couldn't be shown to prevent heart disease in normal children. The data couldn't even show that such a diet helped at-risk children with a genetic predisposition to heart disease. If a low-fat diet were the answer, Cochrane concluded, the evidence didn't exist to make that claim.

Moreover, the diet didn't even appear to be effective in helping children lose weight. In the 1990s, the NIH funded a large, rigorous study on this hypothesis that included some 1,700 elementary schoolchildren. For three years, these children reduced their total fat intake from 34 percent to 27 percent fat of daily calories. They exercised more. Both the children and their families were educated about healthy nutrition. They were doing everything right—indeed, everything we are now counseling our children to do today—yet all these efforts yielded no reduction in body fat.

These results are no doubt startling for American parents who, hoping to give their children the best possible start in life, have dutifully chosen jars of pureed vegetables and fruit for their babies while selecting mainly lean meats and low-fat dairy for lunch boxes and family meals. Disappointingly, a search for further studies on the efficacy of such choices will turn up empty-handed, since mainstream nutrition researchers on the whole stopped questioning the impact of the low-fat diet on children after the AAP's 1998 endorsement.

A degree of skepticism endures in other countries, however, where research continues. The British biochemist and nutrition expert Andrew M. Prentice, for instance, hypothesized that the lack of high-fat animal foods was possibly "the major contributor of growth failure" among babies he studied in Gambia. He compared some 140 Gambian infants to a slightly larger group of relatively affluent babies in Cambridge, England; early on, the Gambians and British infants grew almost equally well. When they started to be weaned off breast milk at six months of age, however, their growth curves steadily diverged. The Gambians ate an equal number of calories as did the Cambridge babies for the first eighteen months of life, but the fat content of their diet steadily declined to just 15 percent of calories by the age of two, and most of that fat was polyunsaturated from nuts and vegetable oils. The Cambridge babies, by contrast, ate a majority of calories from eggs, cow's milk, and meat—a minimum of 37 percent of calories as fat, most of it saturated. By the age of three, the Gambian babies weighed 75 percent less than they should, according to standard growth charts, while the Cambridge babies were growing according to expectations and weighed on average 8 pounds more than the Gambians.*

As an American parent, it's hard to read this study without immediately running to see the fat content of one's own "early weaning" foods—with unsettling results. While rice porridge, the first solid food fed to Gambian infants, was analyzed as containing 5 percent of energy as fat, a jar of Earth Best's Whole Grain Rice Cereal, an organic brand that an American parent might feed a baby, has zero grams of fat. Later on, when Gambian babies were eating rice with groundnut sauce, at 18 percent fat, an American child might get barely 1 percent fat from a salubrious-sounding jar of Earth's

---

*This study echoes the examination by British colonial researchers in the 1920s of the vegetarian Kikuyu tribe in Kenya. Their examinations included 2,500 children who, after weaning, were found to grow far less well than the English or American babies to whom they were compared. These researchers found that the Kenyan children, as well as a group they followed with faltering growth in Scotland, experienced increased growth rates when cod liver oil and whole milk were added to their diets (Orr and Gilks 1931, 30–31 and 49–52).

Best Vegetable Turkey Dinner (and this is one of the few dinner options with meat). Government data shows that American children have reduced their intake of fat, including saturated fat, in recent decades. While a child is still weaning, there's a chance that breast milk or formula can make up for much of the fat deficit in baby foods (with the scary caveat that if a mother eats a lot of carbohydrates, her breast milk will tend to be lower in fat, as some studies have shown), but otherwise the lack of fat in the average American child's diet could very well be a health problem.

The results from Gambia were presented at a major symposium on child nutrition in Houston in 1998, along with a number of papers from other countries. Researchers from Spain and Japan reported that, unlike Americans, children in their countries had been increasing their consumption of fat in recent decades, and that those increases were associated with continued gains in height. Reports from poorer countries in Latin America and Africa, however, revealed that children were eating less fat, with clear implications for nutrition and growth: diets with less than 30 percent of calories as fat started to get nutritionally worrisome, and at 22 percent, they were associated with growth faltering. Those numbers stood in stark contrast to the 40 percent–plus fat that healthy, growing children were reported eating in the wealthier countries of Germany and Spain. However, the Houston symposium summary statement, written by an American expert with close ties to the NIH and principal investigators from the DISC and STRIP studies, concluded conservatively that children should be advised to eat a minimum of 23 percent to 25 percent, a very low amount. The summary did not mention the greater good health and height gains associated with higher-fat diets that had been the subject of many of the conference papers.

Today, the AAP maintains its recommendations for a diet low in fat and saturated fat for all children over the age of two. School districts across the country, including those in New York City and Los Angeles, have banned whole milk and serve low-fat options whenever possible (Bill Clinton's foundation has been a major player in this effort). And ever since the USDA adopted its dietary guidelines in 1980, calling for reductions in fat consumption, the Special Supplemental Nutrition Program for Women, Infants, and Children (WIC) has slowly altered its food packages to contain fewer animal products, replaced by more and more grains. There are fewer eggs today than there were when the program started in 1972. There is now canned fish, tofu, and soy-based beverages, but no meat, and all the milk for women and children above the age of two must be low-fat, 2 percent or less.

Women and the Low-Cholesterol Paradox

Women were another group swept up in the NHLBI endorsement of the low-fat diet, although there was no reason to believe that they would benefit, either, and as a group they had also barely been studied.

Medical research has, of course, historically focused on men as a kind of biological default. And because the heart disease epidemic initially affected more men than women, women were excluded from most clinical trials on heart disease: they represented only 20 percent of participants in those studies until 1990 and only 25 percent thereafter. The result is that all of the National Cholesterol Education Program's cholesterol-lowering targets for the entire US population have been based on studies comprised exclusively of men. As far back as the 1950s, however, researchers had been warning that women responded differently to fat and cholesterol than did men and therefore needed to be studied separately. Atherosclerotic symptoms don't occur in women until ten to twenty years later than men, for instance, and women generally do not suffer high rates of heart disease until after menopause.

Where data existed examining the sexes separately, the disparities were fairly astonishing. In the Framingham Study, one of the few early studies that included women, for example, women over fifty years old showed no significant correlation between total serum cholesterol and coronary mortality. Because heart disease occurs only very rarely in women under fifty, this finding meant that the great majority of American women have been needlessly cutting back on saturated fats these past few decades, since the impact on their blood cholesterol is meaningless for their coronary risk.* Yet this important finding was omitted from the study's conclusions when they were published in 1971. In 1992, an NHLBI expert panel reviewed

---

*Indeed, an analysis of the Framingham data found that women of any age can safely have cholesterol levels up to 294 mg/dL without any increased risk of a heart attack (Kannel 1987).

all the heart disease data on women and found that total mortality was actually *higher* for women with low cholesterol than it was for women with high cholesterol, regardless of age. These results were also ignored. Indeed, how many doctors can you imagine nowadays telling female patients that high cholesterol is no reason to worry?

Framingham was an epidemiological study. As for the clinical trial data on women, the situation was the same as we've seen for children, namely that until nearly the year 2000, there was none. Not until Congress examined gender disparity in scientific funding in a series of hearings in the early 1990s, in fact, did the NHLBI put some money into conducting trials on diet and disease for women.

One of the NHLBI grants went to Robert H. Knopp, a lipid specialist at the University of Washington, who had studied the low-fat diet in men and was concerned about its effects on women. His trial, on 444 male Boeing employees with high cholesterol in Seattle, had yielded some disturbing results. Knopp fed the Boeing men a range of low-fat diets in which the subjects ate from 18 percent to 30 percent of total calories as fat. In 1997, at the end of one year, the men all saw significant changes in their cholesterol levels. Knopp noted that LDL-cholesterol, considered the "bad" kind, went down, and this seemed like a positive outcome. But the men on the lowest-fat diets also saw a troublesome decline in their HDL, known as the "good" cholesterol, along with an unhealthy rise in their triglycerides, which are the fats circulating in the blood. These results have been confirmed by others studies.

The blood markers that Knopp measured reflected the reality that diet-heart research had become far more sophisticated since the 1970s, when only "total" cholesterol could be measured (triglycerides, too, were one of the "old-timer" biomarkers and had been studied since the 1950s by Pete Ahrens and others). By the late 1980s, many more subtleties about cholesterol could be measured. These included HDL- and LDL-cholesterol. But what were these, exactly?

Total cholesterol, it turns out, can be broken down into subsets of different densities, including "high density" HDL-cholesterol and "low-density" LDL-cholesterol. These two biomarkers gained their reputations as "good" and "bad" over many years of studies. Researchers found that

NINA TEICHOLZ

elevated levels of LDL-cholesterol were associated with all kinds of risk factors, such as weighing too much, smoking, not exercising, and high blood pressure, whereas HDL-cholesterol was just the opposite: it goes up when people get more exercise, lose weight, and quit smoking—a kind of Californian epitome of good living.

These cholesterol fractions are unable to dissolve in the blood and cannot travel through veins and arteries on their own. They need to sit inside a little submarine that can zoom along, dissolved in the blood, while safely protecting its cholesterol cargo on the inside. Those submarines are called lipoproteins, and, depending on the type of cholesterol they are carrying, the lipoproteins are called—confusingly—simply HDL and LDL. So, the submarines are named HDL and LDL, and are distinct from their cholesterol *cargo*, which are called HDL-cholesterol and LDL-cholesterol. The theory is that the HDL lipoproteins function by clearing cholesterol from the tissues, including the arterial walls, and transporting it off to the liver. HDL, in other words, rids the body of cholesterol. LDL, meanwhile, does the reverse: LDL lipoproteins fix cholesterol into our artery walls. Hence we should avoid high levels of LDL-cholesterol while seeking to increase our levels of HDL-cholesterol. Whether the cholesterol itself or the lipoproteins can more reliably predict a future heart attack is a matter over which expert opinion is divided.

Nutrition experts became interested in these HDL- and LDL-cholesterol fractions because the Framingham group in 1977, as you might remember, plus a number of other studies, suggested that total cholesterol was not, actually, a good predictor of heart disease for most people. That was not a result anyone wanted to trumpet too loudly, of course, since it thoroughly undermined the diet-heart hypothesis, which had made total cholesterol-lowering the chief target for all its therapies for decades. Hundreds of millions of dollars had been spent in attempting to prove that total cholesterol was the most important risk factor; ten thousand and one journal papers had focused on total cholesterol to the exclusion of every other biological aspect of heart disease. Total cholesterol had been the reason that Americans had been told to cut back on saturated fat in the first place. Now it turned out to be a weak risk factor in the great majority of cases. This reality is still not fully embraced by doctors and health advisories today—although this is not surprising, given total cholesterol's long and prominent legacy. Yet if total cholesterol wasn't a reliable predictor of risk, then what was?

The answer turned out to be a complex mix of other factors measured in the blood, including triglycerides, LDL-cholesterol, and HDL-cholesterol. In fact, one of the big surprises of Framingham's follow-up results had been about the "good" cholesterol. The study leaders reported that in both men and women from ages 40 to 90, "of all the lipoproteins and lipids measured, HDL-cholesterol had the largest impact on risk." People with low HDL-cholesterol levels (below 35 mg/dL) had an eight times higher rate of heart attacks than did people with high HDL-cholesterol levels (65 mg/dL or above).* The correlation was "striking," wrote the authors, and was the "most important finding" from all of their cholesterol data.

And yet, when diet and disease experts finally began to sidle away from total cholesterol, they did not turn to HDL-cholesterol. Instead, they chose to focus on LDL-cholesterol. By 2002, the NCEP was calling elevated LDL-cholesterol a "powerful" risk factor. The AHA and other professional associations agreed.

It was a strange turn of events; if the case for HDL-cholesterol was so compelling, why did the NIH and AHA prefer LDL-cholesterol? There were several explanations. One was that a number of epidemiological studies had linked heart disease victims with LDL-cholesterol levels that were on average a few percentage points higher than those in healthy people. Second, data from animals showed that increased LDL-cholesterol led to sclerotic-looking arteries. And third, there was compelling evidence from two scientists, Michael Brown and Joseph Goldstein, who eventually went on to win the Nobel Prize for their work, showing that people with the genetic disorder familial hypercholesterolemia had defective LDL-cholesterol receptors. These scientists suggested that a similar mechanism might be operating in the rest of us, and experts at the time found this particular bit of evidence especially convincing.

The choice to favor LDL-cholesterol over HDL-cholesterol was also

---

*The AHA currently recommends keeping HDL-cholesterol above 60 mg/dL for both men and women.

NINA TEICHOLZ

probably fueled by the megabillion-dollar pharmaceutical industry, which heavily favored LDL-cholesterol as a target for therapy. Drug companies had made quite a few attempts to find a drug that raised HDL-cholesterol, but those efforts had all failed. Lowering LDL-cholesterol, however, was something they could do—very well. The first such drug, lovastatin, was discovered in the 1970s, and a world of billion-dollar "statin" drugs followed from there: so far, there have been fluvastatin, pitavastatin, pravastatin, rosuvastatin, simvastatin, and atorvastatin. Worldwide, statins earned $956 billion in 2011.

One of the open secrets about statins, however, is that while they do make a difference in preventing coronary deaths, their success is not entirely related to their LDL-lowering ability. Statins work in some other way, perhaps by reducing inflammation; researchers don't really know. These other potential mechanisms are called the "pleiotropic effects" of statins, and they're commonly discussed in the research community. Nonetheless, the public face of statins has until quite recently remained linked exclusively to their power to lower LDL-cholesterol, and they are still, on the whole, marketed on the basis of that benefit.

There was one more, highly compelling rationale for favoring LDL-cholesterol, namely, that diet and disease experts needed it to rescue the diet-heart hypothesis. Results like Knopp's were revealing that the gold-standard diet of the day, low in fat and saturated fat, could improve LDL-cholesterol but would invariably worsen HDL-cholesterol. This was an extremely awkward discovery because it meant that the chosen diet might actually be worsening the risk for heart disease. Experts tried to salvage the situation by simply ignoring HDL-cholesterol. The NIH funded few studies on the relationship between diet and HDL-cholesterol, and researchers omitted it from discussion in scientific papers. Indeed, journal editors were known to sometimes insist that researchers exclude HDL-cholesterol from the discussion section, based on the rationale that it was not an "official" biomarker. "If you don't publish it, you can't talk about it," as one oil chemist described it to me. "If you want the low-fat diet to be good and saturated fats to be bad, then you black out HDL and it's a nice clean story."

Nutrition experts also ignored the research showing that what raised

HDL-cholesterol more effectively than anything else was not red wine or exercise, as we commonly think, but saturated fat. Eating animal fat was found to raise HDL-cholesterol and was the only food known to do so. "This is an important issue. Neglect of the saturated-fat-induced rise in HDL-cholesterol has made saturated fat (in general) look worse than it really is," Meir Stampfer, a nutritional epidemiologist at the Harvard University School of Public Health, wrote in 2004. A growing number of researchers agree with this view, yet in the 1990s, when these highly uncomfortable discoveries by Knopp and others were just coming out, the predominant response to anyone who raised the topic of HDL-cholesterol and the low-fat, high-carbohydrate diet was basically to cough politely and look elsewhere.

The Boeing Women

Knopp was one of the few researchers in those years who was openly interested in HDL-cholesterol. When he began looking at female Boeing employees alongside the men, he discovered that HDL-cholesterol was nearly a symbol of the gender differences in heart disease. Knopp fed his Boeing women diets that had been developed by the National Cholesterol Education Program (NCEP), that NIH bureaucracy created solely to help Americans fight high cholesterol. The NCEP had developed two regimes: Step 1 and Step 2. If you were an "at-risk" man or woman, you first went on the Step 1 diet (10 percent of calories as saturated fat). If that didn't work to lower your cholesterol, then you were told to move on to Step 2 (less than 7 percent saturated fat). Both diets recommend a limit of 30 percent of calories from total fat.

For one year, seven hundred Boeing employees followed the more extreme Step 2 diet. The results showed that their LDL-cholesterol levels dropped—theoretically a good sign—but the Boeing women also saw their HDL-cholesterol levels drop by 7 percent to 17 percent. That's the good cholesterol going down by an amount that researchers calculated implied a 6 percent to 15 percent increase in the risk of heart disease for these women. The changes for men were not nearly so negative, but the women:

they had followed the most stringent NCEP guidelines for an entire year and had apparently increased their risk of having a heart attack.

Knopp was alarmed by how much worse the diet looked for women, but he found that no one wanted to discuss or even acknowledge his study findings when they came out in 2000. The study met with a "mute" reaction by the scientific community," he said. "No one knew what to make of it." No one disputed his results because to do so would have meant having to grapple with the data, and no one had an explanation. Thus, Knopp's so-called BeFIT study, the Boeing Employees Fat Intervention Trial, was largely disregarded, excluded from standard review papers in the field until quite recently.

Yet although these results were unpopular, they were not an anomaly: other trials have also found that women on low-fat diets tend to see their HDL-cholesterol fall by about a third more than do men.* In Knopp's trial, women also saw their triglycerides rise more. And whatever the low-fat diet's benefits—notably, its power to reduce LDL-cholesterol—these tend to happen less in women. Knopp summed up all these gender differences in a review paper in 2005, concluding that the low-fat diet could not really be recommended for women, and that they might consider exploring "alternative dietary interventions" instead. Maybe women need a diet lower in carbohydrates and higher in fat, Knopp suggested.

Knopp's study could very well have been a watershed. After it came out, experts might have alerted women to the possibility, at least, that adopting a low-fat diet was, for them, a premature and inadvertently harmful piece of advice. Women, after all, have been shown to be especially conscientious about reducing calories since the 1970s, and according to government data, have cut back on fat and saturated fat more strictly than have men. Knopp's findings implied that women were actually betraying

---

*On example is a study that fed 103 healthy adults, ages twenty-two to sixty-seven (46 men and 57 women), either an NCEP Step 1 diet (9 percent SFA), a "low-sat-fat diet" (5 percent SFA), or an average American diet for eight weeks. Total cholesterol and LDL-cholesterol fell on the first two diets relative to the third, yet HDL-cholesterol also fell, and more precipitously, especially for the women (Stefanick et al. 2007).

their health by eating a low-fat diet. And yet among the nutrition elite there was no reckoning with these disturbing implications. Most women didn't know—and still don't know—that a low-fat diet may possibly increase their risk for heart disease.

No Findings Connecting Fat and Breast Cancer

Another widely held belief about women's health that turned out not to be supported by the scientific evidence was the notion that dietary fat caused cancer. Since the 1980s, women have been advised by health authorities to reduce their consumption of fat in order to prevent breast cancer—which of course was part of the wider recommendations against dietary fat for all cancers and all people.

The idea that fat might lead to cancer was first aired at the McGovern committee hearings in 1976, when Gio Gori, director of the National Cancer Institute (NCI), testified that men and women in Japan had very low rates of breast and colon cancer and that those rates rose quickly upon emigrating to the United States. Gori showed charts demonstrating the parallel rising lines of fat consumption and cancer rates. "Now I want to emphasize that this is a very strong correlation, but that correlation does not mean causation," he said. "I don't think anybody can go out today, and say that food causes cancer." He urged more research. However, the Senate committee, in its enthusiasm to solve as many of the nations' health problems as possible, overlooked those reservations, and implied in its report that a low-fat diet could help reduce cancer risk. Cancer thus became the second "killer disease" that the Senate pinned on the back of fat consumption. And as with heart disease, the committee's endorsement of a particular hypothesis had a similar ricochet effect all over Washington, DC.

Based on the sort of international comparisons that Gori had made, as well as some data on rats, the fat-cancer hypothesis was soon adopted and incorporated into reports by the National Cancer Institute (1979 and 1984), the National Academy of Sciences (1982), and the American Cancer Society (1984), and in the Surgeon General's Report on Nutrition and Health (1988). They all recommended a low-fat and low-saturated-fat diet to avoid this disease. Indeed, the idea that fat caused cancer was a principal reason that a diet low in fat has been formally recommended by the government since the late 1970s.

For women, the advice was especially compelling, because while heart disease could easily be shrugged off as a middle-aged problem among men, cancer is something that even a young woman can worry about. Breast cancer especially.

It is therefore surprising to learn that as far back as 1987, the epidemiologist Walter Willett at the Harvard School of Public Health had found fat consumption not to be positively linked to breast cancer among the nearly ninety thousand nurses whom he had been following for five years in the Nurses' Health Study. In fact, Willett found just the opposite to be true, namely, that the more fat the nurses ate, particularly the more saturated fat they ate, the less likely they were to get breast cancer. These results held true even as the women aged. After fourteen years of study, Willett reported that his team had found "no evidence" that a reduction in fat overall nor of any particular kind of fat decreased the risk of breast cancer. Saturated fat actually appeared protective. These conclusions were all associations. But although epidemiology cannot demonstrate causation, it *can* be used reliably to show the *absence* of a connection. For instance, if a great many women are eating a relatively high-fat diet and are not getting breast cancer, as was the case here, we can most likely rule out dietary fat as the cause.

The NCI had become very invested in the fat-cancer hypothesis, however, and would not relinquish it so easily. After Willett's results came out, from what was the largest study on women and breast cancer at the time, Peter Greenwald, director of the NCI Division of Cancer Prevention and Control, published a paper in the *Journal of the American Medical Association* (JAMA) entitled, "The Dietary Fat-Breast Cancer Hypothesis Is Alive." He brushed over Willett's study and instead laid down an argument based on data from rats, in which "a high-fat, high-calorie diet" clearly induced mammary tumors. He was right, and there were plenty of rat studies to confirm this effect. Yet what he neglected to mention was that the most effective fats for growing tumors were polyunsaturated—the fats found in vegetable oils that Americans were being counseled to eat. Saturated fats fed to rats had little effect unless supplemented with these vegetable oils.

As for human data, nearly half a million women by 2009 had been observed in studies in Sweden, Greece, France, Spain, and Italy, along with more than forty thousand postmenopausal women in one US study alone. In all of these, researchers have not been able to find an association between breast cancer and animal fat. Even the NCI's own studies came up empty-handed—the most recent of those being the Women's Intervention Nutrition Study in 2006. This trial managed to get women to drop their fat intake to 15 percent or less, thereby answering criticisms that the women in earlier studies had not seen any results because they failed to lower their intake of fat *enough*. But even at 15 percent, the NCI still could not find a statistically significant association between fat reduction—of any kind or amount—and reduced rates of breast cancer.

According to that 500-page report by the World Cancer Research Fund and the American Institute for Cancer Research in 2007, which is the most comprehensive review of the evidence on cancer to date, there was not "convincing," or even "probable" evidence that a fatty diet increased the risk of cancer of any kind. In fact, the results of studies since the mid-1990s have "overall tended to weaken the evidence on fats and oils as direct causes of cancer," wrote the authors.

Even so, as of 2009, the NCI was still favoring the hypothesis that fat causes cancer. Arthur Schatzkin, who was chief of the nutritional epidemiology branch of the NCI before he died of cancer in 2011, told me that while others in his department were starting to lean toward the idea that sugar and refined carbohydrates were the most likely dietary cause of the disease, "My personal view is that the fat-cancer hypothesis is by no means dead." The problem to date, he said, was that epidemiological studies had not used accurate enough diet questionnaires. Schatzkin predicted that, all the evidence to the contrary so far, the hypothesis he favored would eventually be proven true. In 2012, however, when I spoke to the new director of the program, Robert N. Hoover, he readily acknowledged that all the research on the fat-cancer hypothesis had basically gone nowhere. "I think what we're doing now is stepping back from a strong prior hypothesis and starting anew," he told me. Rather than trying to prove the fat-cancer hypothesis, he said, "We're becoming more agnostic." So: on diet and cancer, it's back to square one.

Largest Ever Trial of the Low-Fat Diet

When Knopp got his funds from the NHLBI for his trial on the Boeing women employees in the mid-1990s, the agency also authorized an enormous amount of money—$725 million—for another trial, the largest randomized controlled clinical trial of the low-fat diet ever undertaken. This was the Women's Health Initiative (WHI), which, in addition to testing nearly 49,000 postmenopausal women on the low-fat diet, also assigned intervention groups to hormone replacement therapy and calcium and vitamin D supplementation. WHI researchers promised that the study would be the most definitive trial ever conducted, not just on the low-fat diet but on women's health generally.

The more than twenty thousand women in the low-fat diet group were instructed to cut back on meat, eggs, butter, cream, salad dressings, and other fatty foods. (Another group served as the controls.) *People* magazine quoted one participant, JoAnne Sether Menard, an administrator at the University of Washington, as saying that she gave up chips, doughnuts, fries, cheese, sour cream, and salad dressing, and "I haven't had butter on bread for 10 years." Women were also urged to eat more fruits, vegetables, and whole grains. This is basically the same low-fat, mostly plants diet that the AHA and the USDA recommend today.

When WHI was launched, in 1993, the low-fat diet had been the officially recommended diet of the AHA for more than thirty years and of the USDA for nearly fifteen. Yet WHI was the first large-scale trial ever to study whether this diet actually works. Since cutting back on fat had been considered healthy for so many decades, the results seemed like a foregone conclusion; study participants thought that they just needed to stick with the diet to celebrate the good news they already knew to be true.

Yet to everyone's alarm and bafflement, the results, published in a series of articles in JAMA, did not come out remotely as expected. The women in the study successfully reduced their overall fat from 37 percent to 29 percent of calories and their saturated fat from 12.4 percent to 9.5 percent of calories. They had apparently met all their targets, but after a decade of following this diet, they were no less likely than a control group to contract breast cancer, colorectal cancer, ovarian cancer, endometrial cancer, stroke, or even heart disease. Nor did they lose more weight. As Robert Thun, director of epidemiological research at the American Cancer Society, told the *New York Times*, the results for cancer and heart disease were "completely null."

Finally the low-fat diet had gotten its day in the court of science. WHI was the "Rolls Royce of studies," said Thun, and therefore should be the "final word." Yet had Darwin dropped his *Origin of the Species* into a meeting of the ultra-Catholic group Opus Dei, it might have received a warmer welcome than what met the WHI JAMA papers. "There was a deafening lack of commentary," Robert Knopp told me. Disbelief was really the only option. "We are scratching our heads over some of these results," said Tim Byers, a WHI principal investigator at the University of Colorado Health Sciences Center. After all, everyone already *knew* that eating a lot of fruits and vegetables and cutting back on fat constituted a healthy diet, so the reasoning just had to work back from there.

The study must be flawed, most people agreed. The women must not have stuck to the low-fat diet, and besides, since American women were generally eating less fat anyway by the early 1990s when the trial began, the diet group simply couldn't differ enough from the controls to achieve statistically significant results. Others criticized the study's selection of participants, its failure to distinguish between unsaturated "good" fats and saturated "bad" fats in the women's diets, and the fact that the women didn't get enough physical exercise. Or, just to throw the laundry list at it, as Jacques Rossouw, WHI lead project officer at the NHLBI, did, the study "may have been too short, or studied women who were too old or just too healthy."

Also, one could always blame the media for oversimplifying the message. Newspapers had a heyday with WHI's counterintuitive outcome. "Get Stuffed!" the headlines cried. "Forget all you ever knew about diets!"

"Unfortunately, science never works in sound bites," remarked Marcia Stefanick, a Stanford University School of Medicine professor who led the WHI steering committee. What journalists missed, WHI researchers said, were the subtleties of subgroup analyses, such as the fact that a smaller group of women, who most drastically reduced their fat intake and followed all the trial protocols most faithfully, achieved the lowest rates of breast cancer. While these seem like results pointing in the right direction, it must be noted that these were the so-called "high adherers"—the people who comply in studies and do exactly as doctors or study directors tell them. They are like the vegetarians we discussed in the last chapter, whose health outcomes always look better even if they are taking a placebo. These high adherers look healthier regardless of the intervention and one therefore can't conclude anything from their results.

In any case, scientists generally frown upon singling out subgroups such as these high adherers for analysis because they yield less statistically reliable results. Moreover, when authors pick out a subgroup that seems to prove their hypothesis particularly well at the *end* of their study—well, critics describe this practice as basically like "drawing the target around the bullet-hole."*

So the journalists covering WHI may have been simplistic. They may have been reductive or simply lazy in ignoring the subgroup analyses that WHI press releases tried to steer them toward, but these reductive journalists were right. The WHI had been the largest and longest trial of the low-fat diet ever undertaken, and the diet simply hadn't worked. Knopp's trial before and a number of sizable trials subsequently, as we'll see in Chapter 10, have confirmed WHI's findings. Taken together, these trials have shown that the low-fat diet has at best proved ineffective against disease and at worst aggravated the risk for heart disease, diabetes, and obesity. The standard, AHA-prescribed low-fat diet has consistently failed to produce better results for health than diets higher in fat.

---

*These subgroup analyses can go either way, too. For the subgroup of women diagnosed with heart disease at the start of the study, their risk of developing cardiovascular complications was 26 percent higher on the intervention diet than among those who had not changed their diet, a statistically significant result that was omitted from the table in the report that should have listed it. Moreover, in the subgroup of women at risk for developing diabetes, their risk of contracting that disease increased on the low-fat diet during the study. Neither of these findings was included in the discussion section of the report, however, and have not become part of the scientific discourse (Noakes 2013).

A review in 2008 of all studies of the low-fat diet by the United Nation's Food and Agriculture Organization concluded that there is "no probable or convincing evidence" that a high level of fat in the diet causes heart disease or cancer. And in 2013 in Sweden, an expert health advisory group, after spending two years reviewing 16,000 studies, concluded that a diet low in fat was an ineffective strategy for tackling either obesity or diabetes. Therefore, the inescapable conclusion from numerous trials on this diet, altogether costing more than a billion dollars, can only be that this regime, which became our national diet before being properly tested, has almost certainly been a terrible mistake for American public health.

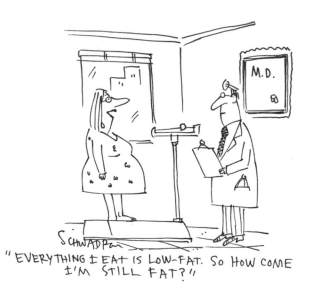

"EVERYTHING I EAT IS LOW-FAT. SO HOW COME I'M STILL FAT?"

"It is increasingly recognized that the low-fat campaign has been based on little scientific evidence and may have caused unintended health consequences," wrote Frank Hu, a nutrition professor at the Harvard School of Public Health, in 2001. With this growing pile of evidence on the table, health authorities clearly see the need to update their advice. Yet they are understandably reluctant to reverse course too loudly on fifty years of nutrition recommendations, and this hesitance has led to a certain vagueness on the subject. The USDA and AHA have both quietly eliminated any specific percent fat targets from their most recent lists of dietary guidelines. Those 30–35 percent fat targets that we've abided by for decades? They're now gone. And so is, actually, any discussion of the topic in their reports. How much fat should we be eating? These groups now don't say, and this silence on the issue—it must be said—does not seem like the clear, confident leadership from our authorities that we might like to see on the subject of how we should eat to fight the major diseases of our time.

Of course many of us who've been paying attention to the science have been welcoming fat back into our diets for some time already. We've given up spraying with Pam, stopped poaching, and started using salad dressings again. And if there's a silver lining to those low-fat years, it's this: we learned that fat is the soul of flavor. Food is tasteless and cooking nearly impossible without fat. Fat is essential in the kitchen to produce crispness and to thicken sauces. It is crucial in conveying flavors. It makes baked goods flaky, moist, and light. And fat has many other, essential functions in cooking and baking. To satisfy all these compelling needs, nutrition experts coming out of the low- to non-fat 1980s and looking for a solution found one apparently perfect candidate: olive oil. And that is one of the reasons why, in the early 1990s, the "Mediterranean Diet" entered the picture.

7

Selling the Mediterranean Diet: What Is the Science?

The Mediterranean diet is now so famous and celebrated that it barely needs introduction. The regime recommends getting most of the body's energy from vegetables, fruits, legumes, and whole grains. Seafood or poultry may be eaten several times a week, along with moderate amounts of yogurt, nuts, eggs, and cheese, while red meat is allowed only rarely, and milk, never. Its main novelty for Americans was the introduction of olive oil, which it advised in abundance. It's been a tasty and well-loved diet in the United States, the subject of hundreds of cookbooks, and more media coverage than a movie star. In recent studies, it has also been shown to be healthier in every way than the low-fat diet. But is the Mediterranean diet really the nutritional ideal, the savior its champions claim it to be?

Of course the diet with a small "d"—the one of bread and branzino eaten by many of the Mediterranean peoples themselves—has obviously existed in Greece, Italy, and Spain for many years, but the Mediterranean Diet with a capital "D," the nutritional concept and program that has been endorsed worldwide by scientists and government bodies alike, didn't really exist before the nutrition experts themselves invented it.

That capital "D" diet began to be developed in the mid-1980s by two smart and ambitious scientists, one from Italy and one from Greece, who took the important first step of establishing the hypothesis that the traditional fare of their homelands might protect against obesity and heart disease. One of these researchers was Antonia Trichopoulou, a professor at the University of Athens Medical School, who is widely known as the "Godmother" of the Mediterranean Diet for having done more than anyone else to shepherd it to global prominence. The idea had a simple origin, she explains. As a young medical doctor working at the hospital of the University of Athens Medical School, Trichopoulou was advising her patients with high cholesterol to eat various vegetable oils, since that was what the WHO, following in the footsteps of the AHA, had been recommending as a way to steer clear of saturated fats in the fight against heart disease.

Antonia Trichopoulou

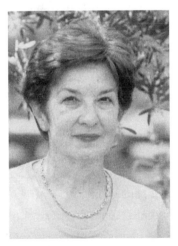

Antonia Trichopoulou, the Greek founder of the "Mediterranean Diet." She felt compelled to act when she saw olive trees being cut down and a traditional way of life disappearing.

Trichopoulou didn't question these dietary precepts until "One day, a very poor man came to the hospital," she explained. "And he said, 'Doctor, they are telling me to eat vegetable oil, but I'm used to olive oil! I cannot eat that!' " Trichopoulou knew that many Greeks still drizzled olive oil over everything, and she respected its traditional place in Greek cuisine going back perhaps thousands of years. Many Greek families still cultivated small plots of olive trees in their backyards to make their own oil. Yet due to the global influence of US-led nutrition policy, which favored polyunsaturated oils such as corn, safflower, and soybean, the consumption of olive oil in Greece was dropping. "We had started cutting down olive trees," lamented Trichopoulou. Given the oil's pedigree in Greek culture, Trichopoulou wondered if it could be any less healthy than the vegetable oils she had been promoting. She had an intuitive sense that something so intertwined in Greek history could not be wrong.

And she asked herself a broader question: Might olive oil not be just one element in a tapestry of Greek dietary traditions that altogether protected against disease? This diet could perhaps explain why, in the 1950s when she was young, the Greeks were found to be second only to the Danish in their life expectancy (among countries with similar statistics, at least). Trichopoulou wondered if she could quantify what her fellow Greeks were eating back then. Researching the topic, she came across the famous Seven Countries study by Ancel Keys, which was a rich source of dietary data for Greece and Italy during those mid-twentieth century years.

Keys had been drawn to Mediterranean countries, of course, because they seemed to be compatible with his hypothesis that saturated fat caused heart disease. The men he had studied during his first trip to the region in 1953 had very low rates of heart disease, and appeared not to eat much meat. Keys was particularly drawn to the island of Crete, because the Greeks living there were reputed to be especially long-lived. When he first visited, he was amazed "to see men of 80 to 100 and more going off to work in the fields with a hoe." To Keys, whose own countrymen were dropping like flies from heart attacks in middle age, the Cretans appeared like some miracle superbreed.

How poetic, too, that Greece, the ancient cradle of art, philosophy, and democracy, might also give to mankind the platonic ideal of a healthy diet! It all seemed to fall into place, with the beautiful, mythic island of Crete coming to radiate a kind of wonderment for Keys and his team. Just the weather alone was a welcome break for Keys, who marveled at his good luck in leaving behind his post as a visiting professor at Oxford University, enduring

Britain's "age of austerity" after the war. "We were freezing in our unheated house and were tired of food rationing," he wrote. As he and his wife, Margaret, drove through Europe, he experienced sheer relief upon leaving the frigid cold of the north for the sunny plazas of southern Italy: "All the way to Switzerland we drove in a snowstorm. . . . On the Italian side the air was mild, the flowers were gay, birds were singing, and we basked at the outdoor table drinking our first espresso coffee at Domodossola. We felt warm all over."

Anyone who has traveled to Italy will instantly recognize this swoon for the warmth, the beauty, the people. And the food! Keys recalled their delight in dining: "Homemade minestrone" and pasta in endless variety, "served with tomato sauce and a sprinkle of cheese," bread fresh out of the oven and "great quantities of fresh vegetables; . . . wine of the type we used to call 'Dago Red,' " and always fresh fruit for dessert. Eventually, Keys built a second home for himself in Italy, a large villa on a cliff overlooking the sea just south of Naples. "Mountains behind and the sea in front, all bathed in shimmering sunshine—that is the Mediterranean to us," he wrote.

Ancel Keys and Colleagues
Touring the Archeological Site of Knossos

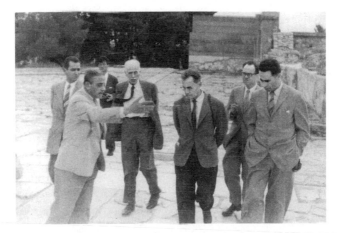

Ancel Keys and colleagues on Crete; the data from their nutritional research on that island became the foundation of the Mediterranean Diet. Ancel Keys is at the center. To the far right is Christos Aravanis, who directed the Greek portion of the Seven Countries study. To the left, with white hair, is Paul Dudley White. The man speaking is a guide.

On the idyllic islands of Crete and Corfu as well as in a town called Crevalcore in southern Italy, Keys collected dietary data for his Seven Countries study. With a low consumption of saturated fat and low rates of heart disease, the population on Crete was the one that fit Keys's hypothesis most perfectly. As we saw in Chapter 1, the saturated fat finding was possibly due to the unreported "Lent problem," but Keys and the Mediterranean diet researchers who followed him nevertheless assumed that, based on this data, the Cretan diet must be preserving life. (The men on Corfu turned out to have high cardiac death rates, despite eating the same amount of saturated fat as the Cretans did, but researchers in the field did not attempt to explain this apparent paradox and have generally ignored that cohort.) For nutrition researchers investigating Mediterranean nutrition, the Cretan islanders became the prized data set. They would become the touchstone of the diet, cited again and again by researchers as holding the key to the secret of long life.

Keys himself did not formally identify a "Mediterranean" cuisine when he published the Seven Countries study in 1970. Only later did he come to view the people of Greece and Italy as having an especially healthy pattern of eating, unique to the region. In 1975, he reissued his 1959 cookbook, *Eat Well and Stay Well,* with few alterations, as *Eat Well and Stay Well the Mediterranean Way.* He was already retired by this time, however, and never did much to advance the idea.

Ultimately, the promotion of the Mediterranean Diet instead came about largely through the efforts of others—Trichopoulou, especially. By unearthing Keys's work on Crete, she brought to light the possibility that this pattern of eating had something to teach the rest of the world, and starting in the mid-1980s, she began organizing the first few scientific conferences on the Mediterranean diet in Greece. "We just wanted to raise the issue" of the diet, she said, to see if it could be discussed in scientific terms "and if anything would come of it." Convened in Delphi and in Athens, these early conferences gave rise to the first academic papers on the Mediterranean diet, by historians, nutrition officials, and scientists.

From Greece to Italy

As Trichopoulou began this work in the late 1980s in Greece, her counterpart, named Anna Ferro-Luzzi, was attempting to do the same thing in Italy. A research director at the National Institute of Nutrition in Rome, Ferro-Luzzi had decades earlier been instrumental in founding the field of nutrition science in her country. "I had to create everything myself," she recalls of the period in the 1960s when nutrition studies barely existed in Italy. It had been an uphill battle, she says, since Italians looked down on the field, which was considered "something for women—to stay in the kitchen and look at food."

Ferro-Luzzi's scientific contributions in creating the "Mediterranean Diet" were twofold: she conducted one of the most important, pioneering studies on the "heart-healthy" effects of olive oil, and she attempted to profile, as rigorously as possible, the exact components of the diet in Mediterranean countries. She and Trichopoulou chose to embrace a regional concept of diet over country-specific ones, because from the start, the conferences were supported by the World Health Organization (WHO), which had a greater interest in working at the regional level. Also, the two women shared a common fear that they were on the front line of a battle to defend an endangered way of life. Their fellow Mediterraneans were starting to eat fast foods at alarming rates, and it seemed that modernization threatened to extinguish the region's traditional cuisine before it had even been properly understood. Both women therefore felt the issue to be pressing. Yet Ferro-Luzzi's task of defining a Mediterranean Diet proved trickier than she had anticipated.

Early on in her efforts, she had to ask herself: Did any single Mediterranean Diet even truly exist? There was so much variation in eating patterns across countries and even within countries that it seemed nearly impossible to define any kind of overarching dietary pattern with any specificity. How could something so vague be evaluated, much less promoted as an ideal? The hope was to demonstrate that the Mediterranean Diet could prevent heart disease, but if the diet itself resisted definition, a proper test would be scientifically impossible.

Even Keys acknowledged in his cookbook that there were "substantial differences" in dietary habits across the region. For example, people in

"France and Spain ate twice as many potatoes than Greece," he wrote, and "the French ate much more butter."* Meat and dairy were consumed much less frequently in southern countries than in the North. Indeed, everywhere in the region he looked, there were differences in the amount and type of dairy consumption, the amount and type of meat, the amount and type of vegetables and nuts—pretty much everything.

Anna Ferro-Luzzi

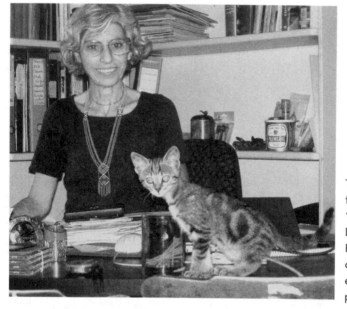

The Italian founder of the "Mediterranean Diet" in Italy, Ferro-Luzzi still questions if it can ever be defined properly.

In a meticulous, landmark paper in 1989, Ferro-Luzzi tried to create a workable definition of the nutritional patterns characterizing European countries bordering the Mediterranean Sea. Hers was the most rigorous attempt ever made, but ultimately she concluded that the project of identifying a Mediterranean diet was an "impossible enterprise, since data are

---

*Keys took a Europe-centered view of the Mediterranean. He focused on Italy, Greece, France, Spain, and Yugoslavia, and did not mention the African and Middle Eastern countries bordering the Mediterranean Sea, which have on the whole been excluded from the Mediterranean diet literature.

lacking, incomplete, or too aggregated." The all-embracing term "Mediterranean diet," "while very attractive," she wrote, "should not be used in scientific literature, until its composition, both in foods, nutrients and non-nutrients, is more clearly defined."

Despite these obstacles, however, Ferro-Luzzi still thought that modern-day, highly processed foods were obviously worse for health, and so she worked assiduously to preserve the traditional cuisine of her homeland. The Mediterranean Diet was a tough sell in those early years, however, since the concept made little sense to her fellow Italians. They did not think of themselves as having a "diet" of any kind, nor did they want to. Italians simply ate. "And bureaucrats didn't like the idea of 'medicalizing' a diet that had always just been a natural way of life," she explains.

Abundance of Olive Oil Confronts the Low-Fat Diet

The fact that the efforts of these two women would eventually lead to the Mediterranean diet being hailed around the world and even granted special status for its "intangible cultural heritage,"* as UNESCO did in 2010, did not seem obvious in these early, scrappy years. Various problems, both political and scientific, seemed likely to prevent the diet from ever attaining the hopes of its early supporters. On the scientific front, the principal challenge that Ferro-Luzzi had tackled—how such disparate eating patterns across different countries could be corralled under a unified concept—remained unresolved. And the ideological obstacles loomed even larger: The main issue was, how could an olive-oil-drenched diet triumph in a world dominated by low-fat dietary guidelines? This question had been present from the start, when Keys observed that the "healthy" Cretan diet was virtually overflowing with fat, representing between 36 percent and 40 percent of daily calories. The fat in question was olive oil, of course: the vegetables, he wrote, were served literally "swimming in oil."

As Ferro-Luzzi and Trichopoulos started to convene European re-

---

*This category of world heritage includes expressions of culture such as mariachi music and wooden movable type in China; the Mediterranean diet is the only nutritional regime on the list.

searchers around the Mediterranean diet idea in the 1980s, most health authorities found the sheer amount of fat in this proposed regime to be more or less preposterous. All that olive oil conflicted with the Western world's dietary guidelines, which limited fat to 20 percent to 30 percent of calories. Mainstream nutrition experts simply could not fathom how these fat-guzzling Greeks could possibly be so healthy. In response to this apparent paradox, Mark Hegsted, the Harvard professor who steered the McGovern committee and then led the USDA to publish its first dietary guidelines, announced, "You can't recommend high-fat diets." That declaration was the sound of the nutrition establishment putting its foot down: it was inconceivable to allow such liberal fat consumption.

In direct opposition to this low-fat monolith, Trichopoulou spearheaded the crusade for the Mediterranean Diet to contain, in its formal definition, 40 percent of calories as fat. This may sound like a relatively high amount, but it's no more than most Western populations ate before adopting the low-fat diet. Trichopoulou, along with other investigators, made a considerable effort to confirm that this 40 percent number was an accurate representation of traditional Greek eating habits. Her research concluded that it was. And she spent even more time fending off the low-fat ideology. "I said this would *destroy* the diet of the region. In Greece, this is the way we have always eaten. You cannot advise less fat!" she told me.

Her most vocal opponent on this score was Ferro-Luzzi, who took the low-fat side of the debate. She knew that in Italy, Keys had found fat consumption to be lower than in Greece, between 22 percent and 27 percent of calories. These numbers aligned more closely with international recommendations and also pertained to her homeland, so naturally she favored them. Ferro-Luzzi also took a magnifying glass to Keys's Greek data expressly to see if she could find some flaw with his 40-percent-fat number. She concluded that his data, like all of those available on the Greek diet of that period, were so scanty and unreliable* that there were "few scientific grounds" for the claim of a traditional Greek diet ever being high in fat.

---

*Anna Ferro-Luzzi identifies many methodological and technical problems with Keys's data, although she did so reluctantly, she says, since she and Keys were friends (Ferro-Luzzi, interview with author).

Ultimately, focusing so incessantly on total fat as the cause of disease turned out to be myopic and misguided, as we know, but this would not be understood for many years. In the meantime, the vast majority of researchers believed that fat made people fat and caused cancer and heart disease, so experts were worried that the Greek arm of the Mediterranean diet might be seriously unhealthy. Not a conference or meeting could pass without the issue being raised, and no one felt casual about it, least of all Ferro-Luzzi and Trichopoulou. "I had to sit in the middle and stop them from fighting," recalls W. Philip T. James, now chairman of the International Obesity Task Force in the United Kingdom.*

Trichopoulou eventually prevailed for the principal reason that she won over two influential Americans to her way of thinking. It turned out that in the same way that the low-fat diet had been catapulted by Keys into the American mainstream, so, too, would the Mediterranean diet depend upon forceful and influential personalities to make it a success. One of those people was Greg Drescher, a founding member of a group in Cambridge, Massachusetts, called the Oldways Preservation and Exchange Trust, which would go on to become the most vigorous promoter of the Mediterranean diet worldwide, and the other was Walter C. Willett, a professor of epidemiology at the Harvard School of Public Health, who would go on to become one of the most powerful nutrition experts in the world. The lines of causation behind success worked in reverse, too. Like Keys, who rode to fame on the low-fat diet, so, too, would Willett rise to prominence with the Mediterranean one.

Drescher and Willett both traveled to Athens in the late 1980s, where they each spent time with Trichopoulos. She and her husband, Dimitrios, who, like Willett, was also an epidemiologist at Harvard, hosted Willett

---

*The argument about fat percentages reached a crescendo among researchers in Europe in the year 2000, at the final planning meeting for a project aimed at establishing a single set of nutritional guidelines for the entire European Union. Called Eurodiet, it involved 150 European nutrition experts over two years, and an agreement seemed in sight until "Anna and Antonia started arguing about the percent of fat that was allowable in the diet," recalls Philip James, a key participant. No agreement could be reached, and the entire Eurodiet project collapsed (James, interview; Willett, interview with author, August 3, 2012).

in Athens and took him to a local tavern, where the menu would have included such fare as stuffed grape leaves and spinach pie. For the son of dairy farmers who grew up in Michigan eating what he called "bland American food," these complex and tasty dishes were a revelation. As Trichopoulos remembers, "I showed him that this simple food is what was contributing to longevity in Greece," and she encouraged him to promote this enticing regime for the good health of Americans, too.

Trichopoulou also played a role in Drescher's Mediterranean-food epiphany. Drescher heard her talk at one of her early conferences, "and everyone in the audience, their jaws dropped," he says. They had not yet heard of Keys's still-obscure Cretan cohort, and Trichopoulos was saying that the "Greeks in the sixties were eating so much fat but had no heart disease. How was that possible?!" wondered Drescher, astonished.

"You have to remember that in the late eighties, the reigning voice on health and wellness was Dean Ornish," Drescher explains, referring to the diet guru who counseled Americans to eat as little fat as possible. Drescher had a culinary background, having previously worked with Julia Child and Robert Mondavi. "Those of us in the culinary community were shocked and horrified [by Ornish's rules], because we knew fat was essential to flavor and a good dining experience," he says. "We were depressed about it. Nobody wanted to be a bad person and serve unhealthy food, but we didn't know how to make it all work." Drescher sought to learn more over coffee with Trichopoulou after her speech, and she recommended that he speak to Willett.

Eventually Drescher and Willett joined forces, and the more they learned, the more they realized that a higher-fat diet, with an appealing heart-healthy promise and wrapped in the bewitching beauty of Italy and Greece, could potentially have a strong appeal in America. Together, they were able to move the Mediterranean diet out of its academic-conference backwater and into prime time.*

---

*The third member of this team was K. Dun Gifford, who had been an aide to both Senator Edward Kennedy and Robert F. Kennedy and then worked in commercial real estate and invested in several restaurants before becoming the founding president of Oldways. Gifford died in 2010.

The Mediterranean Diet in the United States: Building the Pyramid

Drescher and Willett's first task lay in solving the problem that had bedeviled the diet from the start: how to define it in a coherent way. Working with a team that included Marion Nestle, a professor of food policy at New York University, Elisabet Helsing from the WHO, and Antonia's husband, Dimitrios Trichopoulos, they tried to pin down a diet that was literally all over the map.

"Walter Willett was the pivotal figure," said Drescher. "He provided a needed scientific rigor to the diet."

One of the first steps Willett and his team took involved shrinking the map encompassed in the proposed diet down to a more manageable size. It was decided that the great majority of the region would have to be excluded, either because data were lacking or because these countries—France, Portugal, Spain, and even northern Italy—did not fit the model that had emerged from Crete and southern Italy. Only these two locations shared a more or less similar culinary regime and were largely free of heart disease in the 1960s, so for scientific purposes, Willett's team decided that the Mediterranean diet should be based on these places alone.

Willett also settled the score on the total amount of fat to be recommended. He was persuaded by Antonia Trichopoulou's 40 percent number because, according to Keys's data, this amount of daily energy from fat was clearly consistent with the relatively good health of these populations. He wasn't a stickler for olive oil, though. Willett advised using vegetable oils, too, since he believed, as nearly all nutrition experts do, that any fat is fine so long as it is an oil, not a solid.

In 1993, one hundred and fifty of the most prominent nutrition experts from Europe and the United States arrived in Cambridge, Massachusetts, for the first major conference on the Mediterranean Diet. Ancel Keys came out of retirement to attend; Anna Ferro-Luzzi, Antonia Trichopoulou, and even Dean Ornish were there. These experts had long lived in a world where diet was defined by atomized nutrients rather than actual foods; no doubt they were expecting the usual slew of dry scientific slides on HDL- and LDL-cholesterol cross-tabulated with various kinds of dietary fat. Instead, to their delight, over the next few days they were regaled with stories about Italian olive oil and rural life on the islands of Greece.

On the third day, Willett came onstage and unveiled the "Mediterranean Diet Pyramid," to much applause. This pyramid was structurally patterned on the one the USDA had introduced the previous year, and the two pyramids had much in common: the broad middle slab was dedicated to fruits and vegetables, and the giant bottom slab contained grains and potatoes. But for the Mediterranean diet, some of the other horizontal slices were switched around. Whereas the USDA version put fats and oils, "to be used sparingly," in the pyramid tip, Willett's version gave olive oil a generous middle slab. This was the big news: a high-fat diet was okay! (Willett said his pyramid was an improvement on the USDA's because it had "olive oil poured all over it.") The tip of *his* pyramid pictured red meat,

USDA Pyramid

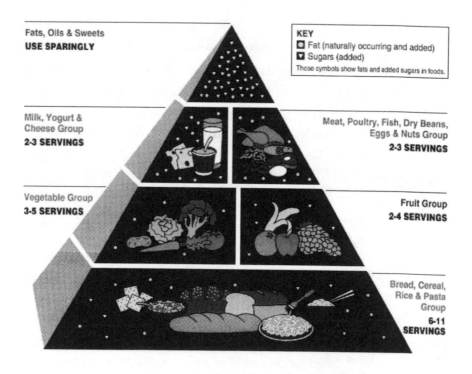

USDA Dietary Guidelines since 1980 have recommended a diet of mainly carbohydrates.

NINA TEICHOLZ

Optimal Traditional Mediterranean Diet
Preliminary Concept

This preliminary concept for a pyramid to represent the Optimal Traditional Mediterranean Diet is based on the dietary traditions of Crete circa 1960, structured in light of 1993 nutrition research. Variations of this optimal diet have traditionally existed in other parts of Greece, parts of the Balkan region, parts of Italy, Spain and Portugal, Southern France, North Africa (esp. Morocco and Tunisia), Turkey, as well as parts of the Middle East (esp. Lebanon and Syria). The geography of the diet is closely tied to the traditional areas of olive cultivation in the Mediterranean region. This is intended for discussion purposes only, and is subject to modification.

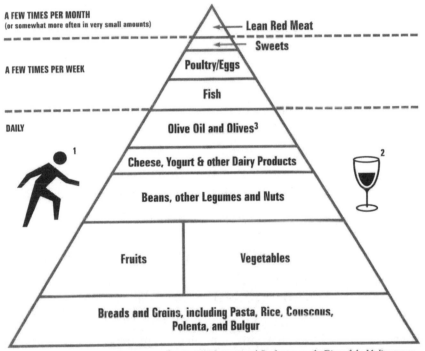

Source: 1993 International Conference on the Diets of the Mediterranean

[1] Indicates the importance of regular physical activity.

[2] Following Mediterranean tradition, wine can be enjoyed in moderation (1-2 glasses/day) primarily with meals; it should be considered optional and avoided whenever consumption would put the individual or others at risk.

[3] Olive oil, high in monounsaturated fat and rich in antioxidants, is the region's principal fat. In the optimal, traditional Mediterranean diet, total fat can be as high as 35-40% of calories, if saturated fat is at or below 7-8% and polyunsaturated fat ranges from 3-8% with the balance coming from monounsaturated fat (in the form of olive oil). Variations of this diet where total fat (again, principally olive oil) is at or below 30% — such as is found in the traditional diet of Southern Italy — may be equally optimal.

The first Mediterranean Diet pyramid, in 1993, was similar to the USDA's but cut back further on red meat while adding a generous allowance of olive oil.

to be eaten only "a few times a month," less often, even, than sweets. Other proteins (fish, poultry, and eggs) in Willett's model could be eaten only a few times a week, versus a few times a day in the USDA pyramid.

Was this truly a representation of the ideal Mediterranean diet? It was difficult to know. Not everyone at the conference was enamored by the underlying science. Marion Nestle, for instance, had worked closely with Willett in the preparations for the conference but ultimately declined to sign her name to the pyramid. "The science just seemed to me too impressionistic," she told me.

By this, she meant that no scientific evaluation of the diet had been done to justify the proportions of the pyramid's various slices. Remember that Ferro-Luzzi had tried to quantify the diet but found it impossible, and since then, no further efforts had been made. Nor had any clinical trials on the Mediterranean Diet been conducted yet. Therefore, like Keys and his diet-heart hypothesis, the Harvard team conveyed their nutritional idea into the world based on epidemiological data only. The evidence was, scientifically speaking, quite premature, hence Nestle's skepticism. Even one of Willett's former graduate students, Lawrence Kushi, who co-authored two papers with Willett justifying the health benefits of the Mediterranean diet, confided to me that Nestle was "correct in that the evidence [in those papers] is a little impressionistic."

The journal articles that Willett's team wrote to establish the pyramid were not subject to the peer-review process that scientific papers normally undergo; they had only one reviewer, not the usual two to three. This was because the papers were published, along with the entire 1993 Cambridge conference proceedings, in a special supplement of the *American Journal of Clinical Nutrition* funded by the olive oil industry. These kinds of journal supplements sponsored by industry are standard in the field of diet and disease research, although a lay reader is unlikely to be aware of this financial backing, because sponsorship is not noted in the articles themselves.*

Yet as the Mediterranean diet took hold among the public and academic researchers alike, it was hard to resist Willett and his distinguished

---

*A supplement is recognizable to the discerning reader by the "S" after the page numbers (page "12S," for instance).

colleagues as they coalesced around an exciting and alluring idea.* A new roster of scientific conferences on the Mediterranean Diet beckoned. Even Ferro-Luzzi, who had previously written sternly of her skepticism about the diet's basic definitional problems, was now serving on a clutch of international boards alongside top experts from around the world. The time for scientific questioning seemed to have passed. "The change came when we moved on from science to policy," Ferro-Luzzi explained to me, describing the shift after the 1993 Cambridge conference. "We put out the Mediterranean diet pyramid, which was rough, imprecise, but gave some connotation of what was compatible with good health. When you get into policy, you forget the minutia. You forget that the ground is not quite solid, a little shaky." Indeed, any uncertainties were soon forgotten. Most people assumed that, after Willett presented the pyramid in Cambridge, all the nitpicky details of the science had already been rigorously worked out, and that the diet was now ready for the wide-angled lens.

The Mediterranean Diet Conference Craze

The Mediterranean Diet ascended rapidly to the apex of the nutrition world, and a legitimate question to ask is: How did that happen? What made it so much more of an enduring success than the other diets that were popular at the time, including the Zone, Ornish, Atkins, and South Beach, which also laid claim to promises of good health? One obvious reason is that only the Mediterranean diet was backed by Harvard professors along with a stack of scientific papers that appeared to offer proof of the diet's disease-fighting properties. But the following step was equally if not more important in the Mediterranean Diet's promotion. Trichopoulou's original allies, Willett and Drescher, continued their efforts on behalf of the Mediterranean Diet, and they developed a whole new strategy that had a tremendous influence on nutrition experts, the media, and, ultimately, the public.

_____

*Later Willett trademarked the Mediterranean diet pyramid as the Harvard Medical School Food Pyramid and used it as the basis for his best-selling book, _Eat, Drink, and Be Healthy: The Harvard Medical School Guide to Healthy Eating_ (New York: Simon & Schuster, 2001).

Walter Willett and Ancel Keys, Cambridge, Massachusetts, 1993

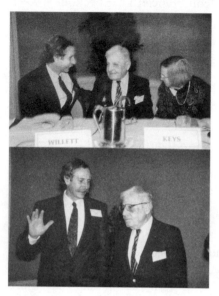

Ancel Keys, who created the Mediterranean Diet concept, with Walter C. Willett, the Harvard professor who made it famous.

The method involved inviting academic researchers, food writers, and health authorities into a slice of paradise: travel, free of charge, to some sun-kissed country around the gorgeous Mediterranean Sea, for the purpose of a scientific conference. In Italy, Greece, and even Tunisia, scientists rubbed elbows with cookbook authors, chefs, journalists, and public officials. Harvard provided the scientific prestige, while Oldways organized the financing. During the 1990s, there was a steady rollout of these conferences, and they effectively served as a nonstop promotion vehicle for the Mediterranean diet.

Oldways calls itself a "food issues think tank," and when it was founded in 1990, there is no doubt that the leadership was motivated by lofty goals. Drescher and his colleagues wanted Americans to understand food in the context of culture and above all wanted to shift the American conversation away from nutrients and the cold, alienating language of public health toward the language of *food*. After all, no one has ever requested "30 percent fat and 25 percent protein, please" for dinner. The average person just asks for a meal, like spaghetti and meatballs. The movement toward whole foods is familiar to us now, through the work of the author

NINA TEICHOLZ

Michael Pollan, among others, but the original idea was pioneered by Old-ways via the Mediterranean diet. The notion was that food, wrapped in the rich complexity of an ancient cuisine, could at once be meaningful and delicious—*and* good for health.

In working to convene people around this profound idea, Oldways organized fifty conferences from 1993 to 2004. And these getaways were an easy sell. The enormous appeal of the Mediterranean had of course been a factor in influencing Keys and his colleagues from the start, and their rapture for the region came even to suffuse their scholarly work. Henry Blackburn, for instance, who worked closely with Keys, wrote a description of the Cretan male who was "free of coronary risk" for the *American Journal of Cardiology* in 1986, using language that is unusually florid for a scientific journal:

> He walks to work daily and labors in the soft light of his Greek Isle, midst the droning of crickets and the bray of distant donkeys, in the peace of his land. . . . In his elder years, he sits in the slanting bronze light of the Greek sun, enveloped in a rich lavender aura from the Aegean sea and sky. He is handsome, rugged, kindly and virile.

The beauty of the landscape and lifestyle, its people, and its diet became united in one, overwhelming swoon. Blackburn admits that he is now embarrassed by this essay. But he says that at the time, "I was feeling very romantic about Crete. I fell in love with it."* Keys himself retired to his villa south of Naples, where he cultivated fruit trees.

Of course, it seems obvious in retrospect that a sustained love affair with the Mediterranean among the twentieth century's most influential nutrition experts helped steered the course of the field. (One has to wonder whether we would know more about the diets of other long-lived peoples,

---

*Keys's neighbors included his colleagues, who also built villas. Together with Seven Countries Study directors Flaminio Fidanza and Martii Karvonen, as well as Jeremiah Stamler, the group formed a cooperative of sorts in the early 1960s and lived part of the year there, becoming a center for scientific meetings and parties (Keys, 1983, 23–24).

such as the Mongolians or Siberians, if researchers were equally drawn to landlocked countries with desert steppes and long, freezing winters. What if they had gone to, say, Germany, which also had low postwar rates of heart disease but possesses fewer sun-drenched conference spots and a likely luncheon menu of *Sauerbraten* and *Blechkuchen*? We shall never know.) The Mediterranean, as a destination, won hands down. And just as Keys and his original group of researchers had been influenced by a love of all things Mediterranean, so, too, was the current crop of experts.

In April 1997, when the island of Crete was flaming with wild lavender irises and electric-purple rockroses, some of the biggest names in food and nutrition were among the 115 people gathered at the Apollonia Beach Hotel in the port town of Heraklion. Walter Willett, Marion Nestle, Serge Renaud (father of the "French paradox"), and Christos Aravanis and Anastasios Dontas, the two original researchers who carried out the Greek portion of the Seven Countries study, all attended, as did National Cancer Institute director Peter Greenwald, famous cooks, and well-known food writers such as Corby Kummer and Mimi Sheraton.

That week, the group led a delectable existence. Serious lectures and discussions on scientific topics such as "50 years of Mediterranean Diet Studies" and "Total Dietary Fat—What Are the Newest Study and Survey Results?" were interspersed with more cultural fare, such as the presentation "At Home with Persephone and Her Mother, Demeter, the Goddess of Grain." There were the trips to museums and ancient palaces as well as a wine tasting and several cooking workshops. One afternoon, women from the nearby prefecture demonstrated how to cook with the traditional ingredients and techniques of Crete. Renaud gave a demonstration on how to prepare snails. Another evening, the group was bused to the top of Mt. Ida, the highest mountain on the island, and ate dinner while the Hale-Bopp comet streaked spectacularly across the night sky.

"It was fabulous. I felt as if I'd died and gone to heaven," says Nestle. "For five years I got invited to absolutely everything they did. . . . We had meetings in the most fabulous places where I never would have been able to go otherwise and under the most lavish circumstances. It was absolutely amazing."

"Every time you sat down there would be eight wine glasses at your setting," remembers Laura Shapiro, then a writer for *Newsweek*, who went on several of the Oldways trips. "It was a level of caretaking and pampering that I had never experienced. Orchids on the pillow, soft air floating in from the balcony, and all that."

Oldways' Drescher was the creative genius behind merging the love of food with nutritional science. "I'm a great believer in trying to create programs that are in some way transformative for people, and not just a bunch of slides and presentations in a lecture hall and having bad food," he said. The educational getaways he organized are widely considered by the scientists, food writers, chefs, and other experts who attended to be some of the greatest food conferences ever. "These kinds of people had never been together at a single conference before. That was, in fact, more dazzling than the hotels," says Shapiro. "To have all those intellectual forces in one room together was just great!" The conferences were a ravishment of wine, scenery, and collegial conversation, and it's easy to see why researchers and food writers made a habit of hopping from one event to the next, all the while passing along glowing reviews about the virtues of the Mediterranean diet to their respective audiences back home.

"Olive Oil Ambassadors"

These endeavors were obviously expensive, however, and required corporate sponsors, which is why, from the start, Oldways had forged a close relationship with the International Olive Oil Council (IOOC). This agency, headquartered in Madrid, was founded by the United Nations to control olive oil quality and to develop the "world olive and olive-oil economy," in countries nearly all of which border the Mediterranean Sea.*

Before becoming involved with Oldways, the IOOC had tried to

---

*In Greece, fully 60 percent of the arable land is devoted to growing olives. Olive oil is the number one agricultural export from Spain and the second, after wine, from Italy.

generate olive-oil-friendly research by funding American scientists.* The academic research community was primarily preoccupied with the effect of various fats on serum cholesterol, and IOOC leaders thought that olive oil might be validated by this type of investigation, since the oil's effect on cholesterol had been shown in preliminary investigations to be neutral overall. Yet clinical trials were a slow-going business, and a positive outcome wasn't a sure thing, so the IOOC was glad to shift gears and assist Oldways in promoting olive oil through the far more efficient and appealing vehicle of the Mediterranean Diet conferences instead.†

Naturally, this meant that olive oil flowed liberally at every event. Samples of olive oil were tucked into flower arrangements and handed out to participants in miniature shopping bags. Olive oil was also, inevitably, the subject of various scientific panels.

"It worked this way," says Drescher, describing how conferences were funded. "We'd start with the IOOC money, but then we'd work with the government, and they're able to absorb hotels. The national airline flies people over. Anytime you can get the government involved, they're able to absorb expenses." Italy, Greece, and Spain all contributed. "It was really about aligning the interests of these countries with the interesting new directions of scientific research," Drescher explained. In other words, nations and their industries promoted themselves by providing lavish perks aimed at buying the good opinion of experts who would ultimately advise the public on nutrition. The strategy clearly worked.

The sway of olive oil money was nothing new in nutrition research. The Greek portion of the Seven Countries study had received funding from

---

*The most important academic researcher funded by the IOOC was Scott M. Grundy, chairman of the department of clinical nutrition at the University of Texas Southwestern Medical Center and one of the most influential experts in the field of diet and disease over the past fifty years. He conducted an experiment on olive oil together with Fred H. Mattson, a chemist who, after a thirty-year career at Procter & Gamble, became a professor of medicine at the University of California, San Diego (the study that resulted was Mattson and Grundy 1985).
†The first conference on the Mediterranean Diet that the IOOC funded was the one in Cambridge, Massachusetts, in 1993, where Willett introduced the pyramid.

the Elais Oil Company in Greece, the International Olive Council, the California State Olive Advisory Board, and the Greek Association of Industries and Processors of Olive Oil. The early part of the study was financed by the NIH, but when those funds ran out, as Henry Blackburn recounts, Christos Aravanis, the principal Greek researcher on the study, "didn't have any problem picking up the phone and collecting oil-company money." And Keys "helped significantly in realizing these funds," too, according to his colleagues. Keys reported only two of these grants when he first came out with his study, and in a later publication, only one.

Beyond the interests of the olive oil industry, which was the first or second most important agricultural product for Italy, Greece, and Spain, each country also had its national fruits or vegetables that could profit from being included in the Oldways' Mediterranean diet menu: tomatoes in Italy, potatoes in Greece.* Sponsoring an Oldways conference was really no different from what these industries were doing in their own countries, anyway: In Italy, for instance, the agricultural sector had early on supported the government's Mediterranean diet public health campaign with posters and TV commercials, urging its citizens to "eat Mediterranean." Ferro-Luzzi had prevailed in convincing authorities that this kind of a campaign was a good idea, based partly on the commercial appeal. "I told them that what was good for commodities was good for the people," she said. Spain and Greece ran similar efforts, as did the European Union as a whole, spending a reported $215 million over roughly a decade on olive-oil-related public relations. These campaigns also targeted European doctors with "scientific" bulletins about olive oil, leading some researchers to complain that their governments were improperly disguising marketing campaigns as scientific advice.

Nothing seemed to influence the scientific elites in Europe and the

---

*Some food industry sponsors, however, clearly pushed the Mediterranean envelope. In Hawaii, for example, where Oldways took Mediterranean diet conference goers to the usually inaccessible Waipi'o Valley ("an unbelievable slice of paradise," says Drescher), the macadamia nut industry was one of the funders, although there are no macadamia nut trees in the Mediterranean.

United States as effectively as the Oldways conferences, however. These heady and luxurious experiences, part science seminar, part foodfest, and part cultural celebration, were a stroke of genius in targeting the nutrition world's most influential people.

Nestle spelled out to me the obvious though unspoken quid pro quo of these sorts of conferences: "Every single journalist who went on one of those trips was expected to write about it, and if they didn't, they weren't invited back. . . . Everyone knew what they were supposed to do. And they were happy to do it! If you're in Morocco and being served a dinner where people come in with flaming platters of whatever, you're going to write about it. There's plenty to write about!"

Looking back, however, Nestle, who wrote *Food Politics*, the seminal work on how the food industry influences nutrition policy, recognizes that the conferences were more of a racket than most participants realized. "At the time it seemed totally benign. But it was so seductive. Oldways was basically a for-hire public relations company. . . . And the purpose was to promote the Mediterranean diet for academics like me who got sucked into that," she told me.

Kushi, the former Willett student who now directs scientific policy for Kaiser Permanente, said he and his colleagues all knew that olive oil money was flowing behind these gatherings, but "the fact that it was laundered through Oldways made it a bit more palatable." The experts invited by Oldways were simply too transported by the whole experience, it seems, to be much concerned about a possible industrial agenda underneath.

Eventually, says *Newsweek*'s Laura Shapiro, she was no longer invited to the Oldways conferences because "I couldn't get with the program." She was going on the free trips without writing stories about them explicitly, and at some point, she says, "Oldways told me they couldn't justify my presence to their sponsors."

But in the meantime, Shapiro says she had written about the health benefits of olive oil and had served the Mediterranean diet agenda quite well. "We, the press, were little olive oil ambassadors, everywhere. That's what Oldways created!"

And although some of these "ambassadors," like Shapiro, fell out of favor with Oldways,* inevitably there were others to replace them. Ten years of conferences organized by Oldways elevated the diet into a stratosphere of success, where it has remained, with continuing attention from the media and academic researchers, for decades. The *New York Times* alone has published more than 650 articles with "Mediterranean diet" in the title since Willett's pyramid came out. And nutrition researchers have given it serious, sustained attention, writing more than a thousand scientific papers on the Mediterranean diet since the early 1990s. Epidemiologists in Willett's department at the Harvard School of Public Health, at least one of whom attended every Oldways' conferences throughout the 1990s, have between them published nearly fifty papers on the Mediterranean diet. By comparison, diets such as South Beach and the Zone, which were not introduced by elite university scientists nor promoted by conferences abroad, have been the subject of only a handful of scientific papers. The Atkins and Ornish diets have received slightly more expert attention than these other popular diets, as we'll see in Chapter 10.

Nancy Harmon Jenkins, one of the founders of Oldways and author of *The Mediterranean Diet Cookbook,* acknowledged to me, "The food world is particularly prey to corruption, because so much money is made on food and so much depends on talk and especially the opinions of experts."†

---

*Ferro-Luzzi believes she was dropped by Oldways because she took an overly critical approach to the science. And Marion Nestle also fell out of favor with Oldways over a dispute involving the financing of the 1993 supplement to the *American Journal of Clinical Nutrition* that the IOOC had funded. Nestle had negotiated the IOOC deal at a luxury hotel in Hawaii, an episode that she writes about in her book *Food Politics,* and which she says she regrets (Ferro-Luzzi, email to author, December 27, 2013; Nestle, interview; Nestle 2002, 114–115).

†For its part, Oldways lost IOOC funding in 2003 and has since put on fewer events. In 2004, in a possibly desperate move, the group picked up the Coca-Cola Company as a major new client and for four years organized conferences called "Managing Sweetness" or "Understanding Sweetness." In the wake of that unfortunate choice, the group unsurprisingly lost some of its stature among nutrition researchers, and its conferences in recent years have been largely devoid of science.

Olive Oil Welcomed in America

Currying the opinions of those experts turned out to be worth every penny. With raves from scientists, food writers, and journalists alike, the Mediterranean Diet swept into magazines, cookbooks, and kitchens around the world, instantly nutrition's Next Big Thing. Health experts loved the diet as a way of delivering the familiar eat-your-fruits-and-vegetables message with a new twist, and also that the Mediterranean diet offered a means of embracing the beauty and deliciousness of food—so much more enticing than the previous nutritional regime based on self-denial and abstinence.

Health-conscious Americans, who had been skipping sautés and forgoing sauces on the USDA- and AHA-recommended low-fat diet for three decades, could not but welcome the permission to indulge in this new way of eating. *Some* fat in the diet could only be an improvement over the tasteless fat-free diets they had so long felt obligated to ingest. The diet soared in popularity because diners were delighted to eat, guilt-free, all those previously banned fatty foods, such as olives, avocados, and nuts. And compared to no fat, foods cooked in oil actually tasted good.

Seductive, sun-kissed, and Harvard-endorsed, the Mediterranean diet splashed into the headlines. One ecstatic food writer, returning from a conference, extolled "All these heavily credentialed men and women" who were confirming that the "cypress-lined roads of the Mediterranean led to a long, low-cholesterol life. . . . Finally, we could have our pasta and eat it, too." The *New York Times*'s Molly O'Neill wrote a long article after the first conference in Cambridge, hoping that the diet would prove to be the next "nutritional eden."

Still, it was hard for low-fat traditionalists to wrap their minds around the idea that a healthy diet could be high in fat. O'Neill initially misreported the Mediterranean breakthrough as nothing more than "a velvet glove around the steely reality of a low-fat regime." It was a common mistake among journalists and others who had followed the low-fat mantra for so long. Nor did the major professional associations—the AHA, the American Medical Association, and others—support the Mediterranean diet at first for the same reason that Mark Hegsted had rejected it: because the diet violated America's long-standing low-fat policy.

Americans were left to make sense of the conflicting advice as best they could, and judging from national consumption statistics, they continued to shift away from animal products, and toward fruits, vegetables, and grains, as advised by both the Mediterranean and USDA pyramids. They ate more fish. They ate more nuts. And they started cooking with olive oil. US consumption of olive oil shot up dramatically, in fact, following the announcement of the Mediterranean diet pyramid, and per capita consumption today is three times what it was in 1990.

No doubt the shift to olive oil represented a healthy step up from the vegetable oils that Americans had been using. One of the known dangers of these oils—peanut, safflower, soybean, sunflower—is that they oxidize easily at high temperatures; this is why their bottles carry warnings about overheating (as we will discuss in Chapter 9). Olive oil, by contrast, is more stable and therefore better for cooking.* Olive oil also had an aesthetic appeal, arriving in tall, alluring glass bottles with the smells and tastes of Italy, which for many cooks, compared favorably to the unsophisticated plastic bottles of relatively taste-free vegetable oils. For all these reasons, drizzling olive oil over a frying pan, onto vegetables, or into a salad dressing was how Americans shifted away from the low-fat diet toward a more "Mediterranean" style of eating.

Olive oil and the Mediterranean diet also seemed like the perfect answer to the question that Americans, longing for more fat, hadn't even known they were asking: Was there a route to good health that could be pleasurable, too? The Mediterranean diet filled this niche nicely.

Yet the question remains: Is the Mediterranean diet an elixir for good health? Starting with the claims for olive oil, it's time to take a look at the science.

---

*Remember that olive oil is a *mono*unsaturated fat, meaning that it has only one double bond along its chain of carbon atoms, whereas vegetable oils are *poly*unsaturated fats, with lots of double bonds, all of which are prone to reacting with oxygen.

A Long Life: Is It the Olive Oil?

The fruit of the olive tree has had many medicinal, religious, and even magical properties assigned to it over the ages. The ancient Greeks used the oil to anoint their bodies, and Hippocrates prescribed its leaves as remedies against numerous ailments, from skin disease to digestive problems. Because olive oil was such a significant part of the diet in Greece and Italy in the mid-twentieth century, and because Antonia Trichopoulou had such a strong feeling for this traditional product of her homeland (and no doubt because the olive oil industry was such a big contributor to the field), researchers from the start assumed that the oil must somehow play a role in the diet's link to longevity.

Anna Ferro-Luzzi was interested in the health effects of the oil, not just because it was a staple of the Italian diet, but also because US researchers had long been focused almost exclusively on fats, so for her, studying olive oil made good professional sense. It was through the study on olive oil, in fact, that Ferro-Luzzi got to meet Keys. "We became good friends," she says, but adds that of all the "tough scientists" (all men) with whom she worked over the years, "Ancel was by far the toughest: he would defend his points to the death." Even so, when Ferro-Luzzi began conducting an experiment on olive oil in the seaside village of Cilento, south of Naples, in the early 1980s, Keys signed on as a study advisor.

For one hundred days, Ferro-Luzzi recorded all the food eaten by fifty men and women. She chose these villagers because they still adhered to their traditional way of life, including the almost exclusive use of olive oil as the only visible fat. Ferro-Luzzi had her team visit each household at least four times per day, and a dietician sat with each family at each meal to make sure everyone ate. Two scales were installed in kitchens to weigh small and large food items. If a family member consumed a meal at a restaurant or a friend's house, a member of the team would visit the place to find out how the food had been prepared. Moreover, because the experiment aimed to see what would happen to blood cholesterol levels upon switching subjects' diets from vegetable to animal fats (with the biggest shift being from olive oil to butter), Ferro-Luzzi provided family members with all the meat and dairy they needed at the beginning of each week. The study was therefore a model of fastidiousness and shows the level of commitment needed to do truly meaningful research in the field of nutrition.

After six weeks, Ferro-Luzzi found that the "bad" LDL-cholesterol shot up a full 19 percent, on average, when villagers switched from olive oil to butter, among other saturated fats. This result was heralded as a stunning point in olive oil's favor, and the study—the first definitive experiment on olive oil's cholesterol effects—served to establish both Ferro-Luzzi in her field professionally and olive oil as a "heart-healthy" oil.*

Focusing on the LDL-cholesterol effects, nutrition researchers lauded olive oil as a salubrious disease-fighting fat, and in the following years, many dozens of papers were published on the oil's possible curative effects. Unfortunately, most of these health benefits have not panned out as hoped. Experts suggested that olive oil might help prevent breast cancer, for instance, but the evidence so far is very weak. It was hoped that olive oil would reduce blood pressure, but various studies on this score have had decidedly mixed results.

In "extra-virgin" olive oil, investigators identified a host of "nonnutrients," such as anthocyanins, flavonoids, and polyphenols, that are believed to work their own minor miracles. They are present in olives because the fruit is dark-colored, a defense developed over thousands of years against exposure to the hot sun. Not all of the effects of these nonnutrients have been adequately explored, but in one case, flavonoids, sizable clinical trials on humans have been unable to show benefits to health.

Some of the more frequently cited data to support olive oil's health claims comes from the Greek cohort of the European Prospective Investigation into Cancer and Nutrition (EPIC), a big epidemiological study of more than 28,000 volunteers, directed by Antonia Trichopoulou. Based on this data, Trichopoulou published a landmark article in the *New England Journal of Medicine* (NEJM) in 2003, in which she concluded that adher-

---

*Ferro-Luzzi's study also showed that the "good" HDL-cholesterol rose when her subjects switched to butter (an effect that was especially pronounced among the women), implying that butter might actually be the healthier option, but as we've seen, experts have been focused on LDL-cholesterol rather than HDL-cholesterol as the biomarker of choice, and this HDL finding by Ferro-Luzzi has been ignored.

ing to a "traditional Mediterranean diet," which includes "a high intake of olive oil" was associated with a "significant and substantial reduction in overall mortality." It is therefore a shock to find out that in this study, Trichopoulou never actually measured the olive oil consumption of her subjects. It was not an item on the food-frequency questionnaire she used, either as a foodstuff eaten directly or as a fat used in cooking. Instead, she "estimated" its use from the questionnaire's list of cooked dishes, making assumptions about how Greeks might cook them.* This shortcoming is not mentioned in the NEJM paper, however, and "olive oil" is listed in the paper without any explanation of its derivation.†

In 2003, the North American Olive Oil Association, which represents olive oil producers, gathered all the available evidence purporting to show that the oil could protect against heart disease and submitted these studies to the FDA. These producers hoped to win the right to a "health claim" that could be used on food package labels—something like "a diet high in olive oil can prevent heart disease."

Yet the FDA was not convinced. Of the seventy-three studies submitted, only four were deemed methodologically sound enough for consideration. (Epidemiological evidence such as the kind that Willett and Trichopoulou published, could not show causation and therefore were not included in the analysis.) The four allowable studies were all clinical trials in which men had been fed olive oil for nearly a month. Taken together, these trials showed that olive oil, compared to other fats, could lower total LDL-cholesterol while leaving HDL-cholesterol intact. But the FDA stated that it could not grant a health claim based on a study sample of only 117 people, all young men. Overall, the evidence reflected "a low level of comfort among qualified scientists" for the hypothesis that olive oil prevented heart disease, ruled the agency. (Since then, a few clinical trials

---

*Trichopoulou also conducted a study on a smaller population to check the validity of these olive oil estimations, but the results provided only "moderate" to "weak" confirmation of the larger survey's accuracy (Katsouyanni et al. 1997, S120).
†In another of Trichopoulou's publications based on this data, the words "olive oil" are in the title (Psaltopoulou et al. 2004).

on olive oil have been performed in the decade since, but they do not add much to the evidence base, since they are small and have had conflicting results. Moreover, a few recent studies on animals suggest that olive oil may even *provoke* heart disease, by stimulating the production of something called cholesterol esters.)

Olive oil producers were therefore only allowed to advertise that "*limited but not conclusive* scientific evidence suggests that eating 2 tablespoons of olive oil daily may reduce the risk of coronary heart disease due to the monounsaturated fat in the olive oil." The statement was hardly a resounding recommendation of olive oil as a fat with special, disease-fighting powers.

The FDA's tepid endorsement, however, did not stop researchers from trying to find other ways that olive oil could indeed be a magic elixir. In 2005, for instance, there was a great deal of excitement over an article in *Nature* about the discovery that olive oil contained a newly discovered anti-inflammatory substance. The biopsychologist Gary Beauchamp had noticed that Lemsip, a pharmaceutical beverage drunk in Britain to fight the flu, irritated the back of his throat in the same way that extra-virgin olive oil did. This "led to the only light-bulb in my head that I've ever had in my life," as he likes to say: that olive oil and ibuprofen must have some ingredient in common. The mystery substance turned out to be oleocanthal. Beauchamp suggested that ibuprofen's anti-inflammatory effects might also be at work in olive oil, yet, as one critic pointed out, a person would have to consume more than two cups of olive oil a day to get an oleocanthal dose equal to that of an adult-sized dose of ibuprofen, and Beauchamp's experiments had been conducted in a lab, not on humans, so the results have to be considered preliminary.

Only because olive oil has been so wildly hyped does the disappointing news about actual scientific findings come as any surprise. Indeed, "surprisingly" is the word that two Spanish researchers used when confronting the data purporting to show olive oil's heart-healthy effect, and concluding, in 2011, that there was "not much evidence."

Homer's "Liquid Gold"?

It is reassuring to think that olive oil, with its presumed four thousand years of human history, must at least be safe, if not beneficial, for human health, perhaps in ways we haven't yet managed to capture through scientific studies. Homer called it "liquid gold," after all.

Or did he? Although "liquid gold" appears on lots of Web sites selling olive oil, the phrase doesn't appear in any translation of Homer's *Odyssey* that I could find. Indeed, the actual passage in the *Odyssey* says something quite different: Odysseus is given "olive oil *in a flask of gold*" to anoint himself with. In fact, nowhere in any of the Hellenic texts is there any mention that olive oil was consumed as a part of the diet. The oil was ancient, true, but—as it turns out—not as a food; it was employed mainly as a cosmetic, for rubbing over the body during ritual activities and athletic contests or simply to enhance physical beauty among gods and mortals alike.

Did the use of olive oil as a food go back much beyond the early twentieth century even? Was it the "dominant item of the diet," going back "at least four thousand years," as Keys claimed? Amazingly, it seems not. "Less than 100 years ago, ordinary people in many parts of Greece ate far less oil than today," wrote a French historian in 1993. Greek archaeologist Yannis Hamilakis, who has researched the subject extensively, looked at Crete in particular and found that the oil was insignificant as a subsistence crop before modern times. The amount of olive oil available to the average medieval Cretan peasant for consumption was, in fact, "very low," and its production expanded only in the mid-seventeenth century, when encouraged by Venetian rulers seeking to respond to a growing industrial demand for the oil—mainly for making soap. As Hamilakis concludes, the historical record shows that "despite conventional wisdom, there is almost no evidence which could indicate with certainty" that olive oil was made for "culinary use" in Greece until the nineteenth century. In Spain, too, olive oil did not appear to be consumed in substantial amounts until the 1880s. And it was apparently the same story in southern Italy, where one scholar found it "doubtful" that olive oil "made a contribution to the diet for over 40 centuries." An analysis of tree cultivation in southern Italy indicates that olive oil "must have been a scare commodity until at least the 16th century and . . .

its principal use in medieval times was in religious rituals." Indeed, in historical accounts going back to antiquity, the fat more commonly used in cooking in the Mediterranean, among peasants and the elite alike, was lard.

So it seems that olive oil is actually a relatively recent addition to the Mediterranean diet and not an ancient foodstuff, despite the best efforts by interested parties to add Homer to the marketing team.

What Is "a Lot" of Vegetables?
Attempting Science on the Mediterranean Diet

But if a Mediterranean Diet prevents heart disease, as Ancel Keys originally proposed, and if olive oil is not the operative element of the diet, then what is? Is it the fruits and vegetables or the diet as a whole? Researchers have wondered if there was a protective element in the folate of the wild greens that the Cretans ate regularly or in the greater content of omega-3 fatty acids in the flesh of the animals eating the wild greens. Research has been done on all these possibilities, but there are no conclusive answers.*

Trichopoulos has even suggested that the Mediterranean pattern of eating and drinking itself might have unquantifiable synergistic effects, including such factors as the "psychosocial environment, mild climatic conditions, preservation of the extended family structure, and even the afternoon siesta habit in the Mediterranean region." †

It's important to identify exactly which part of the Mediterranean diet

---

*The scientific evidence supporting omega-3s is the strongest: the anti-inflammatory effects of these long-chain fatty acids have been well demonstrated, although recent large clinical trials have not successfully confirmed that daily supplements of EPA and DHA can reduce heart attack risk. EPA and DHA are the long-chain omega-3s found in meat, fish, eggs, and other animal foods but not in plants, such as flaxseed and seaweed, which contain shorter-chain omega-3s that cannot easily be converted by humans into the longer-chained versions. Only the longer-chain EPA and DHA omega-3s are thought to be beneficial to health (Galan et al. 2010; Rauch 2010; Kromhout, Giltay, and Gelcijnse 2010; Plourde and Cunnane 2007 on "cannot easily be converted").

†Dimitrios Trichopoulos analyzed the EPIC data on almost twenty-four thousand Greek men and found that the habit of a daily siesta was associated with a *37 percent* lower rate of death from heart disease. However, note that the finding was an associ-

is beneficial for health not just for scientific reasons but for so many seismically important practical ones, too. When Anna Ferro-Luzzi attended an international meeting in Japan in 2008, for instance, experts from around the world who sought to adopt the Mediterranean diet were asking her, "Which fruits and vegetables should we grow? Can you tell us, at least, if we should grow fruits *or* vegetables?" In the end, says Ferro-Luzzi, "We couldn't say what, exactly, was the most important . . . because the research is too vague. Even though we recommend eating more fruits and vegetables, it's not meaningful. It's not possible to know."*

Ferro-Luzzi, of course, had identified the problem of finding a firm definition for the diet from the beginning, and saw it crop up when Willett first formally introduced the diet in 1993. Perhaps the diet was too complicated, with too many factors, ever to be precisely enough defined for meaningful scientific study? These definitional difficulties did not go away, even as Mediterranean countries and interested industries continued to pour funds into research. And there were more research disappointments to come.

Remember that when Walter Willett unveiled the Mediterranean pyramid, no controlled clinical trials of the diet had ever been done. Evidence had therefore been limited to epidemiological studies which, until quite recently, have served as the star players in the diet's evidence base. The first of these studies was, of course, the original Seven Countries study. After that, the largest effort was that EPIC study, with Trichopoulos's Greek cohort. This and smaller such studies were promising, but they could not, by their very design, offer definitive results (since epidemiology can only show associations), and many of the results they did offer were contradictory. Various studies had shown, for instance, that a Mediterranean pattern of eating was associated with diminished rates of diabetes, metabolic syndrome, asthma, Parkinson's disease, and obesity, and these results were encouraging. However, Trichopoulou found, when she combined data from her Greek subjects with that of Europeans from other countries who had also been part

---

ation, and that the same effect might be achieved by getting more sleep during the night, as the study authors observed (Naska et al. 2007, 2143).

*Even fruits, themselves, from bananas to blueberries to avocados, have different compositions of macronutrients, fiber, antioxidants, and sugar.

of the EPIC study, altogether some 74,600 elderly men and women from nine countries, that a Mediterranean Diet was *not* reliably associated with a reduction in coronary risk.*

These epidemiological studies continued to suffer from the diet's fuzzy definition. Yet while Ferro-Luzzi had given up on ever finding a solution to the problem, Trichopoulou kept at it. In 1995, she developed the Mediterranean Diet Score, which boiled the whole diet down to eight factors and assigned a point to each.† A person would earn one point for eating a "high" amount from each of the "protective" food groups (these included 1. vegetables/potatoes; 2. legumes/nuts/seeds; 3. fruits; 4. cereals). That was four possible points, total. Another three points, at a maximum, could be earned by eating a "low" amount from each of the "non-protective" food groups (5. a high ratio of olive oil to animal fats; 6. dairy products; and 7. meat and poultry). Item 8 was alcohol, and a person scored a point for this item by hitting a midrange of consumption.

Trichopoulou's scoring dramatically simplified the study of the Mediterranean diet, and researchers loved it. Two dozen other similar indexes have since been introduced, comprised of anywhere between seven and sixteen food components. But not everyone was convinced of their usefulness. In a comprehensive review of the indexes, a group of professors at the University of Barcelona expressed their considerable doubts. For instance, what is a "lot" of vegetables, and what is a "little" meat?‡ Also, these kinds

---

*Trichopoulou found only a very small reduction in heart attack risk associated with the diet, and in Germany, the association was reversed. Moreover, the diet was defined as "modified" Mediterranean because, as a critic pointed out, it included not just olive oil but also vegetable oils. Trichopoulou explained that the point of the analysis was simply to look at *un*saturated fats, a category that included both of these types of oils. No doubt it was also true that the study did not separate out olive oil because it *could* not (Vos 2005, 1329; "a critic pointed out").

†Trichopoulou based the target amount of each of these items on the consumption patterns of 182 elderly men and women in a remote Greek village, whom she studied in 1995 and assumed they were eating their traditional fare (Trichopoulou et al. 1995).

‡These researchers also doubted whether an index derived from studying elderly Greeks in a mountainside village could be applied to an entirely different group, such as young Spaniards.

of indexes assume, without any scientific basis, that each component contributes equally to heart disease. Yet can we say that someone who eats no vegetables (minus 1 point) and another person who eats no nuts (also minus 1 point) have increased their risk by exactly the same amount? No evidence exists to answer this kind of question.

A more pointed critical voice has been that of Andy R. Ness, chair of the epidemiology department at the University of Bristol, who told me that the indexes, in addition to their other problems, "don't consider total energy intake [calories], whereas with all the other stuff we do in this field, we adjust for the amount of food people eat." Altogether, he said, the critical thinking that has gone into these indexes has been "pretty dire."

In her defense, Trichopoulou replies that her efforts have at least moved the field forward, and that's true. What seems just inevitable is that the diet's persistence in eluding a clear definition has all but necessitated this kind of soft science—and opened the door for passion and bias to enter in.

"We, as a team at Athens Medical School, we want to keep what for generations we have developed. This is our cry!" Trichopoulou once told me, and this statement seems to confirm the opinion of her colleagues that she is motivated as much by "Mother Greece" as by the science. "Antonia is perhaps guilty, as we all were, of thinking with her heart," says her former colleague Elisabet Helsing, who, as the Advisor on Nutrition for WHO-Europe, was involved in all the early work on the Mediterranean diet. "Many of us in this field, we were led not by the head but by our hearts. The evidence was never so good." Or, as Harvard epidemiologist Frank B. Hu wrote in 2003, in a break with his colleagues, the Mediterranean diet "has been surrounded by as much myth as scientific evidence."

India's Mediterranean Coast: Problems with the Clinical Trials

It was still possible that well-conducted clinical trials, which are able to demonstrate causation, might finally show the Mediterranean diet to be superior. Where were those trials? Well, there were a few, but the problem was that they were only Mediterranean-*like*, and yet even so, they would serve as the warhorses of evidence for the diet, repeatedly and widely cited. They are therefore worth looking at briefly, if only to show how far nutrition experts will stretch the evidence to bolster support for a favored hypothesis.

The first, with results in 1994, was the Lyon Diet Heart Study. Researchers at a cardiovascular hospital in Lyon, France, took a group of six hundred middle-aged people (almost all men) who had suffered a heart attack in the previous six months and divided them into two equal groups. People in the control group were left to follow their regular doctors' advice and the others were assigned to follow a Mediterranean-style regime. Researchers had wanted to imitate the 1960s Cretan diet but couldn't see how they could persuade French people, unfamiliar with the taste, to adopt olive oil. So instead, they formulated a special margarine made from canola oil and handed it out to subjects in tubs free of charge every two months. Subjects were also counseled to eat a "Mediterranean-type" diet with more fish, white meat rather than red (and less meat overall), and more fruits and vegetables.

After about two years, the special margarine-eating group had suffered three fatal heart attacks and five nonfatal ones, compared to sixteen fatal and seventeen nonfatal ones in the control group. Deaths from other causes were also lower in the group eating the special margarine (eight compared to twenty among the controls). Survival differences between the two groups were so stark that researchers stopped the experiment prematurely to start prescribing the Mediterranean Diet for everyone. And for nearly two decades, the Lyon study was the star study, cited everywhere as key support for the effectiveness of the diet.

Yet the study had enough methodological problems to give any reasonable person pause: It was small ("hopelessly underpowered," meaning not enough subjects, as one researcher commented). Moreover, aside from the margarine, study participants changed their diet from what they usually ate by only a tiny amount, eating very slightly more fish—about an anchovy-strip's worth a day—as well as a small carrot and half a small apple's worth of additional fruit and vegetables a day, compared to the control group. And these differences might have been nonexistent, given that only a handful of the controls had their diets assessed, which was a huge flaw, given that diet was the variable being studied.*

The big difference between the two groups was the special margarine. What did the margarine contain? Fatally, for the study of the Mediterranean diet, the margarine's fat profile was nothing like olive oil. The margarine was high in alpha-linolenic fatty acid, an omega-3 polyunsaturated fat found in nuts, seeds, and vegetable oils, whereas olive oil contains a mono-unsaturated fat called oleic. These fats are entirely different in their chemical structures and also their biological effects on humans. So whatever the lessons of the Lyon Diet Heart Study, they are therefore clearly not about the Mediterranean Diet.

In addition to the Lyon study, there was one other clinical trial that was promoted widely for many years by experts as vital evidence for the Mediterranean Diet, since it appeared to show the benefits of a diet high in plant foods and low in saturated fats. As in Lyon, researchers intervened in the diets of middle-aged people who had recently suffered a heart attack. One group was put on a diet "containing star gooseberries, grapes, apples,

---

*These problems are described in a paper for the American Heart Association, which found itself in the awkward position of trying to reconcile its own recommended low-fat diet with the success of the relatively high-fat diet used in the Lyon study. The authors concluded that the diet had been "so poorly assessed in both groups" that it "raises questions about the role of diet" in accounting for the "results reported." It's quite possible that the better health outcomes seen in the experimental group were due entirely to what is called the "intervention effect," they wrote. This refers to the positive way that a study subject responds to an intervention, such as a diet counseling class or even just a little added attention from study administrators, which invariably results in better outcomes for these subjects, compared to those who don't. Trials are therefore usually designed to try to provide equal experiences to both the experimental and control groups to avoid this effect. In the case of the Lyon study, however, members of the experimental group initially received personalized, detailed dietary instructions and were then reminded weekly of their participation in the study due to the margarine deliveries, whereas the control group received no parallel interventions. In an early paper on the study, not cited in the final results, investigators acknowledged these significant differences in the experiences of their two study groups (Kris-Etherton et al. 2001, "a paper by the American Heart Association"; de Logheril et al. 1994; de Logheril et al. 1997).

sweet limes, bananas, lemons, raisins, bail, musk melons, onions, garlic, trichosanthes, fenugreek seeds and leaves, mushrooms, bitter and bottle gourds, lotus roots, Bengal and black grams . . . and oils of soya bean and sun flower."

Sound like the Cretan diet of 1960? Not exactly. Ram B. Singh, a private practitioner, apparently performed this experiment in a facility adjacent to his house in Moradabad, India, in the late 1980s. The diet's limits on meat and eggs and abundance of fruits and vegetables somehow justified its characterization as a "Mediterranean type" of diet, which is how scientists have tended to describe it in the literature. The vegetable oils used barely resembled olive oil, and the foods were very different, but these issues were generally overlooked, and the Indo-Mediterranean Heart Study, as the study was suggestively called for many years, has been widely cited as support for the Mediterranean regime.

Eventually, though, it was discovered that Singh's work was so riddled with problems—the daily food diaries by participants appeared to have been fabricated and the serum cholesterol values were calculated using long outdated methods, among many other things—that the prestigious *British Medical Journal* (BMJ), which had published one of his studies in the first place, conducted a lengthy investigation. Ultimately, this was published under the headline "Suspected Research Fraud" along with a statistical investigation which concluded that Singh's data were "either fabricated or falsified." The BMJ editors expressed their serious reservations about the study and stopped just short of retracting it.*

Years later, however, the Singh study was still being included in scientific literature reviews of the Mediterranean Diet, including an influential one by Lluís Serra-Majem in 2006. As the director of the Madrid-based Mediterranean Diet Foundation, the most important international group

---

*It appears that Singh passed off the same data as if coming from different clinical trials and managed to get them published in a number of prestigious journals, including the *Lancet, American Journal of Clinical Nutrition,* and the *American Journal of Cardiology.* Altogether, he was the first author on papers that claimed to be reporting on twenty-five clinical trials between 1990 and 1994, an impossibly high number, and one of the reasons that his work triggered suspicion (White 2005, 281).

promoting the diet today,* Serra-Majem had every reason to emphasize the positive evidence, yet he stressed to me, "We have to take care with what we do, because otherwise we will have no credibility." Indeed, in his literature review he dismissed many studies for being too small or methodologically weak. For instance, some researchers called a diet "Mediterranean" simply if it contained olive oil, a few extra ounces of walnuts, or a couple of glasses of wine. However, when I asked him about his inclusion of the Singh trial, he confided, "I wanted to leave the door open for that study . . . but I did feel a little bad, like when you're in a court, and you realize that one of your witnesses is not so good."

Like many reviewers before him, Serra-Majem also included the GISSI-Prevenzione trial from Italy, which, despite being widely cited in support of the Mediterranean Diet, was really a trial to test the effectiveness of fish oils and vitamin E supplements in which participants happened to eat something *like* a Mediterranean Diet. This was not the intended intervention of the study, however, so researchers had to change the study hypothesis retroactively in order to include conclusions about diet. Yet altering a hypothesis after the fact is not really considered acceptable science, since it introduces the possibility of bias by the investigators, and any resulting conclusions are thus considered to be weak at best.

Serra-Majem is obviously invested in finding support for the Mediterranean diet; he's the one who submitted the application to UNESCO for the diet on behalf of Spain, Greece, Morocco, and Italy. But it wouldn't be fair to single out any one person for overinterpreting the evidence; the dubious citation of these clinical trials simply grew to be the norm among researchers in the field. Collectively, over time, flaws receded from sight and best results came to be emphasized, until a body of evidence that seemed to justify dietary recommendations became etched into the historical record. The same groupthink happened when the vast majority of researchers came

---

*His foundation is funded by the Spanish Institute of Agriculture and interested industries, including Dannon and Kellogg's. Serra-Majem is frank about the motivations: "Their interest is in promoting Mediterranean products," but adds that because government funds are lacking, without industry funding, he would be unable to do research (Serra-Majem, interview with author, August 2, 2008; http://dietamediterranea.com/directorio-mediterraneo/enlaces-mediterraneos/).

to overinterpret the studies on the diet-heart hypothesis in order to endorse the low-fat diet. A tacit agreement to turn a blind eye to the shortcomings of the evidence has been a necessary strategy for the survival of both of these official diets.

A Test of the Real Mediterranean Diet

Nutrition experts were justifiably elated when trial results came out for the *real* diet—not one with specialized margarine, nor with Indian food, but something close to the actual Mediterranean diet itself.

The first such trial, in 2008, was conducted in Israel. It was well designed and rigorous, with an international group of professors on board, including the epidemiologist Meir Stampfer of the Harvard School of Public Health. These researchers selected 322 moderately obese middle-aged people, mostly men, and fed them one of three diets: one low in carbohydrates, one low in fat, and the third, Mediterranean.* Specially prepared meals were served at a workplace cafeteria, allowing for a high degree of control over what and how much foods were eaten. And the experiment lasted two years, a long time for a trial that involves overseeing the preparation and service of food.

During the entire study, those on the Mediterranean diet were found to have a lower risk for heart disease than those on the low-fat diet. Compared to the low-fat group, the Mediterranean dieters maintained lower triglycerides, higher "good" HDL-cholesterol, lower "bad" LDL-cholesterol, lower C-reactive protein (an indicator of chronic inflammation), and lower insulin (a marker for diabetes); they also lost more weight, averaging about 10 pounds over two years, compared to 7 pounds for the low-fat group. The Mediterranean diet therefore looked better than the low-fat diet in every possible way. "So my conservative conclusion is, don't start with a low-fat

---

*The "Mediterranean" diet that the researchers used was based on Walter Willett's pyramid; it was "rich in vegetables and low in red meat, with poultry and fish replacing beef and lamb." It was low-calorie (1,500 per day for women and 1,800 per day for men), with a goal of no more than 35 percent of calories from fat; the main sources of added fat were 30 to 45 grams of olive oil and a handful of nuts (five to seven nuts, or less than 20 grams) per day.

diet," said Stampfer, a pronouncement that would have been unthinkable a decade earlier, in the early 2000s, when the study was conceived.

These are certainly positive results for the much-beloved Mediterranean diet. But do they suggest that the diet is best? Stampfer stresses the point that the people on this diet had the easiest time adhering to it, which is important. But that might be due to the fact that since they were Israeli, it was their local cuisine. Indeed, what Stampfer doesn't like to advertise, and what the study report itself doesn't emphasize, was the notable success of the *third* arm of the study. This was the group eating a low-carbohydrate diet, relatively high in fat. The participants on this diet, it turned out, looked the healthiest of all. They lost even more weight (12 pounds), and their heart disease biomarkers looked even better: their triglycerides were lower and their HDL-cholesterol much higher than the other two groups. Only LDL-cholesterol looked better for Mediterranean dieters, yet this biomarker has proven to be less reliable than previously thought. Therefore, although the finding has received no attention, there's really no doubt that the low-carb diet performed better than both the low-fat and the Mediterranean diets.

Then, in 2013, a large Spanish study came out that grabbed headlines worldwide and seemed to establish the Mediterranean diet's healthfulness once and for all. That study, called Prevención con Dieta Mediterránea, or PREDIMED, was led by a team that included Serra-Majem. The study was a tremendous undertaking, with 7,447 men and women aged fifty-five to eighty, assigned to one of three groups. Two groups were told to eat a Mediterranean diet, for which they were responsible for cooking and preparing meals. In addition, one of the Mediterranean groups received extra allotments of extra-virgin olive oil while the other got extra nuts, provided free to participants. A third group received no free food and served as a control.*

After a median study period of five years, 109 people in the control

---

*This study used a "Mediterranean diet score," of the kind that Trichopoulou had invented (see page 207), to evaluate compliance with the diet. The score was comprised of fourteen items for the Mediterranean dieters and nine items for the controls. The consumption of certain items such as eggs had to be overlooked, because only a limited number of items could be scored (Estruch et al. 2013, 24 and 26).

group had suffered a "cardiovascular event" (a stroke, heart attack, or death related to heart disease), compared to 96 among the extra-virgin olive oil Mediterranean dieters and only 83 in the extra-nuts Mediterranean group. "Mediterranean Diet Shown to Ward Off Heart Attack and Stroke" announced the *New York Times* on the front page of the paper.

However, if you look at PREDIMED's control group, those subjects weren't eating a regular Spanish diet. They were instead on a low-fat diet, because that diet has been the international standard for so many decades. This low-fat group was advised to avoid eggs, nuts, fatty fish, oils, and high-fat foods of all kinds. But that diet, as we know, has now been studied extensively, including in the Women's Health Initiative, the largest dietary trial ever undertaken. And that diet has convincingly been shown to lack any ability to fight heart disease, cancer, or obesity. Therefore PREDIMED, like the Israeli trial, simply demonstrated that the Mediterranean diet was better than the *low-fat diet*.*

If the Israeli trial had never existed, everyone could have assumed that the Mediterranean option in PREDIMED was the best possible regime for health. But that third, low-carb arm in Israel had revealed that an even better option was possible. (Previous shorter trials had found the same thing, as we will see in Chapter 10.)† The Mediterranean diet may very well have outperformed the low-fat diet simply *because* it delivered more dietary fat, since the largest difference between the low-fat and Mediterranean groups was the amount of nuts and olive oil they ate. Was it really much of an accomplishment to be better than that failed AHA-USDA low-fat regime?

It's perfectly possible that any national diet would look better when compared to the low-fat diet. Perhaps the traditional Chilean or Dutch

---

*A few critics noted this point and also observed that the grouping together of various conditions in the "cardiovascular health" end point obscured the fact that there had been no fewer heart attacks among the Mediterranean dieters, compared to controls. The only significant finding had been a drop in strokes, and that was a "minor" absolute reduction seen in the first year of the study only (Opie 2013).

†There was one other long-term (two-year) trial comparing a low-fat to a Mediterranean diet, with results in 2004. It showed that the Mediterranean diet performed better. But the study involved men and women with metabolic syndrome, not a normal population, and could not be generalized (Esposito et al. 2004).

diet, for example—or that of any country eating unrefined, traditional foods—would show fewer cardiovascular events in a comparison with a diet low in fat. We don't know, because such experiments have not been done. Only the Mediterranean diet has been studied so thoroughly. It has monopolized the scientific landscape, with its many days in the Mediterranean sun.

Reconsidering Why the Cretans Were Long-Lived

Although you have to dig into PREDIMED's appendix to find this out, the various arms of the study all ate the same amount of saturated fat. That is, they ate the same amount of fat from meat, eggs, cheese, and the like. "Well, I think saturated fat is not the main problem," Serra-Majem told me, even before the study results came out.

If that's true, then Keys and his team were probably mistaken in concluding that the low disease rates they observed in Greece and Italy were due to the absence of animal fats that they measured. These researchers were predisposed to finding saturated fat to be a problem. Perhaps they overlooked other aspects of the diet that might have better explained the lack of heart disease among these long-lived peoples? It seems worth circling back to the Seven Countries study to take another look.

Aside from the "Lent problem" (see page 40) and the fact that Keys was observing a population during an uncharacteristic period of postwar hardship, his study on Crete had other, equally troubling issues. Notably, its sample size appears to have been a mere handful of people. Keys originally designed his study with two sources of dietary information in mind: written questionnaires from a larger sample of the population—655 men, in the case of the Greeks—and a collection of duplicates of all the actual foods eaten over the course of a week, from a much smaller sample. This collection of foods was intended to check the questionnaire responses. Yet disappointingly, the answers did not line up as expected. The two sources of dietary data gave different results that could not be reconciled. So Keys assumed that the Cretan men must have been giving inaccurate replies to the questionnaires—and he did a rather astonishing thing. Although you have to read carefully between the lines of his papers to figure it out, Keys ended up simply getting rid of the survey data he had collected from the 655 men on Corfu and Crete.* That left only one source of dietary data for his calculations: the food collected from the smaller group of men. These meals were gathered on three separate occasions on Crete and once on Corfu. Keys went to Corfu twice, actually, but had to throw out one set of data because some of the fats had been "destroyed in processing." Other fats were absorbed into the clay containers used to carry the food samples. In the end, it turned out that only thirty to thirty-three men were sampled on Crete and thirty-four on Corfu.

These, then, are the founding men of the Mediterranean Diet, whose meals over the course of a few weeks fifty years ago have influenced the entire course of nutrition history in the Western Hemisphere. Such a small sample size was in no way statistically representative of the 8.375 million Greeks or even the 438,000 Cretans in 1961. According to statistical formulas, Keys would have needed a sample size of 384 people on each island, which he did have, until he discarded the survey data.

Nonetheless, Keys left the overwhelming impression in his early publications that he had based his calculations on dietary data from all the 655 Cretan men he studied, and this erroneous representation has been passed down through the scientific literature.

When I phoned a leading expert on nutritional epidemiology, Sander Greenland at the University of California, Los Angeles, to ask about the sample size of thirty-three men on Crete, I could almost hear his eyebrows

---

*Keys's disaffection with dietary surveys as a tool for nutrition research shows up in papers toward the end of his career: "When people simply are queried about their diets their answers from time to time necessarily reflect their own ideas of their stereotypes; they tend to repeat the same answers whether or not they truly correspond to reality." Without the survey data, however, Keys had no record of the individual foodstuffs eaten. When his colleagues tried to describe the actual Cretan diet for one of Trichopoulou's first conferences on the Mediterranean diet, they wrote that the surveys had been "lost" and that they therefore had to reconstruct the diet as best they could from the text of Keys's original paper on the Greek diet. Among their difficulties was the fact that Keys had made no mention of the consumption of fruits or vegetables on Crete (Keys, Aravanis, and Sdrin 1966, 585; Kromhout et al. 1989; Kromhout and Bloemberg in Kromhout, Menotti, and Blackburn 2002, 63).

go up. "If the thirty-three lined up perfectly with respect to some predicted hypothesis," he told me, "one of the possibilities might be fraud." Small data sets that "look 'too good' are considered signs of possible fraud," he said. "In other words, those Keys data sound as shaky as Jell-O in a Cretan earthquake."

Long after Keys published the data, in the 1980s, the Seven Countries study leaders acknowledged that even in that tiny sample, there was so much variation from one visit to the next that not much about the diet could be concluded from these data. But that qualifier has been lost to history.

Then, atop that shaky data, Walter Willett built his pyramid. And his team of researchers had an even more precarious connection to the original reality of the Cretan diet of the 1960s. For example, their pyramid contains no fresh milk, but this seemed to be a mistake. I asked members of the Harvard team about this oversight at an Oldways meeting in 2008; they were onstage, and I raised my hand from the audience. Keys had published a paper only a few years before the pyramid came out, stating that the average Cretan consumed 8 ounces (1 cup) of fresh milk every day, mainly from goats but also from cows, which was more than the US cohort was drinking. Why did this information not make it into the pyramid? I asked. Willett even cited this paper by Keys* but then explained that he is nevertheless excluding milk because it is so "high in saturated fatty acids, which are believed to cause CHD." A fear of saturated fat appeared to trump all other considerations, even the actual data on milk consumption itself. And in answering my question, the team onstage in Cambridge remembered only Willett's assertion from fifteen years earlier: milk was "not generally consumed," they replied.

Another historical inaccuracy of the Mediterranean diet pyramid is the near-absence of red meat. This is ironic because the Cretans actually *preferred* red meat. "In Crete the meat is mostly goat, beef, and mutton, with an occasional chicken or rabbit. In Corfu, the meat is mostly beef and veal," Keys wrote. An earlier survey of the Cretan diet also found the same

---

*Indeed, Keys's paper is the *only* one that Willett's team cites to document milk consumption from that period (their other principal source was a study that lumped together "milk and cheese") (Kushi, Lenart, and Willett 1995, 1410S).

thing. And it's hard to find a cookbook or historical text on Italy, Spain, or Greece that does not make clear how the populations in these countries favored lamb, goat, and oxen over fowl. Nor were the ancient Greeks feasting on chicken. *The Iliad* describes the dinner given by Achilles for Odysseus this way: "Patrokles put a big bench in the firelight and laid on it the backs of a sheep and a fat goat and the chine of a great wild hog rich in lard."

So how is it that the Mediterranean Diet pyramid recommends the reverse: poultry several times per week and red meat only a few times a *month*? After all, the dramatically lower red meat recommendation was, as Willett wrote, a "major hallmark" of his pyramid.

Part of the answer is that Keys simply ground up all the food that the Cretans ate and sent the mixture back to his lab in Minnesota to have it analyzed. The resulting data that scrolled out of his printer were not a list of food items like snails, mutton, liver. Instead it was a list of macronutrients: saturated fat, monounsaturated fat, protein, carbohydrate, and so on. The saturated-fat content turned out to be low, probably because Keys collected a third of his Cretan data during the fasting holiday of Lent, when animal foods are greatly restricted. Yet in their paper on meat, Willett and his colleagues don't cite any of Keys's original reports about the actual foods eaten. Willett told me that he relied on his own epidemiological findings about red meat instead and that to the extent that he consulted Keys's work, he simply looked at the macronutrient profile and selected poultry as the meat that would best fit the low-saturated-fat specification.*

It was quite a leap. Not only did the selection of chicken as the dominant meat source have no basis in the history of the Mediterranean diet, but one could reasonably question whether chicken has the same effect on health as do Cretan goats or kids or lamb. Red meat, for example, has a far

---

*Willett's team cites only one study to support the chicken recommendation: his own Nurses' Health Study, which showed an association between lower heart disease rates and a higher consumption of a category called "chicken and fish." The observed association could therefore have been due to the fish rather than the chicken. The rest of the evidence that Willett and his team used to support the choice of chicken is not pro-chicken but rather anti–red meat, and almost all the studies employed to support this case were epidemiological.

greater abundance of vitamins B12 and B6, as well as the nutrients selenium, thiamine, riboflavin, and iron, than does chicken.

So it seems that Willett and his team selected chicken because they were already convinced that red meat was unhealthy, and they took for granted that it couldn't be part of an ideal diet. Recommending lamb and beef, much less goat, would have been inconceivable, whereas promoting chicken fell within acceptable norms.

It therefore appears that in following the Mediterranean Diet, we are relying on data collected by Keys in postwar Greece from a mere handful of men, partly during Lent, and then distorted by Willett's team who, like so many experts, were biased against saturated fat. Cretans in the 1960s clearly drank more milk and ate more red meat than we've been led to believe. Even so, it's curious that this diet in its day, on Crete, was not widely beloved.

It turns out that before Keys arrived on Crete he had been preceded by another epidemiologist, named Leland G. Allbaugh, who was employed by the Rockefeller Foundation in New York to improve its understanding of "underdevelopment." Crete was selected for its pre-industrialized economy, which had suffered gravely during the war. Allbaugh, seeking to understand the human toll of these recent hardships, conducted a thorough study of the Cretan diet, and like Keys, found that their fare "consisted chiefly of foods of vegetable origin, with cereals, vegetables, fruits, and olive oil predominating," with only "small amounts" of meat, fish, and eggs. Yet far from adoring this perfect example of the Mediterranean Diet, Allbaugh reveals a startling reality: the Cretans were openly miserable with their daily fare. "We are hungry most of the time," said one. When asked how their diet could be improved, "Meat alone or with cereal was mentioned as a 'favorite food' by 72% of the families questioned." They had evidently eaten more meat before the war and were now suffering without it.

It was the same for peasants in Calabria, in the boot of Italy, whom, Ferro-Luzzi had visited in the 1970s and described as eating nearly an "ideal" Mediterranean diet, ample in greens and olive oil, with very little meat. Yet according to Vito Teti, a local historian who wrote on this period, the Calabrian peasants and farm laborers considered this diet to be the scourge of poverty and expressed relentless scorn for vegetables, which were considered "not very nourishing." It went beyond simple dislike. A diet of mainly plants was considered nonnutritious—unhealthy, even, which was the main reason that Lent was so disfavored. A rigorous review of survey data led Teti to conclude that Calabrians "considered the lack of food . . . almost entirely vegetarian, as the cause . . . of general mortality for cases linked to nutrition, the low stature of individuals, their physical weakness, their low ability to work and psychological debility. Indeed, in the 1960s, 18 percent of men in southern Italy were of "low stature" (under 5 feet 2 inches), compared to only 5 percent in the north, where more animal foods were eaten. Men from Calabria who were measured when they turned up for military service from 1920 to 1960, were the shortest men in the entire country. To improve their lot, the Calabrians, like the Cretans, desired mainly one thing, as Teti described: "Meat is what these peasants craved, above all else. . . . The robust man, tall and 'erotic,' was the man who had eaten meat."

Of course it's possible that these peasants were misguided in craving meat. If they were of short stature, hungry, and ill much of the time, as Teti documents, then who knows if meat was the magic ingredient that could have solved those problems or if better medical care, more hygiene, or some other kind of food might have served them better?*

A modern-day nutrition expert would say that these cravings by the poor, if satisfied, would lead to even greater ill-health. Yet historical trends suggest that these peasants were probably right. As Italy and Greece slowly grew more prosperous following the war, they started to leave the near-vegetarian diet behind. From 1960 to 1990, Italian men came to eat ten times more meat on average, which was by far the biggest change in the Italian diet, yet the sizable spike in heart disease rates that might have been expected did not occur; in fact, they declined. And the height of the average Italian male during this time increased by almost three inches.

It was the same in Spain: since 1960, meat and fat consumption have

---

*One clue from history is that the Mediterranean's meat-loving tradition seems to have quite a pedigree going back to the Romans and Ancient Greeks. Hellenic heroes dined almost exclusively on meat, served with lots of bread and wine, according to scholars who have analyzed the writings of Homer. Only rarely does Homer mention vegetables and fruits, which were "considered beneath the dignity of the gods and heroes" (Yonge 1854, 41).

skyrocketed, while at the same time deaths from heart disease have plummeted. In fact, coronary mortality over the past three decades has halved in Spain, while saturated fat consumption during roughly this period increased by more than 50 percent.

The trends are the same in France and Switzerland, whose populations have long eaten a great deal of saturated fat yet never suffered much from heart disease. The Swiss ate 20 percent more animal fats in 1976 than in 1951 while deaths from heart disease and hypertension fell by 13 percent for men and 40 percent for women.

This apparent contradiction holds true even on the island of Crete. When the lead researcher for the Greek portion of the Seven Countries study, Christos Aravanis, went back to Crete in 1980, two decades after his initial research, he found that the farmers were eating 54 percent more saturated fat, yet heart attack rates remained extraordinarily low.

To his considerable credit, Lluís Serra-Majem of the Mediterranean Diet Foundation has tried to deal with these facts, which are inconvenient for the diet he promotes. He acknowledges that despite the "spectacular" rise in meat intake, as well as the drop in wine and olive oil consumption, the Spaniards are definitely healthier today than they were thirty years ago.* In a 2004 paper entitled "Does the Definition of the Mediterranean Diet Need to Be Updated?" Serra-Majem gingerly concluded, "The evidence for . . . certain types of meat, traditionally presented in a less favorable light, warrants reassessment of recommendations for these products."

In the end, when Keys focused on the low consumption of animal fat as the reason for good health among the Cretans, he found what he had hoped to find, but he was unlikely to have been right. His observation that a diet low in saturated fat was consistent with minimal heart disease was possibly accurate in 1960 but was no longer true in 1990. And this original

---

*Serra-Majem has suggested that reduced salt intake or smoking among men might be factors, or that better medical care might be helping people survive heart attacks. On this last point, however, Simon Capewell, a professor of clinical epidemiology at the University of Liverpool, has conducted detailed analyses and found that only a quarter to a half of the declines in heart disease deaths in recent decades can be explained by improved medical care in most countries, including Italy (Palmieri et al. 2010; Capewell and O'Flaherty 2008; Serra-Majem, interview with author).

mistake seems to have been compounded a thousand times over during the next decades by scientists who inherited Keys's dietary biases. No doubt a Cretan or Calabrian peasant might find it ironic that New York socialites and Hollywood movie stars—indeed, nearly all the wealthy peoples on the planet—are now trying to replicate the diet of an impoverished post-war population desperate to improve its lot.

These apparent paradoxes would be vexing, except that an alternative explanation for the relative absence of heart disease on Crete had always been at hand: the near complete absence of sugar in the Cretan diet. As Allbaugh described, the Cretans "do not serve desserts—except for fresh fruit in season. . . . Cake is seldom served, and pie almost never." The consumption of "sweets" in the Seven Countries study, as you might remember, correlated more closely with heart disease rates than did any other kind of food: they were abundant in Finland and the Netherlands, where heart disease rates were highest, while study leaders observed that "hardly any pastries were eaten in Yugoslavia, Greece, and Japan," where heart disease rates were low. And these observations have held true over time. From 1960 to 1990 in Spain, for example, the intake of sugar and other carbohydrates fell dramatically, right along with heart disease rates, as meat consumption rose. Italian sugar consumption, always very low, also dropped during those years.

All of this makes one wonder if the Mediterranean diet is associated with good health because it is low in sugar. The additional red meat consumed in the region over recent decades seems not to have been a factor in determining disease, whereas sugar is a possible—plausible, even—explanation, and it fits the observations.

Should We All Be Mediterranean?

International researchers from outside the Mediterranean studied the diet because they hoped to learn the secret to good health, and because they were drawn to the beauty and romance of the region. Olive oil money greased their wheels. And researchers from *within* the Mediterranean studied the diet because they hoped to save their health along with their treasured, disappearing traditions. As Serra-Majem told me, "For us, it's very important, because it's not a nutritional recipe but also a way of living. The Mediterranean diet is not just nutrients but a whole culture." It's a beautiful sentiment, and one can easily sympathize with the feelings of people who fear the homogenization and destruction of their heritage. But we might also ask ourselves: Should other societies not be able to transmit their own cultures through their own cuisines, too? Should a Swede abandon her grandmother's butter-based recipes? Should a German give up sausage? Should the Chileans or Dutch or their descendants in the US give up their own national diets because international experts are telling them to eat like the Greeks and Italians? With some study, other national diets might also outperform a low-fat diet, as the Mediterranean diet did, and these would be worth exploring, too, for the compelling reason that a person's food tradition encompasses generations of recipes and a unique cultural inheritance.

Because America is a nation of immigrants, and so many of us have lost our connections to the original cuisines of our homelands, we are probably more susceptible to the guidance of nutrition experts. These experts have suggested to us a delicious way of eating, but we can also ask ourselves: Should we all be Mediterranean?

The Mediterranean diet *has* been a boon in certain ways. It offered relief during a particularly austere and restrictive period of American cuisine. It offered a corrective to mistaken low-fat policies. It demonstrated a more relaxed attitude toward dietary fat. And even if olive oil's ancient provenance falls apart under scrutiny, it is a relatively stable oil that doesn't oxidize easily and therefore has no doubt been a healthier alternative to the more unstable oils made from soybeans, corn, and the like. Humans *do* have more years of experience consuming this oil than the vegetable oils that line the aisles of our supermarkets today. In fact, one of the more disturbing aspects of the Mediterranean diet pyramid is that it has intensified America's phobia about animal fats, accelerating our flight from these ancient foods to using vegetable oils instead. And this result may have harmed health in ways that appear serious but have not yet been well researched—because experts have for so long been focused exclusively on the supposed dangers of eating meat and dairy instead.

8

Exit Saturated Fats, Enter Trans Fats

Olive oil was the great solution for home cooks seeing a way out of their restricted-fat diets. For food manufacturers making packaged goods, however, olive oil was expensive, so when Big Food faced the government-driven imperative to get saturated fats out of their products, they turned to using vegetable oils instead. In replacing saturated fats, such as lard, suet, and tallow, which are solids at room temperature, these vegetable oils had to be hardened. And the only way to do that was by hydrogenation. The process of hydrogenation was the alchemy that turned a liquid into a solid, and it opened up a vast new range of possibilities for these oils, which could now be used wherever solid animal fats had been used. We saw how margarine became a substitute for butter, for instance, and how Crisco, an entirely new animal-fat substitute, entered the US market in 1911. Margarine and Crisco were both huge sellers in the first half of the twentieth century.

Yet you might also remember that the process of hydrogenation produces trans-fatty acids. It took ninety years after hydrogenated oils were introduced for these trans fats to be recognized by the FDA as questionable for human health. And while we are perhaps accustomed to that federal agency working at a glacial pace to protect the nation's food supply, one could argue that hydrogenated oils should have been fully examined more expeditiously, since they grew to be a sizable 8 percent of all calories consumed by Americans by the late 1980s. Why did we understand so little about hydrogenated oils for so long? In looking at how food companies and vegetable oil producers influenced the scientific research on trans fats, we can learn a lot about how the food industry works as it attempts to steer expert understanding and ultimately public opinion on the subject of dietary fats. The International Olive Oil Council's work in influencing our perceptions of olive oil were actually fairly unsophisticated compared to the high-level tactics routinely employed by the large edible oil companies.

From the late 1970s on, due to the success of Keys's diet-heart hypothesis, the drive to oust saturated fats from the US food supply intensified. And as a result, hydrogenated oils came to be used to make not only Crisco and margarine but virtually all manufactured food products. By the late 1980s, in fact, these hardened oils had become the backbone of the entire food industry, used in most cookies, crackers, chips, margarines, and shortenings, as well as fried, frozen, and baked goods. They were in supermarkets and restaurants, bakeries, school cafeterias, sports stadia, amusement parks, and so on.*

Food manufacturers, from Big Food to the corner bakery, came to rely upon hydrogenated oils because they're cheaper than butter and lard and also because they're highly versatile. Depending on the level of hydrogenation in the oil, they can be tailored to a wide variety of food products.

For instance, hardened oils perform superbly well in creating crisp-crumbly cookies, crunchy crackers, moist cupcakes, and flaky pastries. Their relatively smaller fat crystals means that shortenings made from these oils can trap smaller air bubbles that stay in the batter longer and produce reliably fluffy cakes. A chocolate candy could be customized to melt in the

---

*Remember that only a portion of the oil is hydrogenated, and so it is called "*partially* hydrogenated oil." The more hydrogenation used, the more solid the oil, and the more trans fats it contains. Although the terms "trans fats," "trans fatty acids," "partially hydrogenated oil," and "hydrogenated oil" are not synonymous, we will use them interchangeably, for sake of ease.

mouth, not in the hands. Less hydrogenation would produce a softer type of chocolate for, say, a donut topping, while a more highly hydrogenated oil would make the "coating fat" of individual boxed chocolates harder. While cooking with vegetable oils would cause pastry layers to collapse and give them a greasy feel, a hydrogenated product would keep the pastry layers separated, making them airy and crisp. In margarines, partially hydrogenated oils are spreadable at cool or warm temperatures without being greasy or soggy. In muffins and other baked goods, hydrogenated oils make them long-lasting and moist.

Hydrogenated oils are also great for frying foods such as doughnuts, potato chips, chicken nuggets, and french fries. The oils don't smoke up at normal frying temperatures (because they don't oxidize easily), and they could be reused many times over in batch frying.

Partially hydrogenated oils were, in sum, the food industry's endlessly adaptable Zelig. They became the backbone of Big Food.

More and More Trans Fats

As in most of the nutrition stories we've explored, many of the people and institutions behind the ramp-up of trans fats in America had the best possible intentions, based on the official version of the best available knowledge. In this case, because the National Institutes of Health had declared saturated fat to be the main dietary culprit, what could be more well-intentioned than doing everything possible to eradicate these fats from the US diet? Encouraging food manufacturers to abandon animal fats for hydrogenated oils seemed like the optimal idea. After all, the health implications of using trans fats at the time were little known.

One of the best-intentioned forces driving people away from saturated fats and toward trans fats was the Center for Science in the Public Interest (CSPI), based in Washington, DC, which is the most powerful food-focused consumer group in the country. With Michael Jacobson, a microbiologist, at its helm, CSPI has long been a leader in pushing the FDA to do a better job overseeing America's food. Jacobson is so powerful that food companies will even drop by his office to "ok" a new food product even before introducing it on the market—a level of servility seen as necessary since the late 1980s, when CSPI single-handedly destroyed the prospects of a substitute fat (called Olestra) that Procter & Gamble had spent more than a decade developing. CSPI lobbied the FDA to require that products containing Olestra carry a warning about possible "anal leakage"—no doubt a requiem for any foodstuff.

When it came to saturated fats, CSPI, like every other health-oriented group in America, was squarely on board with the idea that these fats caused heart disease. Indeed, Jacobson made the elimination of saturated fats one of his top priorities when calling on federal agencies in Washington, and in 1984 launched an enormous media and letter-writing campaign called "Saturated Fat Attack." CSPI encouraged fast-food companies such as Burger King and McDonald's to abandon beef tallow for partially hydrogenated soybean oil in their french-fry operations. Saturated fats should be replaced by "healthy" hydrogenated oils, CSPI asserted, citing evidence that hydrogenated oils had a relatively benign effect on cholesterol, compared to saturated fats. Hydrogenated oils were therefore "not a bad bargain" when it came to heart disease, the group concluded. Due to CSPI's persistent and public urgings throughout the 1980s, all the major fast-food chains removed tallow, lard, or palm oil from their french-fry operations and converted them over to partially hydrogenated soybean oil instead.

Another CSPI campaign successfully convinced movie theaters across America to switch from butter and coconut oil to partially hydrogenated oils in their popcorn poppers. This was "a great boon to American arteries" CSPI judged. Not much was known about these hydrogenated oils when CSPI was recommending them, but in the 1980s, everyone had been living with the diet-heart hypothesis for so many decades that the great majority of nutrition experts firmly believed that any kind of fat would be better than one that was saturated.

Another force pushing food companies to ditch saturated fats for hydrogenated oils was a lone multimillionaire in Omaha, Nebraska, Philip Sokolof, who had an outsized impact on the US food industry. Sokolof was neither a scientist nor an expert in the field, but after suffering a near-fatal heart attack in his forties, made it his mission in his retirement to inform Americans about the dangers of saturated fats. His target was not animal fats so much as the coconut and palm oils that were being widely used by

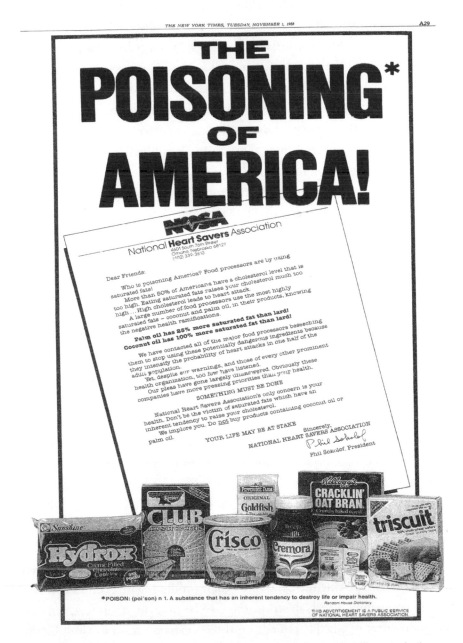

A series of 1980s ads in national newspapers inaccurately portrayed tropical oils as a threat to health.

food companies in their packaged foods. These tropical oils are very high in saturated fats—very very high, as it turned out. Fully half of palm oil is composed of saturated fats, as is 86 percent of the oil from the kernel of that palm fruit and 92 percent of coconut oil. (Palm oil is extracted from the pulp of the oil palm fruit and is different from palm *kernel* oil, which is extracted from the kernel of that fruit.) These numbers were scary to a public that had long been assured of saturated fat's dangers. And if they didn't currently know enough to be scared, then Sokolof made it his job to inform them. (The science on these oils has since evolved, and the cardiac risk associated with them is now thought to be minimal.)

Sokolof founded a group called the National Heart Saver Association, funded by his own millions, and ran it mostly by himself. Starting in 1988, he ran a series of full-page ads in major newspapers with the alarming, all-capitals headline, "THE POISONING OF AMERICA!" Who was poisoning America? "The food processors . . . by using saturated fats!" stated the ads. They went on: "We have contacted all the major food processors beseeching them to stop using these potentially dangerous ingredients because they intensify the probability of heart attacks. . . . Our pleas have gone unanswered. . . . Something MUST BE DONE."

Sokolof's ad pictured items that at the time contained coconut or palm oil: a can of Crisco shortening, Kellogg's Cracklin' Oat Bran, Triscuit by Nabisco, Sunshine Hydrox Cookies, Club crackers by Keebler, Cremora Non-dairy creamer, Carnation Coffee-mate, and Pepperidge Farm's famous Goldfish.

Sokolof says he placed the ads because he had mailed "thousands of letters" to food manufacturers urging them to eliminate tropical oils from their products but received "only a few replies." Company executives— unsurprisingly—did not return his phone calls, so an irritated Sokolof decided that a campaign to shame these manufacturers publicly was his best option. After the ads ran, Sokolof reported that his calls "went straight through to the vice president." More importantly, food companies started to respond by replacing the palm oil in their products with trans fats. When certain companies, like Nabisco, seemed to be dragging their feet, Sokolof ran another set of ads. He ran ads on three separate occasions, and, by the end, there's no doubt that his message was heard: tropical oils were nationally understood to be a threat. The ads, he said, were his "greatest triumph."

American Soybeans Take up Arms Against Tropical Oils

Though theatrical in his tactics, Sokolof was channeling the prevailing expert opinion against saturated fats; he merely infused the government's dietary guidelines with a dose of post-heart-attack passion. By all accounts, Sokolof was a lone crusader and, like CSPI, motivated by high-minded motives. What he probably didn't know, however, was that his efforts operated against the backdrop of a much larger and more pernicious crusade against tropical oils guided not by the public good but by profit. This far more complex campaign was quietly being run by the American Soybean Association (ASA), representing the industry that stood to gain the most from the promotion of hydrogenated oils.

Vegetable Oil Consumption in the United States, 1909-1999

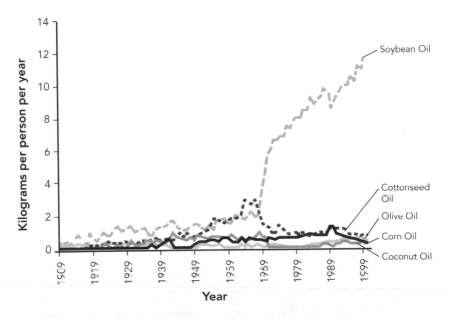

Source: Tanya L. Blasbalg et al., "Changes in Consumption of Omega-3 and Omega-6 Fatty Acids in the United States During the 20th Century," *American Journal of Clinical Nutrition* 93, no. 5 (May 2011): Figure 1C, 954.

Americans now eat over a thousand times more soybean oil than they did in 1909, the biggest change in the American diet.

The vast majority of hydrogenated oils consumed by Americans are made from soybeans, and this has been true since the 1960s (a mechanized way to press soybeans into oil was discovered in 1911). The farmers who grow soybeans and the companies that process them into oils are, like all industries, always on the lookout for competitive threats. Rivals in the form of tropical oils—coconut oil from the Philippines and palm oil from Malaysia—have long been on the industry radar. In the 1930s, these foreign oils made inroads enough that the ASA had mobilized to try to kick them out, which it did by persuading Congress to pass ruinous taxes on them. This had been the first "tropical oil war," and when it was over, in 1948, David G. Wing, president of the ASA, declared, "We want to hold this market." The ASA successfully did so for almost forty years, until the 1980s, when tropical oil imports started to creep up in the United States again, and the ASA went back to war.

The motive was, as ever, financial: "Our real concern was that it [these imports] was eating into our profits," remembers Steven Drake, a top executive at the ASA in the mid-1980s. The amount imported was small; palm and coconut oil together represented only 4 percent to 10 percent of the fats and oils consumed in the United States in the mid-1980s, according to various estimates. Yet the ASA still felt it needed to defend its own product, soybean oil, which was so widely used in packaged goods and in food service operations (restaurants, cafeterias, etc.) in the United States.

Palm oil imported from Malaysia was terrifying to the American soybean industry because palm oil could do everything that soybean oil did, but 15 percent more cheaply. Palm oil was therefore a formidable threat—indeed, the only real threat—to the soybean industry.

In order to drive tropical oils out of the market once again, Drake ran what amounted to a slander campaign from 1986 to 1989 out of ASA headquarters in St. Louis. Under his guidance, ASA distributed speeches and leaflets, put ads and cartoons in newspapers, and launched letter-writing efforts aimed at food companies and government officials, to drive home the same point that Sokolof was making: tropical oils, because they were high in saturated fats, should not be used by American food manufacturers.*

---

*Drake states that the ASA worked independently from Sokolof and the CSPI.

The ASA's other main point was that since tropical "oils" were actually solids at room temperature, calling them oils could be seen as deceptive marketing. "One of our guys, he came up with the name 'tree lard' for it," Drake recalled.

Part of the ASA's so-called "Fat Fighter" kits, distributed around the country, included a leaflet with the alarming title, "What You Don't Know About Tropical Fats Can Kill You!" next to a picture of a lighted fuse attached to the top of a coconut. Another ad announced, "Meet the Man Who's Trying to Put You Out of Business," and showed, as the *Wall Street Journal* described it, "a surly looking tropical fat cat," with a cigar and coconut drink in hand, sitting beside a black barrel labeled "palm oil." With a white suit and wide-brimmed hat, "his hefty expanse fills his rattan peacock-shaped chair." The point was: this devious Asian character with his tropical-oil excesses represented a threat to the American soybean farmer. The image was so offensive that when it arrived on the shores of Malaysia in 1987, protestors turned up in front of the US Embassy. "It was viewed as a racist picture," Drake acknowledges. "We didn't even think about it, to tell you the truth."

The ASA stayed focused on its audience in the United States. Throughout the late 1980s, Drake and his colleagues put a lot of time into lobbying various agencies in Washington, especially those that had the power to regulate or tax palm oils. The aim was to get Congress or the FDA to label tropical oils as "saturated fats." It was hoped that this would be the kiss of death in a nutrition-conscious, animal-fat-phobic society.

In Defense of Tropical Oils

In Malaysia panic struck, since palm oil producers knew that being considered a "saturated fat" would taint their product in the worst possible way. Palm oil in Malaysia was like olive oil in Greece: revered for the sheen of riches that it had brought to the country, and a vital national commodity, with a high level of government involvement in its production. Only 5 percent to 10 percent of Malaysia's exports went to the United States in the late 1980s, but American nutrition policy was so influential internationally that the Malaysians justly feared an American food-labeling law would have a chilling effect on palm sales around the globe.

"We decided to fight for palm oil based on the science," said Tan Sri Augustine Ong, director general of the quasi-governmental Palm Oil Research Institute of Malaysia (PORIM), in charge of defending his country's product worldwide. Ong had a degree in organic chemistry from King's College, London, and was a professor of chemistry at the University of Malaysia before joining PORIM. A man of science, Ong therefore embraced the somewhat naïve belief that a simple presentation of the scientific facts on palm oil would win the day.

The facts, as Ong knew them, were these: palm oil was a rich source of vitamin E, tocopherols, and beta-carotene, which are all considered healthy in their natural form. In preliminary studies, palm oil seemed to protect against blood clots. And most important for a research community obsessed with the cholesterol effects of fats, palm oil had been shown in early clinical trials to act like other vegetable oils in lowering total blood cholesterol. For this reason, the editors of the journal *Nutrition Reviews* wrote in 1987 that palm oil does "not behave" like other saturated fats, which typically raise total cholesterol. Ong emphasized this positive cholesterol finding on palm oil, which he knew to be important for his American colleagues.

Ong also made the simple point that the possibility of palm or coconut oil contributing to heart disease seemed unlikely, given that these saturated fats had been the dietary mainstay for largely disease-free Southeast Asian populations for thousands of years. Researchers had discovered in 1981, for instance, that heart disease was almost unknown among groups of Polynesian atoll dwellers who derived an enormous portion of their calories from coconuts and nearly *two thirds* of daily calories from coconut oil—without significant signs of heart disease. In Malaysia and the Philippines, too, where people ate large amounts of both palm and coconut oils, heart disease rates were lower than in Western nations.

Armed with this data, Ong led a delegation of six Malaysians from PORIM across the United States in 1987, visiting half a dozen cities where they delivered seminars to audiences of journalists, government officials, scientists, and food-company executives. Ong rolled out his scientific talking points, wrapped in a larger message that this whole debate was "a trade issue under the guise of a health issue."

Though his reception in the United States wasn't always friendly, Ong was able to win over one key person: Richard J. Ronk, an administrator of the FDA's Center for Food Safety and Applied Nutrition. Ronk's testimony to Congress in 1987 was widely credited with persuading both the Senate and the House to drop the bills they had been considering that would have labeled tropical oils as saturated fats. Ong therefore briefly won the battle, but the war was far from over. The ASA was not giving up, nor was CSPI or Sokolof. And not only the Malaysians, but the entire US food industry, were trembling at their impact.

From the perspective of Big Food, the negative publicity about tropical oils, a vital ingredient in their packaged goods, was nearly unprecedented. The Sokolof ads, the Congressional hearings, the letter-writing campaigns, and various other anti-tropical-oil tactics all added up to a tsunami of bad news. "We are getting piles of mail every day, from everywhere," a spokesman for the Keebler Company told the *New York Times*. "American consumers and their health is our concern, and they are telling us they don't want it [tropical oils]." So food companies caved: by 1989, General Mills, Quaker Oats, Borden, Pepperidge Farm, Keebler, Purina, and Pillsbury all declared that they would eliminate tropical oils from their product lines.

Indeed, companies were so afraid of being stuck with these now-unpopular oils in their food that they practically pleaded with the American public for patience. "We are trying to remove it from as many cookies and crackers as possible," said a Nabisco spokeswoman in 1989, yet some products, such as Triscuits, which contained palm oil, were just not easy to change without sacrificing quality and taste. Nor could Bugles, the cornucopia-shaped snack made by General Mills, be easily reformulated without coconut oil. "When you take out one component, like coconut oil, you are probably tampering with two or three hundred of those flavors," Stephen Garthwaite, the vice president for research and development at General Mills, tried to explain. "The chances of matching that exactly on a chemical basis is essentially zero. You hope you can come close enough that the whole taste and sensory system will think they are the same." In the end, Nabisco did succeed in eliminating tropical oils from nearly all of its products.

The consequence for the American public was that in every company, for nearly every food item, the replacement fat for these tropical oils was partially hydrogenated soybean oil. Executives in food companies from that time say that almost all of the nearly 2 billion pounds of tropical oils removed from annual use in the US food supply in the late 1980s was replaced, pound for pound, by hydrogenated oils containing trans fats.

Once US companies gave in to the ASA, Sokolof, and CSPI, the only defenders of tropical oils left fighting were the Malaysians. But they were foreigners, with a clear commercial agenda, so it seemed a foregone conclusion that they would not prevail. More dark clouds gathered for Ong and his team in 1989, when Congress reopened the question of labeling tropical oils as saturated fats. Ong was desperate, he says. He decided to deploy a weapon that he'd apparently been reluctant to use. He called it his "nuclear" option—his "hydrogen bomb."

The "hydrogen," of course, referred to hydrogenated oil, or trans fats. Copying Sokolof's tactic, Ong ran full-page ads in major newspapers in 1989, stating that palm oil did "not require artificial hardening or hydrogenation," which "seems to promote saturation and creates transfatty acids." The ads continued: "Approximately 70% of the soybean oil consumed in the USA is hydrogenated." What the American public knew about hydrogenation at that point was precisely nothing, but, as the ASA was well-aware, it didn't sound good, and the Malaysians could easily do more than drop a hint. Researchers in the field knew that some studies had raised disturbing questions about the trans fats found in hydrogenated oils; this evidence had not been much publicized, but it could be. The ads were a shot across the bow.

Drake described the Malaysian ads to me as "pretty scary" for the ASA. Another event that "really shook us up," he added, was that he and fellow ASA officers were called in to meet with Procter & Gamble executives. "They hammered us about being negative about knocking one oil," says Drake. "The bottom line was that they wanted the flexibility to use whatever oil they wanted in their products, and they didn't like the idea that we were attacking one oil."

Ultimately, the ASA backed down. The whole ASA campaign had been "technically unsound and represented bad manners from the start," recalls Lars Wiedermann, an oil chemist who was working for ASA in Asia at the time. In the end, during the summer of 1989, the two sides sat down at a hotel in Hawaii and struck a truce. The Malaysians would keep quiet about hydrogenation, while the ASA would stop its efforts to lobby officials in Washington against tropical oils as well as any publicity efforts aimed at portraying palm oil as a saturated fat. Following this agreement, an ASA spokesman made a statement that the group's "efforts to inform" the public about tropical oils were over, and that "it was time to get on to something more positive about [the merits of] soybean oil." He also expressed regret that the ASA had "stirred up an awful lot of emotions" in Southeast Asian countries. As the *Wall Street Journal* reported, it was finally the end of a "bitter, two-year feud."

Yet it all came too late for palm oil, which was well on its way to being virtually eliminated from American foods. No one trusted palm or coconut oil anymore. And the result for the public of all these efforts by CSPI, the ASA, and Sokolof was that every packaged food product on supermarket aisles, every serving of french fries and chicken fingers in every major fast-food restaurant, and every tub of movie popcorn were now made with partially hydrogenated oil, which contained trans fats. The usurpation of saturated fats—tallow, lard, butter, and now, palm oil—was complete.

In the following years, use of these adaptable and cheap hydrogenated oils continued to grow. "Believe it or not, we actually wanted to create *more* trans so we could get a sharper melting point, which is better for some products, like flakey pastry," explained Ron Harris, a retired oil chemist who had worked at Anderson, Clayton & Co. as well as Kraft and Nabisco. "For thirty to forty years, industry cranked up trans all it could," confirmed a trans-fat expert at the USDA. And Walter Farr, an executive for Kraft Foods and Wesson Oils, among many other food companies, told me, "We intentionally upped trans fats because it made the best shortenings and tub margarines . . . and also coating fats, like butter-cream icings of chocolate coatings." Farr, who started working in the field in the mid-1960s, says, "Over my career, I saw tremendous growth in the food industry, and all that growth was a result of hydrogenation! It was household use, yes, but even more so for food service industrial use. It was just growing by leaps and bounds!"

Americans came to consume more than 18 billion pounds of soybean oil by 2001—more than 80 percent of all oils eaten in the United States—and most of that soybean oil was partially hydrogenated, containing a hefty load of trans fats.

"Scientific" Smokescreen:
Obscuring the Truth about Trans Fats

Even such a huge quantity was for a long time assumed to be of no health concern, since any disturbing scientific findings on these fats had largely been buried. In the 1920s and thirties, when nutrition science was still in its infancy, food scientists had no particular opinion about partially hydrogenated oil. In fact, they didn't even discover that Crisco contained something called trans-fatty acids until 1929, a decade after the product had been launched.

The scientific findings that did get published, moreover, were conflicting. In 1933, for instance, one study looked at how hydrogenated oils were metabolized by rats and concluded that trans fats were "in no way objectionable as a constituent of foodstuffs." In other words, they weren't good, but they weren't bad, either. That same year, however, another researcher found that rats eating margarine containing trans fats grew more slowly than did those on a diet of unhydrogenated soybean oil or butter. A couple of other studies over the next few years had the same yin-yang of conflicting results. There was evidence on both sides.

What settled the score and established the overall early perception that trans fats were benign, thereby allowing hydrogenated oils to flow freely into the food supply for the next forty years, was a 1944 study. That trial concluded that rats fed margarine for three months were not impaired in their growth or fertility, nor in their ability to lactate. Even though the study was sponsored by Best Foods, a manufacturer of margarines, these apparently positive findings stamped trans fats with a clean bill of health. The point was driven home by the study leader himself, Harry J. Deuel, who had been funded by Best Foods. He stated in an opinion piece that not only was margarine healthy but it could be seen as the nutritional equivalent of butter—an extraordinary stretch of the science because even then it was known that the fatty-acid profiles of the two fats were entirely different.

By 1952, the invention of gas chromatography had made it possible to analyze the fatty-acid composition of hydrogenated oils far more precisely, but even then, food companies didn't appear to be interested in gaining a better understanding of their products—at least publicly. The only published analysis of trans fats using this new method at the time was by an Egyptian doctoral student, Ahmed Fahmy Mabrouk, at Ohio State University in 1956. He wrote that hydrogenated oils contained an "almost hopelessly complex" mixture of known and unknown fatty acids. "We are consuming nearly a billion pounds of trans fatty acids," Mabrouk stated in his conclusion. "It is indeed fortunate that at present there is no evidence to indicate that these unique acids are in any sense deleterious." Fortunate indeed.

In 1961, Ancel Keys turned his attention to trans fats. In one of his mental hospital trials on men, he found that hydrogenated oils not only raised total cholesterol, an assumed risk factor for heart disease, but also increased triglycerides quite dramatically, which, as we saw in Chapter 3, had been found to be linked to heart disease and diabetes. These were disquieting findings, to say the least, and Procter & Gamble, which had first introduced hydrogenated oils to America in the form of Crisco in 1911, leapt to the challenge of defending its prize ingredient. P&G did what Best Foods had done more than a decade earlier and what came to be a standard operating practice by large food companies in the field of nutrition science: When negative findings emerged about some important ingredient, companies would fund studies to counter them. As Joseph T. Judd, a USDA biochemist and a central figure in trans-fat research, explains, "The scientific literature would be flooded with enough contradictory studies so that no one could conclude anything for certain." One study would show a bad effect of trans, "but for every study showing bad effects, there was one showing the opposite—something from industry," he said. Generating a lot of conflicting scientific findings was a tactic that industry has employed to great effect, since uncertainty is a climate in which a questionable ingredient can thrive.

This strategy also seemed to be P&G's objective in 1962 when it ran a study out of its company lab in Cincinnati, Ohio, in response to Keys's negative findings. The P&G experiment contradicted Keys's results and came to be the last word on hydrogenated oil for the next fifteen years. Researchers, including Keys, were drawn away from the subject of trans fats toward other directions. The year was 1962, after all, just after the AHA had come out with its first low-fat diet recommendation, and the diet and disease research community became entirely focused on saturated fats, not on the potentially unhealthy aspects of the vegetable oils that Americans were now being encouraged to eat in ever-greater amounts.

The Lonely World of Trans-Fats Research

That left pretty much only one academic researcher in the trans-fat field for the next twenty years: Fred A. Kummerow, a professor of biochemistry at the University of Illinois in Urbana-Champaign, who would publish more than seventy papers on trans fats over the course of his career, more than any other scientist worldwide. These included some important and highly unsettling findings on the subject of trans fats and health, and in their day, they made the food industry quake. In order for food companies to continue using their most-favored ingredient, it was clear that they would have to discredit Kummerow and his discoveries, and this is precisely what happened.

Kummerow published his first study in *Science* magazine in 1957. He reported that he had examined autopsy materials from twenty-four human subjects and found that trans fats accumulated in tissues all over the body: in the liver, the arteries, the fat tissue, and a good deal in the heart. Fatty acids lodged in tissue are a sign that they're not being fully metabolized. "It would seem necessary" to determine what effect trans fats have on the normal metabolic process, Kummerow's article concluded.*

---

*Kummerow's suspicion about trans fats stemmed from the belief that they simply weren't natural—literally, not found in nature. Some do occur naturally in the meat and milk of ruminant animals like deer and cows. These are the so-called "ruminant trans fats." They are comprised of exactly the same atoms as the trans fats found in

Early in his career Kummerow was, as he likes to say, a "big wheel" in the diet-heart research community. He was president of the Illinois Heart Association, active in the AHA at a national level, and an officer in the American Oil Chemists' Society (AOCS), the most prestigious group in the field of edible oil chemistry. The NIH regularly funded his work. Kummerow was clearly on his way up, yet when he waded into the trans fats issue, he didn't realize the power of the industry that he was taking on. Although Kummerow was self-confident, he was a political innocent. He knew that the AHA received millions of dollars in support from the food industry whose seed oils the group endorsed. Kummerow had even criticized the AHA medical director, Campbell Moses, for posing with a bottle of Crisco oil in an AHA educational film in 1969. What Kummerow failed to comprehend, however, was the deep-seated strength of that alliance and how quickly he would be thrown over for challenging it.

Remember that the AHA had started recommending the "prudent diet," low in saturated fats and high in vegetable oils, in 1961. And for food companies, it didn't matter whether those oils were regular liquid oils or the ones hardened by hydrogenation; on packages they were all just listed in the same way, as "liquid oil." This simplification benefited the food industry greatly, since hydrogenated oil could masquerade as one of the highly desirable, AHA-endorsed polyunsaturated oils, the use of which was advised to prevent heart disease. Skipping over the "hydrogenated" part of the name on the label effectively hid these trans fats from consumers for many years.

---

hydrogenated oil, but there is a tiny difference—a matter of one double bond on a different side of the molecule—and this bit of geometry is not reflected in the chemical formula. This tiny distinction is probably enough to make ruminant trans fats behave differently in the body. Kummerow first demonstrated this difference in a 1979 experiment, and subsequent research has shown these ruminant fats to be largely free of the damaging health effects that occur with industrially produced trans fats. However, the FDA, when regulating trans fats, rejected arguments by the dairy and cattle industries seeking an exclusion for ruminant trans fats from the FDA rule, explaining that the agency's standards were strictly tied to chemical formulas (Lawson and Kummerow 1979; Bendsen et al. 2011).

Kummerow proposed bringing trans fats out into the open by including a warning about them in the next set of AHA dietary guidelines, due out in 1968. He wanted to let the public know two things: first, simply that margarines *contained* partially hydrogenated oil, and second, that these hardened oils had not been shown to lower total cholesterol (the liquid form of the oils *did* lower total cholesterol, even though, as we now know, total cholesterol did not ultimately turn out to be a good predictor for heart disease in most people). Moses, who oversaw the AHA committee on which Kummerow served, agreed with him about the trans-fat language and had 150,000 dietary-guideline pamphlets printed up for distribution.

Then came an astonishing about-face. Moses had sent a preliminary copy of the guidelines to the Institute for Shortening and Edible Oils (ISEO), the lobbying group for the edible-oil industry, and, for obvious reasons, the group objected. It didn't want anything revealed about the existence of this potentially unhealthy ingredient. Moses was clearly close to industry (he had posed for that Crisco ad, after all), and it seems that he now chose to have the entire run of 150,000 pamphlets destroyed and a new batch of guidelines printed up instead. In any case, there are two versions of the 1968 guidelines, one with the hydrogenated oils warning and one without. It was another example of the food industry's ability to influence scientific opinion at its very origin.

For the AHA, which said not another word about the possible health effects of partially hydrogenated oils for almost forty years, long after every other major health group had started warning against trans fats, this retraction could be seen as craven. A warning about the cholesterol effects of trans fats may have been premature, since the data were not yet entirely clear. But shouldn't the guardians of cardiovascular health have at least supported the push for the full disclosure of ingredients?

Kummerow was now persona non grata at the AHA. "After that, I never got back on any of the heart association committees," he told me. The group had been an integral part of his career, giving him money to help build his lab in 1959, "But I didn't think the way they did," he mourned. Yet impelled to continue his quixotic crusade despite the obvious costs to his own career, Kummerow proceeded to do important research on trans fats—virtually alone among edible-oil experts for decades. And during this time, he and a few colleagues discovered a number of unsettling things.

First, they confirmed Kummerow's original 1957 study about how trans fats "accumulated" in the fat tissue, meaning that these artificial fatty acids were supplanting normal fatty acids in all of the body's cells. It's worth understanding that fatty acids are not just stored as fat; they are also used as building blocks in every cell membrane. And those membranes are not simply containers, like ziplock bags. Instead, they are more like patrol sentries on a highly trafficked border, carefully regulating everything going in and out of the cell. They also control what hangs out right on the border, *inside* the membrane. Kummerow found that when trans-fatty acids occupy cell-membrane positions, they are like foreign agents who do not operate according to the normal plan.

Kummerow also showed that unnatural fatty acids in the cell membrane have a negative effect on calcification. Kummerow marinated cells from umbilical cords in different kinds of fats and found that those in hydrogenated oil ramped up their uptake of calcium. Calcium is a fine ingredient in milk, but inside cells it can lead to calcification, which is not a desirable condition in the arteries. Elevated levels of calcium in blood vessels are closely associated with heart disease.

Finally, in 1977, Kummerow's colleague, the biochemist Randall Wood, made the important discovery that hydrogenating an oil does not just produce trans fats; it removes four naturally occurring fatty acids from the oil and replaces them with some fifty unnatural ones. "We don't know—some of these cis-isomers that you get with partial hydrogenation could be worse than the trans! They could very well be the culprits!" Wood told me.*

"No one has experimented with these," echoed David Kritchevsky, an organic chemist who was one of the twentieth century's most influential researchers on diet and health, and whom I interviewed before he died

---

*Isomers are molecules that contain the same number and type of atoms (they have the same chemical formula), but their atoms are arranged differently. The difference between "cis" and "trans" isomers lies in the type of their double bond: the "cis" bond produces a U-shaped molecule, while the "trans" produces a zigzag, as described earlier.

in 2006. "We don't know which of these fatty acids is bad or what about them is bad. Randall Wood tried for years to get a grant to study that, but he never could. It may be that one kind of these isomers kills you, but we don't know which."

All these findings were significant and worrisome. They did not prove any link to disease in humans, but they showed that basic cell functioning and therefore normal physiology could be altered by trans fats. Saturated fats had been convicted in the court of scientific opinion on far weaker biological evidence. Kummerow's work therefore should have spread alarm and prompted more studies. Instead, Kummerow and Wood met a virtual wall of silence. For forty years, from the late 1950s through the early 1990s, few colleagues would even engage in correspondence with them. The two men could barely get their papers published. Nor could Kummerow raise funds for scientific meetings to discuss trans fats—though he certainly tried—for the obvious reason that the usual underwriters of such gatherings were members of industry, and they didn't want to touch the topic with a ten-foot pole. Even the American Dairy Association would not fund research on trans fats, because some of the group's members made margarine, too. In fact, from the day hydrogenated oil was introduced as Crisco in 1911 right up until the year 2005, nearly a century later, not one major scientific conference was devoted to the discussion of trans fats.*

Big Food Fights Back

The giant companies that made and used hydrogenated oils were so much in control of the science on trans fats that Kummerow never had a chance. These companies included the margarine manufacturers as well as the big edible-oil producers such as P&G, Anderson, Clayton & Co., and the Corn Products Company. They all had labs and oil chemists. The most influential among them were invited to serve on the prestigious technical

---

*A closed, day-long meeting was held at Kraft General Foods in Toronto, Ontario, in 1991, and no doubt there were others, but the first major scientific conference open to the public was hosted near Copenhagen by the Danish Nutrition Society in 2005. In 2006, the AHA convened the first US conference devoted to trans fats.

committee of the ISEO, the industry lobbying group that had influenced Moses at the AHA. It was a small but important committee that served as the scientific guardian of the entire fats-and-oils industry. And defending the reputation of hydrogenated oils, one of the industry's largest commodities, topped its priority list for decades.

"Preserving trans fats from the taint of negative scientific findings *was* our charge," explained Lars H. Wiedermann, a senior oil chemist at the food giant Swift & Co., who served on the ISEO committee in the 1970s. Another committee member was Thomas H. Applewhite, an organic chemist and plant physiologist who was the director of research at Kraft for many years and who told me defiantly after he'd retired, "No question, I was the ringleader on trans."

With Applewhite directing, the committee had the job of watching out for scholarly articles like Kummerow's that could damage the reputation of trans fats. Applewhite and team would then fire back scholarly rebuttals. They also attended conferences and asked pointed questions during the question-and-answer period, intending to cast doubt on every aspect of any research on trans fats that was even remotely critical. Wiedermann remembers going after Kummerow: "We chased him at three or four conferences. Our objective was to sit in the audience, and when he stopped talking, to raise a lot of questions."

Kummerow found them intimidating—especially Applewhite, a tall man with a booming voice. "He would jump up and make points. He was very aggressive," Kummerow remembers. In his opinion, this went "beyond the sort of standard respectful exchange that you'd expect among scientists." Randall Wood had the same experience. "Applewhite and Hunter . . . their main effect was at meetings, where the abstract had been put in a long time before, so they knew what you were going to say," he recalls. "So sometimes, in the question period, they would blindside you with something that was, in many cases, not even related to what you were saying." Having encountered this acutely negative criticism, both at conferences and in scientific journals, Wood eventually gave up studying trans fats altogether. "This was a very unrewarding area of study. It was just so hard to make any progress without any support," he lamented.

The moment that Kummerow found himself at real loggerheads with the ISEO came in 1974, when he presented results from a study he had conducted on miniature pigs. He had chosen these animals because they, like humans, are omnivores and are therefore considered adequate models for studying the development of atherosclerosis. Kummerow found that when he fed trans fats to a group of pigs, their arterial lesions grew faster than they did in a group fed butterfat, beef tallow, or a trans-fat-free vegetable oil. The group on trans fats also had more cholesterol and fats deposited in the linings of their arteries. Unsurprisingly, when Kummerow presented this data at a conference in 1974, "the industry went into convulsions," as a USDA chemist who attended the meetings described it to me. "Industry realized that if trans fats were linked to heart disease, the jig was up."

Kummerow's study had some flaws, which the ISEO's technical committee took every opportunity to accentuate.* "We spent lots of time, and lots of money and energy, refuting this work," Wiedermann told me, explaining that "Shoddy research, once published, became part of the record and could do irrevocable damage." He elaborates that it's not "like we were some sort of bogey-men going around terrorizing poor defenseless researchers working on a shoe string." He had seen a lot of sloppy work done in the name of science, which is why he saw "nothing either wrong or immoral to 'challenge' [it]."

For his part, Kummerow never gave up. In 2013, at the age of ninety-eight, he was still publishing papers and pressuring the FDA to ban trans fats from the food supply altogether and in 2014, partly in response to his petition, the FDA appears to be on the verge of doing this.

Aside from Kummerow, there was one other principal trans fats re-

---

*The critique of Kummerow's swine study was that his high-trans diet had been lacking in one of the essential fatty acids (linoleic oil) needed for normal growth. When Swift & Co. replicated the study at the University of Wisconsin, this time with more linoleic acid, the atherosclerotic effect of trans fat disappeared. It's not clear if this second study better reflected the reality of the American diet, however, since diets of the kind that Kummerow fed his pigs seemed possible, if not common, in the United States, especially because the process of hydrogenation destroys the linoleic content of the oil (margarines high in trans fats are therefore "naturally" low in linoleic acid). Kummerow's experiment may have identified a real danger to Americans, yet the general consensus has been against his experiment's findings.

searcher in the scientific wilderness for many years. This was Mary G. Enig, a nutritional biochemist from the University of Maryland, who from the late 1970s, had been studying trans fats quite separately from Kummerow. In 1978, she managed to set off "alarm bells" at the ISEO by publishing a paper documenting a correlation between trans fat consumption and cancer rates. This was an association, not proof of causation, and Enig was only a part-time faculty member at a second-tier university, but the ISEO still perceived her as a potential threat to the oil industry. (The link between trans fats and cancer has subsequently been studied in more depth, but no cause-and-effect connection has ever been found.)

To rebut her paper on cancer, Applewhite managed to get *three* highly critical Letters to the Editor published in reply. He and a few colleagues paid her a visit, too. Enig recalled, "These guys from ISEO came to see me, and, boy, were they angry." Aside from Applewhite, those "guys" included Siert Frederick Riepma, chairman of the National Association of Margarine Manufacturers, and officials from Lever Brothers and Central Soya, both soybean-oil producers. As Enig describes, "They said that they'd been keeping a careful watch to prevent articles like mine from coming out in the literature, and didn't know how this horse had gotten out of the barn."

Although she may not have had a lot of professional clout, Enig refused to play the role of a shrinking violet. Instead, she seemed to relish taking unorthodox positions and arguing them to the point of obstinacy. She lacked subtlety and had no interest in endearing herself to her colleagues, perhaps because she knew that she would never be invited to join the ranks of the all-male club of oil chemists, anyway. And most of them took her point. Although many acknowledged that she was right to question the accuracy of the data on trans fats, industry oil chemists considered her to be radicalized. Some words they used when describing her to me were "nutso," "paranoid," "off-the-wall," and "a zealot." Applewhite, by contrast, had worked in the vegetable oil industry since the 1960s and was a leader among his peers.*

Through the 1980s and nineties, as trans fats became more openly

---

*Among other things, Thomas Applewhite served as president of the AOCS in 1977 and was selected by John Wiley & Sons in 1985 to edit a volume of *Bailey's*

discussed and studied, the debate over the science seemed increasingly to boil down to Enig versus Applewhite. At any conference where the topic was discussed, each would counter nearly everything the other person said. She would parry and he'd bark back. At a 1995 conference in San Antonio, Texas, this went on for a hot five or ten minutes. "It was agonizing to watch. We were all uncomfortable," said one attendee. "Their interaction went way beyond the normal back-and-forth of scientific disagreement that we were used to," commented another.

An important standoff came in 1985, at a meeting that represented one of the first times the government had ever seriously reckoned with the existence of hydrogenated oils and their possible health effects. For most of the twentieth century, the government had taken a hands-off approach to this ingredient: the NIH was instead focused on saturated fats and cholesterol, while the FDA never took much of an interest, perhaps because the ISEO made a point of keeping especially close relations with that agency: for decades, the fats-and-oils group even hired its presidents straight out of the FDA legal office.*

Eventually, however, hydrogenated oils got swept up in President Richard Nixon's effort in 1969 to establish a list of food ingredients "Generally Recognized as Safe." The FDA, in response, commissioned its first review of hydrogenated soybean oil in 1976, and handed the job over to the Federation of American Societies for Experimental Biology (FASEB), a nonprofit federation now comprised of twenty-one societies for biomedical research. The selected panel of experts had very little experience in lipid science, and the review, perhaps predictably, found "no evidence" that these oils posed any "hazard to the public." The authors did take note of Kummerow's disturbing finding that "membrane functions could be affected by the incorporation of trans-fatty acids." They also described the five out of

---

Industrial Oil and Fat Products, the most important reference book in the field of oil chemistry.

*Malcolm R. Stephens, an FDA assistant commissioner, became ISEO president from 1966 to 1971, and William W. Goodrich, chief counsel at the FDA, went on to be ISEO president from 1971 to 1984. Both had more than thirty years of experience at the FDA before moving over to the ISEO.

eight experiments showing that hydrogenated oil raised total cholesterol more than did regular oils. Without explanation, however, they swept these concerns aside.

In 1985, when the FDA asked FASEB to revisit the topic, Enig was concerned that the job would be similarly superficial. Just as a start, for instance, neither she nor Kummerow had been invited to serve on the review panel, even though Kummerow was one of the most knowledgeable trans fat researchers to date.

The panel *did* have more relevant expertise this time, however, including scientists with a variety of views on trans fats. There were both the former Procter & Gamble powerhouse, Fred Mattson, and the trans fat critic, Randall Wood. These experts reviewed many of the same critical findings as the previous panel had and also covered some growing worries, such as the fact that hydrogenation didn't create just trans fats but also those dozens of other artificial fatty acids that Wood had identified. But in the end, the FASEB report again swept past these concerns to conclude that trans fats in the diet had no ill effect on health.

Since she wasn't on the committee, Enig had to confine her comments to the public question period at one of the panel's meetings. She was most concerned that the FASEB panel might not recognize just how much of these trans fats Americans were actually eating. The expert group had been grappling with this question because some of the negative health effects linked to trans fats depended heavily on the quantity consumed. Armed with her own interpretation of the data, Enig told assembled experts that there were "serious errors" in the national food database they were relying upon to ascertain the quantity. Her own analyses of food had found the trans fat content to be two to four times higher than was officially recognized, meaning that Americans would be eating far more of these fats than the experts realized.*

---

*Enig had been hired to measure the trans fat content of foods by the USDA, which agreed with her that the principal government database on food consumption patterns, called the National Health and Nutrition Examination Surveys (NHANES), was problematic regarding trans fats. Until the early 1990s, Enig and her team at the

Applewhite continued to criticize Enig's work sharply to his colleagues. It was a "fallacy," he wrote, "replete with misstatements and glaring errors as well as biased selections of 'fact.' " His dismissive tone can be seen as an echo of Ancel Keys's. He had successfully crushed any questioning of the diet-heart hypothesis a decade earlier, and the effect now was similar. Enig, Kummerow, and a few others in the field had unquestionably been beaten down by Applewhite and his ISEO colleagues. The multiple letters of critique, unrelenting questioning, and endless challenges were a wholly successful tactic, and the paucity of research on trans fats from the 1960s to the nineties was likely in large part due to the ISEO's efforts.

Thus all the early ideas about trans fats from Kummerow and others that should have been debated and dissected through the back-and-forth of lively minds, instead died in the water. "One can think of an idea almost as one thinks of a living organism. It has to be continually nourished with the resources that permit it to grow and reproduce," David Ozonoff, an environmental scientist at Boston University, once observed. "In a hostile environment that denies it the material necessities, scientific ideas tend to languish and die." This slow asphyxiation of scientific research is no doubt what happened to the early research on trans fats.

How Much Trans Fats Were We Eating?

The point that Enig had argued with the FASEB panel turned out to be the issue of greatest debate for these researchers in the 1980s: Just how much trans fats were Americans actually eating? At the FASEB meeting, the food industry's case had been made by Applewhite's close colleague, the longtime Procter & Gamble chemist J. Edward Hunter. He submitted a paper stating that based on his analyses, one could realistically assume each American was consuming only 3 to 7 grams of trans fats per day. Enig claimed that Hunter's calculations must be in error, because the food-consumption numbers from the government's NHANES database, upon which Hunter had based his calculations, were hopelessly flawed. For instance, as she

---

University of Maryland were among the only academic researchers trying to obtain accurate numbers for the trans fat content of foods.

pointed out, NHANES listed Crisco and margarine as having zero trans fat, when the reality was 22 percent of the calorie content or more. According to her measurements, a snack-sized bag of cheese puffs had 3 to 6 grams of trans fats; a bran muffin had nearly 4 grams, and depending on the brand, a snack-pack of chocolate chip cookies had 11.5 grams.

"In a study I did on breast milk," says Enig's colleague, Beverly B. Teter, "I gave one mother two Dunkin's doughnuts, a pack of cheese curls, and a small package of Pepperidge Farm cookies. If she ate the whole thing, that would have been twenty-plus grams of trans fat just from that. And there are a lot of people who would eat that way! So you know that there were a lot of people who were eating even more than the three to seven grams that the industry folks came up with." Teter found that these trans fats appeared in breast milk in amounts proportional to what was consumed in the mother's diet.

Enig's best estimate for trans fat consumption was 12 grams a day for the average American, which was two-to-four times more than Hunter's estimate. Faced with these divergent views, the FASEB panel simply chose to ignore Enig's submission. Without explanation, the panel appended Hunter's analysis on the subject to its official report in 1985 but not Enig's.

These consumption numbers were hotly disputed and became the focus of yet another expert panel. This one was set up by FASEB in 1986 to review trans fats for Congress, which was considering the labeling of all fats on packaged foods. The stakes were therefore high. In an exchange of letters with FASEB, Enig insisted that the NHANES database needed to be corrected before any intelligent policy could be enacted. Applewhite and Hunter, representing the ISEO, attempted to portray her as a nutty lone ranger: "No one other than Enig has raised questions about the validity of the . . . data," they wrote. Enig appeared to raise "unwarranted and unsubstantiated concerns" about the "imagined" physiological effects of trans fats, and they emphasized that "trans fatty acids do not pose any harm to humans or animals consuming a balanced diet."

Enig, for her part, publicly wondered in a letter published in a small trade journal why the ISEO was so concerned about the level of trans fat consumption if its scientists truly believed that the ingredient posed no harm. The answer was that trans fats *do* have negative health consequences, which anyone reviewing even the scant scientific literature could see, but for the food industry, the issue was a Pandora's box, if possible, never to be opened.

Pandora's Box Is Opened

The beginning of the end for trans fats came not from any American scientist, since critics of trans fats in the US research community had effectively been marginalized. Instead, it came from Holland: from Martijn B. Katan, a molecular biologist and nutrition professor at Wageningen University, and his graduate student, Ronald Mensink. "Mensink and Katan were the start of the whole ruckus," grumbled Hunter of Procter & Gamble.

Katan is one of the more highly respected and influential European scientists in the nutrition world, with strong connections to researchers in the United States. In the mid-1980s, officials at the Netherlands Heart Foundation had read and been troubled by Enig and Kummerow's work and asked Katan to look into it.

Katan visited his friend Onno Korver, the head of nutrition at the consumer-brand giant Unilever, whose headquarters are in Rotterdam, and asked him to fund an experiment on how trans fats affect cholesterol markers. Earlier studies had measured the impact of trans fats only on total cholesterol, but now it was possible to measure LDL- and HDL-cholesterol as well. Korver explains that he took an interest because "we started to realize that the scientific data on trans fats was scanty and contradictory. So under the slogan, 'know your product,' we started to think, how do we get more data?" Even so, says Korver, "It took some persuasion to convince Unilever to pay for this, because things were quiet about trans, and why take the risk to stir it up?"

Katan conducted a feeding trial on thirty-four women and twenty-five men, varying the fat content of their diets. One diet had 10 percent of energy as trans fats; another had 10 percent as olive oil,* and a third group

---

*Olive oil was chosen because it has relatively neutral effects on HDL- and LDL-cholesterol.

had a special margarine high in saturated fat. Subjects rotated through all the diets for three weeks each.

Mensink and Katan found that the diet high in trans fat not only raised LDL-cholesterol compared to olive oil, but also lowered HDL-cholesterol. "I thought the HDL-effect must be incorrect, because no fat *lowers* HDL-cholesterol," Katan told me. (Saturated fat, the kind found mainly in animal foods, *raises* HDL-cholesterol, but nutrition experts had been assiduously ignoring that effect for years, since saturated fats are considered generally unhealthy.) This potential HDL-cholesterol-lowering effect of trans fats could not ultimately be confirmed but early on appeared to be a significant strike against them.

To the dismay of food manufacturers and the edible-oil industry, major newspapers across the United States reported on Mensink and Katan's study, interpreting it as a major indictment of hydrogenated oils; "Margarine's Fatty Acids Raise Concern," read the Associated Press headline in 1990. These findings came as a shock to everyone, especially the major health groups, which had been recommending margarine as a healthier alternative to butter for decades.

Predictably, the ISEO attacked Mensink and Katan's work. The group's president wrote a letter to the editor of the *New England Journal of Medicine*, criticizing various aspects of the study methodology and suggesting that the level of trans fats eaten by the subjects was too high to be representative. But industry scientists weren't overly alarmed—not yet, at least. "A collection of knowledge about the effect had to build up. One study is not totally convincing," said Hunter.

"I could sense that my American colleagues, especially those from industry, wouldn't believe any of this stuff" about the LDL- and HDL-cholesterol effects, says Katan. "But we were proper scientists with no strong biases, and they should have realized that something was going on here."

That "something" was confirmed by a number of follow-up studies over the next five years conducted by Katan as well as others, although doubts about methodologies persisted. For instance, as ISEO experts pointed out, several studies fed their subjects partially hydrogenated oil rather than pure trans fats, so any LDL-cholesterol effect that was observed could very well have been caused by those other artificial fatty-acid isomers created during hydrogenation. This is a crucial point, because the process of hydrogenating oil, as we've seen, produces dozens of additional fatty-acid isomers along with trans fats. Little is known about these additional fatty acids, and most of the scientific research to date has made no attempt to isolate the effects of trans fats from these other isomers.

This and other, significant doubts about the evidence against trans fats posed real questions about whether their damaging impact on health was due to their cholesterol effects or something else; industry oil chemists therefore continued to defend hydrogenated oils on what appeared to be legitimate scientific grounds.

By 1992, the number of studies on trans fats and cholesterol amounted only to a handful, yet the accumulated evidence was sufficient for Unilever to announce that it would remove partially hydrogenated oils from most of its products within three years. "We had seven large hydrogenation plants at margarine-production sites across Europe, and we had to close all of them," says Korver. Unilever is such a significant leader in the European food industry that many other companies soon followed suit, switching over to palm oil. In Europe, "industry was open to change," observes Katan. "In the US, industry really dug in its heels."

The American food industry instead decided that it would fund its own study to refute the damaging findings by Katan and others. Most industry scientists still genuinely believed that trans fats were not unhealthy (the LDL- and HDL-cholesterol effects weren't so dramatic, after all), and they sought to regain control of the scientific narrative on the subject. A collection hat went around, and more than a million dollars were raised from various food manufacturers, soybean associations, and, of course, the ISEO.*

---

*Those contributing included Nabisco Foods Group, the National Association of Margarine Manufacturers, the Snack Food Association, Mallinckrodt Specialty Chemicals, the United Soybean Board, state soybean boards in Maryland, Ohio, North Carolina, Illinois, Michigan, Minnesota, and Indiana, and the National Cottonseed Products Association.

Here is yet another common tactic that food companies have used to steer scientific understanding of food: they pay reputable scientists at prestigious institutions to conduct studies that are intended to find positive results on behalf of their products. Best Foods played this game, funding studies to establish the safety of hydrogenated oils in the first place, and Unilever and other oil giants have influenced the science on vegetable oils this way ever since. From the researcher's perspective, receipt of these funds is, of course, awkward, but since funds for nutrition research are so scarce and the practice of nutrition science so expensive, the practice is considered a necessary evil. "All of us get industry money," Robert J. Nicolosi, a biochemist and trans fat researcher at the University of Massachusetts Lowell, told me. "But we all sign agreements saying that in no way can industry influence the way we publish our results. The problem you have is public perception, but we disclose it, and that's all we can do."

However, when a food company funds a university scientist, it expects to get results that will favor the company's product. Gerald McNeill, who directs research at the edible-oils giant Loders Croklaan, spelled this out for me. "Let's say I'm a big margarine company, and I want to make a health claim about my product," he explained. The company would look for one of nutrition's elite: a university professor who is well connected at the AHA or NIH, and fund him or her to conduct a trial. Company scientists sometimes help academic researchers design study methods to assure positive outcomes or at least no negative outcomes. "You can be absolutely sure, for two hundred and fifty thousand dollars, that you're going to get the results that you want!" McNeill exclaims. And in fact, a number of reviews have shown that industry-funded trials are far more likely to have positive outcomes that favor industry, compared to those without such funding. Big Food also creates relationships with academic researchers by paying for their travel expenses to conferences as well as honoraria for speaking. Said McNeill, "Every company does it, because if you don't play the game, you're out."

In this case, in their effort to refute Mensink and Katan's results, the edible-oil industry chose to fund an experiment at the USDA's well-regarded lipid lab, where the biochemist Joseph T. Judd was in charge. He was a rigorous scientist, and one thing that everyone could agree upon was that Judd's results would be unimpeachable.

Judd undertook several clinical trials on trans fats, but the first, in 1994, was the most important. At the USDA cafeteria, Judd provided specially prepared meals to twenty-nine men and twenty-nine women on four different diets, which they rotated through for six weeks each. One diet was high in olive oil; the second had "moderate" trans (3.8 percent of energy); the third had "high" trans (6.6 percent of energy); and the last was high in saturated fats. Outcome measures were HDL-, LDL-, and total cholesterol markers. And Kraft provided all the fats, courtesy of Thomas Applewhite.

Judd was aware that everyone hoped his findings would contradict Katan's and "therefore neutralize them." This was just how the food industry worked. Seeking to obtain an outcome that everyone would be obligated to accept, Judd took the unusual step of allowing industry scientists to help design the study protocol even prior to their decisions to fund it.

However, when the results came in, to everyone's astonishment, they did not refute Katan's findings. Instead, Judd confirmed them. The diet high in trans fats caused a "minor reduction" in HDL-cholesterol, though somewhat less than what Katan had found, and a significant rise in LDL-cholesterol. Unfortunately for the extensive list of companies supporting this effort, the "Judd studies" became the food industry's most famous example of shooting itself in the foot. "When I submitted my report, all I got was dead silence!" recalled Judd. "They knew this was a good study. They wanted to know the truth, and I think that's what they got . . . but of course it was not what they hoped would be found."

The Judd studies are a unique, treasured memory for many scientists. They represent a rare David-and-Goliath episode, a triumph of science over commerce. "Industry had even designed the study, and boom! They got slapped in the face!" relished K. C. Hayes, a nutritional biologist at Brandeis University who has been researching fats and oils for thirty-five years. By contrast, industry insiders were, quite naturally, sobered. "There was concern in the industry," acknowledged Hunter. He had pushed hard for the Judd studies and, when the findings were not in Procter & Gamble's favor, found himself transferred to another department.

"Concern is putting it mildly," said Michael Mudd, then vice president of corporate affairs at Kraft, which at that time produced a great many products high in trans fats, including Ritz crackers and Triscuits. "There was a panic in the industry, especially in companies that were heavy-duty into baked goods." In the mid-1990s, after the Judd studies came out, trans fats were "the most riveting topic du jour for a while," Mudd told me. "It got our absolute focus and concentration." Industry lay in wait for a trans fat backlash. Would Congress or the FDA pounce on the fats? "There was speculation about when government labeling would kick in and exacerbate things," said Mudd. "But those things didn't happen. Public outrage didn't materialize."

Because the effects on LDL- and HDL-cholesterol weren't so dramatic,* food companies thought that industry could still conceivably win on the playing field of scientific opinion. Toward that end, industry paid for yet another review of trans fats, this time by the International Life Sciences Institute (ILSI), an industry-funded group. And this time the results were more in line with industry desires, with the report concluding that because the evidence was minimal and conflicting, trans fats could still be considered safe. It was written "from an *industry* perspective," said Penny Kris-Etherton, a co-chair of the review and an influential nutrition professor at Penn State University: Food companies wanted to know if the evidence on trans fat merited changing their products. Nevertheless, she and other elite academic experts lent their names to this effort, and the report was consequently taken by others to be a solid, reliable source of data exonerating trans fats from causing ill effects. Indeed, it was cited to that effect by members of the ILSI panel themselves. Katan, by contrast, considered the report just "part of the industry's damage control," and thought it "didn't do justice" to the data.

In the end, the reason trans fats became infamous, banned from cities and states across the nation and the subject of the most important FDA ruling on food in recent history, was not, paradoxically, because new data emerged. Instead, the advocacy against these fats mounted. A number of forces lined up against trans fats and pushed them into the spotlight as our

---

*The HDL-cholesterol effect was never shown to occur with any reliability, and the LDL-cholesterol effect was small: a rise of 7.5 mg/dL for every 5 percent increase in trans fats as a portion of daily calories, or only about a 7 percent increase in LDL-cholesterol for the average American (FDA 2003, 41448 "a rise of 7.5 mg/dL").

number one fats villain. Among these forces was another lone guy, this one in San Francisco. There was the CSPI. And there was a familiar member of the nutrition elite, a researcher who, like Ancel Keys, sat atop a mountain of epidemiological data and used this data to change the course of nutrition history—just as Keys had done with saturated fats. This was the Harvard University nutrition professor Walter C. Willett, who had became famous in the nutrition world by introducing the Mediterranean diet, and he would now further boost his profile with trans fats. By establishing these fats as an officially vilified ingredient, Willett would set them down the path toward their near-total eradication from the food supply. And this might have been a good outcome if what replaced trans fats, in terms of the impact on health, had not been potentially so much worse.

9

Exit Trans Fats,
Enter Something Worse?

In some ways, Harvard epidemiologist Walter Willett could not be a more different personality from Ancel Keys. Willett is soft-spoken and mild-mannered, a gentle, willowy man with a walrus mustache whose unfailing cordiality makes him an unlikely candidate to rise to the apex of the nutrition world. Yet Willett's voice has been one of the most influential in the field for two decades. He was, as we've seen, the main force behind the Mediterranean diet, introducing the pyramid in Cambridge in 1993. And in that same year, Willett had a big announcement to make about trans fats.

It would be based on data from his Nurses' Health Study, which has been collecting dietary data on some 100,000 nurses since 1976—the largest epidemiological undertaking in the history of nutrition. Like Keys, Willett derives his power from being the director of a study that produces more data than anyone else in the field—even though, as with any observational study, it can show only association, not causation. And like Keys, Willett has always tended to express that caveat in sotto voce while announcing his positive findings with a far more confident voice. Willett's voice is also amplified by the authoritative vehicle of the Harvard University press office.

In this way, Willett has promoted a number of ideas that became adopted as public health recommendations based largely on his nurses' study findings. Most significantly, his nurses' findings led to advice that postmenopausal women should use hormone replacement therapy (HRT) and that the entire population should take vitamin E supplements. Both these widely adopted recommendations had to be retracted later, when clinical trials were performed and demonstrated that the associations found in the nurses' study could not be confirmed; both HRT and vitamin E supplements, in fact, when properly tested in trials, were found to be *dangerous* for health. It appeared that the nurses' data had been used prematurely to issue these health recommendations. When Willett made an announcement about trans fats, a clinical trial *had* been performed—the one by Mensink and Katan—but it had not yet been replicated. Willett thus relied primarily on his Nurses' Health Study data in making the case against trans fats, too.

Tipped off by Mary Enig's work, Willett had started collecting data on trans fat consumption for ninety thousand of his subjects back in 1980. A dozen years later, he looked at the data and found that eating trans fats was correlated with an increased risk of heart disease. Willett published this finding in *The Lancet* in 1993, but his paper didn't get much play. The next year, Willett and a colleague followed up with an opinion piece: according to their calculations, trans fats were causing an astonishing thirty thousand American deaths a year from heart disease. The Harvard press release that accompanied the article carried the real punch: it stated that a woman who ate four or more teaspoons of margarine per day had a 50 percent higher risk of heart disease. That got everyone's attention. Newspapers quickly picked up those numbers in front-page articles, and news stories ran around the world. Willett's article hadn't been peer-reviewed because it was an opinion piece rather than a scientific paper, and this led to some legitimate complaints about the methodology he used in calculating the thirty thousand number. But those concerns were barely a footnote to the alarming headlines.

"I'll never forget as long as I live," said Michael Mudd, the retired Kraft vice president. "I was watching ABC News on a Sunday night. Walter Willett was on, and there he was saying that margarine kills thirty thousand people a year. It was an earthquake in the industry!"

"It's a month that will live with me in infamy. Everything went downhill from there," recalls Rick Cristol, former president of the National Association of Margarine Manufacturers. "The industry went nuclear over it," says Katan.

In Denmark, one day after the thirty thousand number came out, the quasi-governmental Danish Nutrition Council held an emergency meeting to announce Willett's shocking results, an unprecedented move that, in itself, generated a huge amount of publicity. From that day on, this group became a world leader in raising the profile of trans fats as a health danger, and the Danish Parliament was persuaded to pass the world's first trans fat ban: beginning in 2003, no foods were allowed to contain more than 2 percent trans fats as a percent of total fat.* This is the most comprehensive measure taken by any national government worldwide.

The actions in Denmark were triggered by Willett's thirty thousand number. The number also spurred CSPI to petition the FDA to put trans fats on the food label, which eventually led to an FDA labeling rule in 2003. The thirty thousand number was what put trans fats on the map; it changed the public perception of these fats, and it was the explosion that triggered their demise.

"He Articulately and Enthusiastically Ran Past His Own Data"

Far more than the public realizes, however, Willett was out on a limb with his data. His number was based on the ability of trans fats to raise LDL-cholesterol while marginally lowering HDL-cholesterol, but his paper did not go into the calculations in any detail. And Willett's support among his fellow scientists for his work, it turns out, is rather slim.

A few months after publishing his thirty thousand number, Willett was

---

*Publicity about trans fats in Denmark has continued to blaze bright. In 2004, when a 7-Eleven store was found to be selling a doughnut containing 6 percent of its fat as trans, the manager of the entire 7-Eleven franchise appeared on national television to assure the public that all the doughnuts in his stores would be removed from the shelves within twenty-four hours (L'Abbé, Stender, and Skeaff 2009, S53).

invited to a meeting of the Toxicology Forum, a not-for-profit group that simply aims to hold intelligent discussions about potential toxins. The meetings are private and tend to be small, with a mixture of high-level industry representatives and scientists from both government and academia. The July 1994 group, which met in Aspen, Colorado, had the goal of dissecting the evidence behind Willett's assertion that trans fats caused heart disease.

After Willett presented his epidemiological findings at length to the group, Samuel Shapiro, the director of the Slone Epidemiology Center at Boston University, rose to argue against them. Shapiro's main point was that any number of study subjects who thought they might have heart disease would be more likely to have switched from butter to margarine, because this had been the advice of medical professionals for at-risk patients since the 1960s. So when a study subject eating a lot of trans fat died, how could investigators know whether it was the trans fats that had caused the heart disease, or if the person already had heart disease and that this condition had impelled him or her to eat more margarine in the first place? In other words, eating margarine might be the *result* of heart disease, not the cause. This problem is called "confounding by indication," and Shapiro said it was "a central dilemma" in trying to use epidemiology to establish cause and effect.

Further, there had always been basic problems with Willett's Nurses' Health Study, according to numerous critics over the years, familiar to any epidemiologist, and Shapiro also addressed these issues. He expounded on how difficult it is to adjust fully for various "confounders"—other aspects of diet and lifestyle that can confuse the results—such as multivitamin use, vigorous exercise, or sugar intake. No one really knows exactly how much any of these factors affect heart disease, said Shapiro, so even if the study authors claim they are "adjusting for them," those adjustments cannot truly be accurate.

Moreover, just measuring any one of those lifestyle factors with any degree of precision is enormously difficult. This is the reason that the Food Frequency Questionnaire (FFQ), used to query the nurses about their diets, has long been a source of controversy in the field. The idea that every one of those nurses could accurately recall or record what she'd eaten over the past year seems questionable, even to a layperson. For example, how often do you think you ate "peaches, apricots or plums" over the past year?

Twenty times? Fifty? Put down your estimate. Then move on to one of the next two hundred or so such questions.

In fact, when researchers have tried to validate the FFQ, the results have generally been unimpressive. Even Willett's own team found that a person's ability to record most of the types of fat he or she had eaten on the questionnaire to be "weak" to "very weak." In 2003, an international team led by the National Cancer Institute concluded that Willett's FFQ "cannot be recommended" for evaluating the relationship between calories or protein intake and disease.

Beyond this problem, there are many other possible sources of error in the FFQ: estimation of food quantities, estimation of frequency of consumption, bias toward under- or overcounting to make one's diet look better, and errors in the food tables that convert foods to nutrients. Which is hardly the full list of concerns.

Every item filled out on one of those questionnaires is what statisticians call a "predictor variable," and, as any statistician will tell you, for any of these variables to be reliably linked to health outcomes, it needs to be measured without error. A large number of imprecise predictor variables with more than one outcome variable (the various health problems; Willett collects about fifty of these) spells near-certain disaster on the statistical-reliability front.

These flaws could more readily be overlooked, said Shapiro, if trans fats had a giant impact, causing a thirtyfold increase in risk, for instance, which is the magnitude of the difference seen between heavy smokers and nonsmokers with regard to their risk for lung cancer. Errors of bias and confounding would then fade away against the enormity of such an association, and the relationship would be relatively undeniable. But the effect of trans fats seen in the Nurses' Health Study was small, noted Shapiro, not even a twofold increase in risk.*

Shapiro concluded that Willett's study had "failed" to rule out plausible sources of bias and confounding, and that the epidemiological evidence

---

*Indeed, one year after Willett published his trans fat findings, two large observational studies conducted in Europe showed *no* relationship between trans fats and rates of heart attacks or sudden cardiac death (Aro et al. 1995; Roberts et al. 1995).

did not, on its own, give "any justification" for Willett's statement that trans fats cause coronary disease.

Willett rose to defend himself. He pointed out that he had controlled for "a huge array of confounders . . . including life-style factors as well as known risk factors for coronary heart disease" and that the effect of trans fat remained the same. This result, he said, gave him confidence that any residual confounding effect would be small. Also, he pointed out that a lot of the trans fats he measured were in cookies, which are "not something that you would start eating a lot of if you thought you had coronary heart disease."*

People in the room were not convinced. Richard Hall, an organic chemist and longtime employee of the spice and herb manufacturer Mc-Cormick & Company, recalled, "We were all used to harder data than what epidemiology usually produces. Walter Willett is a very articulate, persuasive guy, until you really stop and say, to what extent do his data firmly support his conclusions? My impression was that he articulately and enthusiastically ran past his own data." The chair of the meeting, Michael Pariza, director of the Food Research Institute at the University of Wisconsin-Madison, said, "I think a lot of people walked out of the room thinking that Willett had overstated the case."

Yet Willett prevailed. Just as Ancel Keys became famous by making saturated fat a villain, so too did Willett gain publicity with his case against trans fats. And there are other similarities. Like Keys, Willett frequently appears in news media; he has authored a cover story for *Newsweek* magazine and is often on television. He also has close relationships with top scientific journals. In the case of trans fats, the *New England Journal of Medicine*, which is headquartered in Willett's hometown of Boston, has kept up the pressure by publishing multiple articles on the issue over the years, a majority of them written by Willett and his colleagues. And like Keys, Willett publishes papers—a lot. In 1993, for instance, the same year that Willett's

---

*Interestingly, Willett found that the trans fats from junk food—cookies, etc.—and bread were the *most* responsible for the increased risk of heart disease that he observed, and because he could not control for carbohydrate intake, the overall effect he saw may well have been due, at least in part, to carbohydrates.

trans fats article came out, he published thirty-two additional papers based on his nurses' study—an astonishing number. (A clinical trial, by contrast, will generate only one or two papers after many months or even years of work.)

What allows Willett to write so many papers is simply the enormous number of variables in his database. Willett can cross-calculate every one of his food and lifestyle variables against death rates from different ailments. This exercise can generate a huge number of speculations relatively effortlessly about what may or may not cause disease. Just as a matter of probability, a result will inevitably pop up. Ask one hundred questions and five of those are bound to turn up as statistically significant—simply by random. Statisticians call this problem "multiple comparisons," or "multiple testing." "The sheer number of questions you ask means you're guaranteed to have results," said S. Stanley Young, a statistician at the National Institute of Statistical Sciences who has written on the subject. "But many of them will be spurious."

Some scientists have even run data as a joke to show just how easy it is to produce these kinds of false associations. Looking at the astrological signs of 10.6 million Ontario residents, for instance, researchers found that people born under Leo had a higher probability of gastrointestinal hemorrhage, while Sagittarians were more susceptible to arm fractures. These associations met the traditional mathematical standard for "statistical significance" but were completely random and disappeared when a statistical adjustment was made for the problem of "multiple comparisons."

For all these reasons, many nutrition experts are critical of Willett's work. "He did a very poor job of justifying his thirty thousand number," said Bob Nicolosi, who chaired the ILSI review. "But he carried the day because he loves to carry the day." Epidemiologists can provide important clues, but many researchers believe that Willett takes his studies a step too far by using them, effectively, to demonstrate cause and effect.

Nevertheless, Willett changed the game on trans fats in America. By having these fats in the food supply, he told the expert group in Aspen, "We are really conducting a very large human-scale, uncontrolled, unmonitored national experiment." The same could have been said about the massively increased consumption of vegetable oils over the twentieth century—or, for that matter, the low-fat diet. Both of these were recommended to Americans as the best possible prevention against heart disease without first being properly tested. But these had been part of the official dietary advice for so many decades that reversing course on them was far less plausible. Only the hardened version of these oils, containing trans fats, was questioned.

Trans Fats Become the Next Dietary Evil

In campaigning against trans fats, Willett became, literally, a campaigner. In 2006, I saw him at a rally in downtown New York City, close to where lawmakers were debating a citywide ban on trans fats in restaurants. It was a cold, windy day in late October, and I was surprised to see him ascend to a podium. Willett bobbed, and the crowd drew in close. "Trans fats are a kind of metabolic poison!" he declared. A cheer went up. It wasn't just heart disease that Willett claimed resulted from eating trans fats. "There's probably a diabetes dimension, and the evidence is quite strong that there's a link with overweight and obesity," he informed the audience—even though these claims had very little science to support them then and still do not. "So this is a very important step. Congratulations to the New York City Department of Health," he concluded.

The trans-fat-free rally organizer was Michael Jacobson's group, CSPI. Although CSPI had originally been a major force in pushing food manufacturers *toward* trans fats in the 1980s while fanning the flames of the tropical-oil scare, a decade later the group had reversed course entirely. CSPI had gone from calling trans fats "not a bad bargain" to headlining them as "Trans: The Phantom Fat" on the cover of the group's widely circulated newsletter.

Jacobson was a powerhouse in whichever direction he turned, and trans fats, in their new incarnation as the bad fats, were the perfect fuel for his organization. Teaming up with a Harvard professor rendered CSPI nearly invincible on this issue. "Walter Willett played a *very* significant role" in getting trans fats on the food label, said Jacobson. "He has been continually outspoken. He's articulate and knowledgeable. So he was key."

CSPI's 1994 petition to the FDA against trans fats yielded results. In

1999, the FDA issued a "proposed rule" to add trans fats to the list of ingredients that must be identified on food labels. Every food company and food association, from the ISEO to the National Confectioners Association and the National Association of Margarine Manufacturers, from McDonald's to ConAgra Foods, sent in letters in response, mostly opposing the regulation. Fred Kummerow, Mary Enig, and other scientists and health advocacy groups also sent in letters; altogether, the FDA received 2,020 of them.

Seeking expert guidance, the FDA asked the Institute of Medicine (IOM), which is part of the National Academy of Sciences, to come up with a recommended limit for trans fat consumption.* Because studies had consistently shown that trans fats raise LDL-cholesterol (the HDL effects were less clear), the IOM expert panel recommended that an upper limit of intake be set at "zero."† Willett heavily lobbied the FDA to use the zero intake level, but the FDA rejected this idea, explaining that doing so would have excessively disparaged trans fats on the food label. Willett and the CSPI were also disappointed in their effort to get trans fats listed as a type of saturated fat. Ruling against that idea, the FDA sided with the majority of experts who said that combining the two would be "scientifically inaccurate and misleading, because *trans* and saturated fats are chemically, functionally, and physiologically different."

In 2003, the rule finally came out. It mandated that, as of January 1, 2006, trans fats would have their own separate line of the Nutrition Facts

---

*This "daily value intake" was the work of a standing IOM committee made up of the nutrition world's elite, including Ronald Krauss, Penny Kris-Etherton, Alice Lichtenstein, Scott Grundy, and Eric Rimm.

†Industry scientists attacked the "zero" intake proposal, since no clinical studies had examined trans fat consumption at levels below 4 percent of total calories. The IOM panel had relied on a chart drawn by a member of Willett's team, the nutritional epidemiologist Alberto Ascherio, who had simply plotted all the studies conducted at higher levels of trans fat consumption and then drawn a line backward to zero. Ascherio assumed a stepwise, linear relationship between the amount of trans fats eaten and their cholesterol effects—an assumption that the food industry, quite reasonably, challenged. (Ascherio et al. 1999; for a critique of Ascherio, see Hunter 2006.)

Panel on the back of all packaged foods. The FDA had considered the scientific evidence "sufficient" to conclude that trans fats contributed to heart disease. The fact that trans fats raise LDL-cholesterol was the main point of evidence against them, since that was the risk factor of choice for mainstream diet and disease experts. Other lines of evidence—Willett's epidemiological findings and Kummerow's work on cell-membrane interference—were deemed secondary.*†

There's no doubt that the FDA's labeling rule was a major event for that agency—because although the FDA is America's main line of defense against dangerous or tainted foods, it has long suffered from a lack of money and skilled scientists to do its job properly. Now, the agency had issued a landmark ruling that was nothing less than transformative for the industry. It's fair to say that there are few things more likely to compel change within the food industry than putting an ingredient on the food label. I understood this vividly when I sat one day in the office of Mark Matlock, senior vice president at Archer Daniels Midland (ADM), and he described to me how new food products are designed. "It begins with what a company wants to have on the food facts panel," he said. "Do they want a 'low in saturated fat' claim, for instance?"‡ That claim requires 1 gram or less of saturated fat on the food label. From there, a food is reverse engineered. For instance, when I saw Matlock, he was working with a food manufacturer that wanted a certain fat content and a "low in cholesterol"

_____

*The rule states that it excluded studies on the HDL-lowering effect of trans fats from its lineup of evidence because the National Institutes of Health favored LDL-cholesterol over HDL-cholesterol as a risk factor for heart disease.

†One of the lasting problems with the rule is that it allows food packages to list "zero grams" for any serving size that contains up to 0.5 grams of trans fats. Many food companies reduced the serving sizes of their products to slide in just under the 0.5 gram limit. "Serving size was key," Bob Wainright, a vice president at Cargill, a major edible-oils manufacturer, told me. The FDA defended its 0.5 gram limit with the rationale that it was consistent with the way other fats were labeled, which seems fair enough (FDA 2003, 41463).

‡These kinds of health claims on food packages have been regulated by the FDA since 1990. In 2003, the FDA lowered its standard of evidence for such claims. They could now be based on "inconclusive evidence." Previously, a "significant scientific consensus" had to be demonstrated before a claim could be made.

NINA TEICHOLZ

claim for a new dessert, and from those criteria, his team developed a nondairy chocolate pudding that would fit the bill.

Without the FDA rule on trans fats, the vast majority of companies would have likely done precisely nothing. Even after Willett's thirty thousand number, food companies didn't see the point in an expensive swap-out of trans fats for some unknown ingredient in all their products if no one was forcing their hand. "The effort to get rid of trans was not serious at all," said Farr, the industry consultant who had worked at Kraft and Wesson Oil. "They didn't know what would happen. So they were just going to wait until they needed to do it." With few exceptions, this is the story I've heard across the food industry. Perhaps Bruce Holub, a nutritional scientist at the University of Guelph in Canada, who worked intensively on the trans fat issue, put it most eloquently: "Some companies started avoiding trans fats when they learned the science many years ago. Other companies waited until they had to confess them." Whatever their path, food companies facing the FDA mandate had a big job ahead of them.

The day the FDA rule came out, there were partially hydrogenated oils in some 42,720 packaged food products, including 100 percent of crackers, 95 percent of cookies, 85 percent of breading and croutons, 75 percent of baking mixes, 70 percent of chip-type snacks, 65 percent of margarines, and 65 percent of pie shells, frosting, and chocolate chips. The changeover would be a Herculean task, the biggest the American food industry had ever confronted.

Big Fat Reformulation

When trans fats had to be removed from food products, the fundamental problem encountered by the industry was that it had no solid-fat option to use in its products. It could not go back to using saturated fats because, after decades of training, many people in supermarket aisles had customarily come to flip over packages to look at the saturated-fat content, and food companies knew that any upwards tick in these fats by even just 0.5 grams might alienate their customers. "Everyone is so sensitive to saturated-fat content. That's just our basic reality," said ADM's Mark Matlock, reflecting the industry view.

Yet without a hard fat, as we've seen, it's nearly impossible to make most processed food products. When Marie Callender tried using liquid soybean oil in its frozen dinners, for instance, the oil puddled under the roasted potatoes and caused the sauce to slip right off the meat, leaving it barren and dry. "It wasn't very appealing," said Pat Verduin, senior vice president for product quality and development at ConAgra. Hard fats are needed for structure, texture, and longevity. For cooking and baking, a hard fat is essential.

Historically, lard, butter, suet, and tallow had been widely used in domestic kitchens for cooking and baking. And these were what large food manufacturers had originally used, too, plus some palm and coconut oil. But then the industry switched over almost entirely to partially hydrogenated oils. And now that the trans fats in these oils were found to be a problem for health, food companies were left without options. They had no acceptable solid fat with which to make many of their products.

Food companies in Europe faced the same dilemma, but at least they could shift over to tropical oils, since Europeans had not been exposed to so much negative publicity as Americans had about those foreign imports. Said Martijn Katan, the Dutch biochemist, "In the US, companies shot themselves in the foot, because they could have used some palm oil to give a bit of solid in the fat. But in the US, palm oil was like arsenic."

Fearing palm oil and barred from returning to animal fats, the food industry faced a giant challenge. They had to figure out how to fry and cook without hard fats, and this challenge sent many of them back to the same company labs that had invented trans fats to begin with—to find a new kind of fat altogether.

For food companies, the complexities were enormous and the risk to every reformulated food item nerve-racking. "You notice the difference when you change the oil!" exclaimed Gill Leveille, the former vice president of research technical services at Nabisco, who participated in overseeing the company's changeover from palm oil to hydrogenated oils in the 1980s and remembers what it was like to face that same reformulation challenge fifteen years later: "The vision of doing that all over again to get rid of trans, and fewer options this time, was a nightmare, for us and every company."

"You don't just have to take the trans fat out. You need to know what new ingredients to put in," pointed out Au Bon Pain's Master Baker Harold Midttun. "And you have to do it without the customer noticing." In the company's plain muffin batter, for instance, Midttun replaced hydrogenated oil shortening with liquid canola oil, but that changed the resulting texture and reduced the batter's nine-week freezer life. Midttun used a monoglyceride to restore freezer life, added soy protein, oat bran, and ground flax for texture, and changed the method of leavening. Each step was a matter of trial and error. Said Midttun, "We removed one ingredient—the shortening—and had to add six to replace it." These kinds of complex solutions, involving artificial stews of multiple ingredients, were necessary for most food product reformulations but, it must be said, they would not have been if the food industry had just been using butter, lard, or tallow all along.

The Oreo cookie was a particular headache for Kraft Nabisco.* With its creamy white middle sandwiched between two crisp chocolate wafers, the Oreo cookie is what is known in the business as a "marquee" or "heritage" brand. Messing with such a product incurs the risk of alienating customers. Change can be dangerous (remember New Coke!). "An Oreo has to taste like an Oreo," said Kris Charles, an executive at the company. The creamy white filling had originally been made with lard, but the campaigns against animal fats in the mid-1990s had pushed the company to use partially hydrogenated oils instead. Now Kraft was having difficulty removing that oil without the option of returning to lard. With one recipe they tried, the creamy middle melted during shipping. And the chocolate wafers tended to break.

Reformulating the Oreo cookie was especially stressful for another reason: On May 1, 2003, it became the subject of a lawsuit, a gutsy move by a San Francisco lawyer named Stephen Joseph, who decided, all on his own, to sue Kraft Foods North America. Like Sokolof before him, he wasn't worried about money; what he wanted was an injunction against the sale and marketing of Oreos to children in California, because the cookies contained trans fats, a fact that was not widely known by the public (the

---

*Kraft Foods and Nabisco were merged as one company from 2000 to 2011 under the ownership of the Philip Morris Companies.

FDA labeling law would not go into effect for another three years). Joseph's lawsuit generated widespread national and even international publicity. A hundred thousand people visited Joseph's Web site, bantransfats.com, and he received thousands of emails, mainly from women who, he said, were "deeply concerned and angry about trans fat and the lack of labeling." Two weeks after all that publicity, Joseph concluded he could no longer tell a judge that the existence and danger of trans fat were not common knowledge, and for that reason, he dropped his suit.

In those two weeks, however, Joseph had single-handedly made trans fat a household word. And although Kraft had already begun reformulating the Oreo cookie before the lawsuit, the company now stepped up its efforts. In the end, the company used a mixture of fats to make the creamy middle, including some palm oil. And overall, Kraft reportedly spent more than thirty thousand hours and conducted 125 plant trials just to reformulate the Oreo cookie and get it right.

The Oils That Replaced Trans Fats

Amazingly, considering all the work involved in this huge industry changeover, it's not clear that Americans are now eating oils that are any healthier. A good portion of the trans fat alternatives are simply vegetable oils, including some new, untested varieties that could very well be even less healthy than the partially hydrogenated kind we are now ushering out.

The onus of finding trans-free alternatives fell not on the food manufacturers, nor on fast-food restaurants, who don't make their own ingredients, but rather on the big edible-oils suppliers: Cargill, Archer Daniels Midland, Dow Chemical Company, Loders Croklaan, Unilever, and Bungee. Unlike the food manufacturers, which took a wait-and-see attitude toward the trans fat regulations, the big oil companies had instead tried to get out ahead of the curve years before the FDA ruling.

The industry faced the same problem that it had one hundred years earlier: how to harden an oil so that it would be functional in cooking and baking and also not oxidize easily? Hydrogenation had solved those problems for the twentieth century; now, with partial hydrogenation off the table, new solutions were needed.

One new fat that came out of industry labs was made through a process called interesterification, a word that itself possibly spares the arteries by clogging the palate. Oil chemists had been working on this type of new fat on and off for decades and had stepped up efforts in the late 1970s when Kummerow's work first exposed the potential health dangers of trans fats.*

To understand interesterification, there's yet another detail about fat chemistry to know. All fatty acid chains are bound in packs of three, bound together by a "glycerol" molecule at their base, like a pitchfork. These pitchforks are the triglycerides that we've learned about: the fats floating around in our blood stream which, at high levels, are a risk factor for heart disease. Interesterification works by swapping around the order of the tines (fatty acid chains) on the pitchfork. But it's an inexact science, as Gil Leveille explained. "Interesterification is akin to hitting something with a sledgehammer, because you randomly distribute all the fatty acids on the glycerol. It produces a lot of new triglycerides," many of which we know nothing about. As of 2013, the process of interesterifying fats was still too expensive to be the preferred option for most food operations, but they are now being widely used. Leveille and others are therefore nervous about the health implications: "We just don't know," he judges. "It could be another trans lurking; we really need to look at it and understand it." And of course, in the same way that consumers didn't know that they were eating trans fats, they now don't know they're eating interesterified fats, because they are listed on the food label simply as "oil" (usually "soybean oil").

Rancidity in vegetable oils is caused by one type of fatty acid called linolenic, which the process of hydrogenation was able to reduce. One intriguing idea for minimizing linoleic involved altering the oil at its source by breeding soybeans that would produce oils *naturally* low in that type of fatty acid. Walter Fehr, a plant breeder at Iowa State University, has been working on this idea since the 1960s. Yet even after the FDA rule went into effect and companies desperately needed new oils, only 1 percent of

---

*Some of the work on interesterified fats was done by the USDA, foreseeing the day when a replacement might be needed (Gary List, interview with author, February 15, 2008).

soybean acres in the United States had been planted with "low-linolenic" beans. They just weren't particularly profitable for farmers and required extra work keeping them separated from regular soybeans to avoid contamination. So, overall, these low-linolenic soybeans have not yet enjoyed their day in the sun.

More recently, some companies have genetically engineered soybeans to be not only low in linolenic but also high in oleic acid (the fatty acid in olive oil), and the oils pressed from these beans are quite stable, but they, too, as of 2013, were in short supply.

Then there are chemically complex solutions that are not fats but can act like fats (the "fat replacers"). There are, for instance, lecithin and sorbitan tristearate mixtures, which form gels that act as emulsifiers, as well as crystal habit modifiers. And the Danish company Danisco created a trans-free shortening by using a combination of emulsifiers and an oil to create a "gel system" that mimics the functionality of a shortening for cookies, crackers, and tortillas. These solutions are obviously not natural, and perhaps the best thing that can be said about them is that they appear to work.

Finally, there was sunflower oil. Sunflower seeds were a small crop in the United States, grown mainly for birdseed and snacks. In the early 1990s, edible-oils companies started working with farmers who were planting new sunflower seeds bred to be high in oleic fatty acid, which made their oil stable enough for frying. By 2007, nearly 90 percent of the American sunflower crop was given over to the new breed of seed, which produces an oil called NuSun. This was an extraordinarily fast transformation of the sunflower crop, but the amount of oil it produces is still tiny, by industrial standards, and Frito-Lay, the 800-pound gorilla of the snack industry, buys up most of it. (To its credit, Frito-Lay, which makes Lay's, Ruffles, Fritos, Rold Gold, Cheetos, Doritos, and Tostitos, was a leader in getting trans fats out of its products even before the FDA rule took effect.)

The main problem with all these newly developed fats and fat replacers coming out of food company laboratories is that their effects on health have barely been studied. In some cases, trials have been performed to confirm that the new oils have no adverse effects on LDL- and HDL-cholesterol markers, yet cholesterol is just one small part of a much more complicated set of physiological effects that food has on human bodies.

Moreover, because each of these new oils has, in its own way, been disappointing—either too expensive or rare or too difficult to use—food companies are compensating in several ways. In some cases, they are *fully* hydrogenating oils (compared to the usual method of *partial* hydrogenation). This creates a hard fat which, ironically, eliminates all the trans fats. It can be blended with oil to make a more malleable product, but the result is waxy tasting, which is obviously unappetizing. In other cases, food manufacturers are quietly sneaking the familiar standby, palm oil, back into their products. Research over the past twenty years has allayed the health concerns raised about palm oil during the "tropical oil wars"; the oil may actually be beneficial for health in some ways, but the public perception left over from those wars remains negative. Because manufacturers have few other viable options, however, they are using palm oil anyway, and imports have grown rapidly. American companies were importing 2.5 billion pounds in 2012, about five times more than they were in the 1980s when American soybean growers launched their anti-tropical-oil campaign.

A third inexpensive trans-fat-free option for food companies are regular liquid oils. These oils are greasy and turn rancid easily, as we know, and for these reasons cannot be employed in most packaged foods. But they can be used for frying and cooking in restaurants, cafeterias, and other food-service operations, and since the mid-2000s, when the health dangers of trans fats became nationally known, liquid oils began to be used in these settings.

The troubled history of these regular oils has, unfortunately, never been resolved. Remember that the NIH held a series of workshops in the 1980s to address the fact that the early clinical trials using diets high in soybean oil showed subjects dying of cancer at alarmingly elevated rates. Gallstones were also associated with diets high in vegetable oils. And a large body of subsequent research has demonstrated that these types of oils, which are high in a type of fatty acid called omega-6, compete with the healthier omega-3s, found in fish oils, for vitally important spots in every cell membrane throughout the body, including those in the brain. The tsunami of omega-6s that have entered our diets via vegetable oils appears to have literally swamped the omega-3s (the supply of which has remained relatively constant over the past century).

A large body of literature has now documented the apparent results:

while omega-3s fight the kind of inflammation that is implicated in heart disease, omega-6s are largely proinflammatory. More speculatively, research over the past decades has shown that omega-6s are related to depression and mood disorders. Remember that subjects in the early clinical trials who were eating a lot of soybean oil also had higher rates of death due to suicides and violence, which have never been explained. Because those trials were not well controlled, all their results, both positive and negative, have to be viewed with some skepticism. But it remains an astonishing fact that although vegetable oils constitute around 8 percent of all calories consumed by Americans, a large, well-controlled clinical trial testing their impact on health beyond just their cholesterol effects has never been conducted.* And the AHA's most recent dietary review of vegetable oils in 2009 encouraged the public to eat more of them ("at least" 5 percent to 10 percent of all calories), owing to their ability to lower total and LDL-cholesterol.†

These cholesterol markers have not proven to be strong predictors of heart attacks for most people, as we've discussed in Chapter 3 and will revisit in the next chapter. Cholesterol, moreover, is just one aspect of the health effects of omega-6s or any other kind of fat. Inflammation and the functioning of cell membranes may be equally if not more important to our health, and the evidence to date suggests these are negatively affected by vegetable oils. The unexplained clinical trial findings about violence are an additional worrisome data point. A full accounting of the influence of vegetable oils on health is vitally important because Americans are eating a lot of them, and the potential impact of vegetable oils—interesterified, hydrogenated, or even as just plain oils—is obviously huge.

Toxic Heated Oils

In late 2012, as I was researching the latest news on trans fat replacements, Gerald McNeill, vice president of Loders Croklaan, which is one

---

*The first such trial is now being conducted at the NIH by Christopher E. Ramsden.
†William S. Harris, the chair of the AHA committee that wrote the review, was at the time receiving "significant" research funds from Monsanto, one of the biggest producers of soybean oil in the world (Harris et al. 2009, 4).

of the country's largest suppliers of edible oil, told me something scary. He explained that fast-food chains including McDonald's, Burger King, and Wendy's have swapped out hydrogenated oils and started using regular vegetable oil instead. "As those oils are heated, you're creating toxic oxidative breakdown products," he said. "One of those products is a compound called an aldehyde, which interferes with DNA. Another is formaldehyde, which is extremely toxic."

Aldehydes? Formaldehyde? Isn't that the stuff that's used to preserve dead bodies?

He went on to tell me how these heated, oxidized oils form polymers that create "a thick gunk" on the bottom of the fryer and clog up the drains. "It's sticky, horrible! Like a witches' brew!" he exclaimed. Partially hydrogenated oils, by contrast, were long-lasting and stable in fryers, which is of course why they were favored. And beef tallow, McDonald's original frying fat, was even more stable.

McNeill's company was a subsidiary of a giant Malaysian corporation that sold palm oil, so I wondered at first if he wasn't just vilifying the competition. Then I called Robert Ryther, a senior scientist at Ecolab, the giant industrial cleaning company that services nearly all the major national fast-food restaurants, and he confirmed the "gunk" issue. "It builds up on everything. It's like paint shellac . . . anywhere from a real hard, clear coating to a thick, gooey material, like a white silicone lubricant that you use on car engines, with a Crisco-type feel to it." The gunk, he said, is the result of a hot oil mist coming off the fryer and then collecting on cold surfaces all over the restaurant—in mixers, ovens, and vents and on the floors and walls. Within a day, it would start building up. "Literally," says Ryther, "we'd go into [restaurants], and people would say that we've been trying to get rid of this stuff for three weeks using sand blasters or hand scraping."

Ryther told me that these unstable products from oils would also accumulate on the uniforms of fast-food workers, which, when heated in clothes dryers, had been known to spontaneously combust. And fires would start in the back of the trucks carrying the uniforms to be cleaned. Even after the laundry was clean and folded, it would sometimes catch fire, Ryther told me, "because the oxidation products are continuing to react in very small amounts. You're never going to get it all out, and they will generate heat." Ryther started seeing this problem in 2007, shortly after restaurants went trans-free and converted their frying operations over to regular vegetable oils.

Ryther developed a product called Exelerate ZTF, which converts the shellac-like substance back into oil so that it can be cleaned off. The process is more expensive than previous solutions, however, and also uses stronger chemicals, so it's not a job for untrained employees. And pretty much all restaurants, large and small, are dealing with this, says Ryther. "McDonald's had this problem. Anybody that has a fryer has this problem."[*]

An obvious health question is whether these substance might also damage the lungs of patrons and restaurant workers.[†] And in fact, rates of cancers of the respiratory tract have been found to be higher among chefs and restaurant workers in Britain and Switzerland, where the subject has been studied.[‡] However, these studies did not track the type of cooking fat used and were confounded by the fact that the stoves themselves also emit damaging microparticles. Nevertheless, the highest-level report on cancer and heated oils to date, published in 2010 by the International Agency for Research on Cancer (IARC), which is part of the World Health Organization, determined that emissions from frying oils at the temperatures typically used in restaurants are "probably" carcinogenic to humans.

The problem, as we know, is that these regular vegetable oils oxidize easily, and heat speeds up the reaction, especially when heated over periods of hours, as typically occurs when these oils are used in restaurant fryers.

---

[*]McDonald's and Burger King list these oils as ingredients on their websites but would not confirm the cleaning problems.

[†]Even though people spend on average only 1.8 percent of their time in restaurants, they get about 11 percent of their exposure to tiny, potentially damaging airborne particles during this time, according to one analysis (Wallace and Ott 2011).

[‡]A team in Taiwan, which includes molecular biologists, toxicologists, and chemists, was formed due to concern about high rates of lung cancer among women living in Shanghai, Singapore, Hong Kong, and Taiwan. The team began investigating the possibility that heated cooking oils might be playing a role, since wok cooking with vegetable oils in unventilated space is common in Taiwan. (Some analyses show that in the United States, too, women who have never smoked have higher rates of lung cancer than do men) (Zhong et al. September 1999; Zhong et al. August 1999; Young et al. 2010).

NINA TEICHOLZ

The linoleic fatty acid in these oils starts a snowballing chain of reactions. Linoleic fatty acid comprises 30 percent of peanut oil, 52 percent of soybean oil, and 60 percent of corn oil, and it degrades into oxidation products such as free radicals, degraded triglycerides, and others; in one analysis, a total of 130 volatile compounds were isolated from a piece of fried chicken alone.* And while the IARC report looked only at the effects of particles that were airborne, it said nothing about those absorbed into foods fried in these oils. And it seems likely that the impact of these oxidation products is far greater when they are eaten—and digested.

Oil chemists began discovering these compounds in the mid-1940s, when vegetable oils first came to be widely used, and published a large body of work showing that heated linseed, corn, and especially soybean oil were toxic to rats, causing them to grow poorly, suffer diarrhea, have enlarged livers, gastric ulcers, and heart damage, and die prematurely. In one experiment, a "varnish-like" substance was found in the rat feces—which caused the animals themselves to be "stuck to the wire floor" of the cages. The oil in some of these experiments was heated to temperatures higher than those typically used in restaurant fryers, but the "varnish" was likely to have been an oxidation product in the same family as those shellac-like substances turning up in fast-food restaurants of late.

One would think that these disturbing early findings would have generated a great deal more research and discussion, especially since the AHA started recommending these polyunsaturated oils to the public in 1961. However, one of the only US researchers warning authorities not to jump into embracing the oils so quickly was the chemist Denham Harman, a founder of the hypothesis that free radicals cause aging. The scientific literature on the negative effects of these oxidation products was convincing enough, wrote Harman in a letter to *The Lancet* in 1957 that "the present

---

*The unnatural oxidation products of heated oils are still being discovered. In addition to free radicals and aldehydes, these compounds include sterol derivatives, a plethora of products formed from degraded triglycerides, and other oxidized decomposition compounds. There are other unnatural chemical compounds, too, created by processes other than oxidation, including hydrolysis, isomerization, and polymerization (Zhang et al. 2012).

enthusiasm" for these unsaturated oils should "be curbed" pending additional study of the possible adverse health effects of this dietary change.

Yet since then, publications and international meetings on the topic have been rare, even as research continued to turn up worrisome results. At a symposium on the topic attended by industry scientists in 1972, for instance, teams of food chemists from Japan reported that heated soybean oil produced compounds that were "highly toxic" to mice. A pathologist from Columbia University also reported that rats fed "mildly oxidized" oils suffered liver damage and heart lesions, compared to rats fed tallow, lard, dairy fats, and chicken fat, which showed no such damage. Most of this research was published in obscure, highly technical journals that nutrition experts rarely read, however; and in the US, diet-and-disease researchers were instead focused almost exclusively on cholesterol, anyway.

Interest in these oxidation products picked up in the 1990s, when an especially toxic one, called 4-hydroxynonenal (HNE), was identified by a group of researchers at the University of Siena, Italy. This was one of those aldehydes that Gerald McNeill had mentioned to me. Hermann Esterbauer, an Austrian biochemist, is credited with discovering the general category of aldehydes as peroxidation products in 1964, and in 1991, he took stock of the field. His review is considered a landmark, and it is, frankly, a little terrifying to read. Esterbauer goes through the evidence that aldehydes are extremely chemically reactive, causing "rapid cell death," interfering with DNA and RNA, and disturbing basic cell functioning. He meticulously lists all the research to date showing that aldehydes cause extreme oxidative stress to every possible kind of tissue, with a "great diversity of deleterious effects" to health, all of which were "rather likely" to occur at levels normally consumed by humans.

Aldehydes are "*very* reactive compounds," says the Hungarian-born biochemist A. Saari Csallany, who studied with Esterbauer and is the main researcher of these compounds in the United States. "They are reacting constantly. From one minute to the next, they have decomposed and changed into something else." In fact, one of the reasons that aldehydes were not more studied until relatively recently is that they were hard to measure accurately, and researchers therefore did not know that they occurred in such large amounts. Csallany refined the ability to detect HNEs and showed that they were produced by a range of vegetable oils, at temperatures well below those regularly used for frying and long before the oils start to smoke or smell, which are the alarm bells normally employed to signal that the oils are going bad.* Many oxidation products, including HNEs, are not detected by the standard tests restaurants use to monitor their oils.

One of Csallany's recent projects involved buying fries at six fast-food restaurants in Minneapolis near her office at the University of Minnesota, which led to the discovery that people could easily eat "quite a lot" of these toxic compounds (13.52 μg HNE per 100 grams of fries). She would like to do more studies, but she says the NIH and USDA have shown minimal interest in funding this topic.

The proliferation of research has mostly been in Europe over the past decade. The strongest evidence now points to HNE's role in atherosclerosis, says Giuseppi Poli, a biochemist at the University of Turin who co-founded of the International 4-HNE Club in 2002, which now meets every two years. HNEs cause LDL-cholesterol to oxidize, which is thought to be what makes that kind of cholesterol dangerous. And the evidence implicating HNEs in the development of neurodegenerative diseases like Alzheimer's is also strong, he says. Moreover, HNEs so reliably create oxidative stress in the body that they are used as a formal marker for the process.

This kind of stress was observed in an experiment on mice fed a type of aldehyde called acrolein, named for its acrid smell when produced by overheated oils. It is also present in cigarette smoke. The effect on mice fed acrolein was dramatic: they suffered injuries to their gastrointestinal tracts as well as a whole-body response called "acute phase response," a dramatic attempt by the body to avoid septic shock.† Markers of inflammation and other signs of acute infection also went up dramatically—sometimes by a hundred fold. Daniel J. Conklin, the cardiovascular physiologist who did this work, told me he was "stunned" to find that the dose required to

---

*The recommended frying temperature is 180 degrees Centigrade, but a study conducted by a leading biochemist found that restaurants almost always fry at higher temperatures (Firestone 1993).

†While the outward symptoms of the shock are few, significant changes take place inside the body, causing a dramatic increase in proinflammatory markers, a rise in some kinds of cholesterol, and a drop in serum total protein and albumin.

provoke some version of this response was entirely possible from the levels of acrolein typically consumed on a daily basis, especially among people eating fried foods.

Aldehydes have not yet been officially classified as a toxin, but even so, there have been fewer experiments on humans to date.* One exception was a trial in New Zealand on diabetic patients. Those who were fed "thermally stressed" safflower oil had a significantly higher level of markers for oxidative stress than those consuming olive oil. In fact, olive oil has consistently been shown to produce fewer oxidation products than do polyunsaturated oils like soybean and corn. Olive oil, a monounsaturated fat, as you might remember, has only one double bond to react with oxygen, whereas vegetable oils are polyunsaturated, with many double bonds. However, the fats that produce the fewest oxidation products are those without any double bonds: the saturated fats found in tallow, suet, lard, coconut oil, and butter.

In 2008, Csallany presented her findings to her colleagues, mostly industry employees, at a meeting of the American Oil Chemists' Society (AOCS) in Salt Lake City. "First they were alarmed and then nothing," she said. And in London, a team of researchers have repeatedly tried to alert people of the problem through the news media and at professional conferences. The team wrote a letter to the journal *Food Chemistry* in 1999 entitled, "Warning: Thermally-Stressed Polyunsaturates Are Damaging to Health," followed by a paper directed to "alert the foodservice industry" to health problems. Yet they, too, found little interest. Other researchers in the field are molecular biologists or biochemists, a world away from studying actual food items or making nutrition policy; as Rudolf Jörg Schaur, another of the HNE Club founders, wrote to me when I asked him if scientists were concerned about the increasing use of trans-free liquid oils in restaurants, "Since I am not a food chemist, I do not know."

In 2006, the European Union formed a group of international researchers to better understand these lipid oxidation products and their

---

*Determination of a toxin is usually drawn from animal experiments. Human data may come from epidemiological studies, but epidemiologists have yet to study the issue of heated polyunsaturated oils in restaurant fryers, since usage only became common after the FDA enacted its labeling rule in 2006.

implications for health. However, ADM's Mark Matlock told me that there was nothing the industry could do about the production of aldehydes in their oils. Some restaurants were using specialized low-linoleic or high-oleic oils, but regular oil (usually soybean or canola) was still the cheapest option. Kathleen Warner, a oil chemist who worked with the USDA for more than three decades and also directed the committee on heated oils for the AOCS for many years, told me that the best solution was simply to "hope" that restaurants filtered and changed their frying oils frequently and had good ventilation systems. Large fast-food chains also employ sophisticated techniques such as replacing the air over fryers with a "nitrogen blanket" and using micro-electric fields to minimize oxidation products. Warner confirmed that the aldehydes were "toxic," however, and therefore a problem. Poli, the HNE Club co-founder, said he couldn't understand why nutrition experts were so preoccupied with cholesterol, a vital molecule for many basic biological functions in the body, while ignoring HNE, a potential "killer" molecule. Another longtime oil chemist, Lars Wiedermann, who worked for many different food companies including Kraft and Swift & Co. from the early 1950s, told me that aldehydes and other toxic products need more mainstream attention: "Someone will surely discover how deadly used frying oils are," he said.

Mark Matlock at ADM told me that the industry is waiting to see if the FDA takes an interest, since the FDA is the only agency that can formally designate something a "toxin." So I asked to speak to scientists there. After months of delay, the FDA press office finally responded that while the agency was aware that oxidation products such as "alpha-beta unsaturated aldehydes" can form in heated polyunsaturated oils, there wasn't yet enough information about their health effects. Is the agency working toward finding more information? Not yet. For now, it appears that the agency isn't interested in knowing more about the oils that are a principal alternative to trans fats in baked and fried foods, billions of pounds of which are consumed by Americans each year.*

---

*The day that the FDA proposed banning all trans fats in late 2013, partly in response to a petition by Fred Kummerow, he told me that he knew about the problem of oxidation products produced by heated polyunsaturated oils; in fact, he had

However, the FDA *has* been investigating other strange compounds that pop up in vegetable oils during processing: monochlorpropane diols and glycidol esters (MCPDs), which are also produced by heat and have been targeted by the European Food and Safety Authority for regulation due to their potential to cause cancer and kidney disease, among other things. Even though they occur only in trace amounts, Matlock told me that companies such as ADM are still working to get rid of them. Sound familiar? We are once more confronted by the unknown health consequences of vegetable oils, a century after they were first introduced into the United States.

From the earliest clinical trials in the 1940s, in which diets high in polyunsaturated fats were found to raise mortality from cancer, to these more recent "discoveries" that they contain highly toxic oxidation products, polyunsaturated oils have been problematic for health. They have nevertheless multiplied in use more than any other single foodstuff over the course of the twentieth century, fueled in large part by expert recommendations to eat more of them.

For more than sixty years, Americans have been told to eat polyunsaturated vegetable oils instead of saturated fats. This advice has been based on the simple reality that vegetable oils lower total cholesterol (and LDL-cholesterol, too, as later discovered). The fact that vegetable oils also create toxic oxidation products when heated and trigger inflammatory effects linked to heart disease, are, it seems, less important to mainstream nutrition experts, whose focus hasn't wavered from cholesterol. Most Americans don't realize that their nutritional advice is based on such a narrow set of health concerns, nor that large edible-oil companies have been contributing funds to their trusted, guiding institutions, such as the AHA, as well as to schools of medicine and public health. And while the scientists at large food manufacturers might understand the problems of unsaturated oils, they have not had alternatives to work with, due to the prevailing stigma

---

done some of the original research on them himself in the 1950s. He said it was "unfortunate" that companies were now using regular oils for their frying operations and suggested that perhaps McDonald's and Burger King could start broiling their french fries instead (Kummerow, interview with author, November 7, 2013).

against saturated fats. Everyone has therefore gotten on board with the advice to use vegetable oils in both the home and industrial kitchens alike.

Our consumption has moved from saturated fats at the beginning of the twentieth century to partially hydrogenated oils to polyunsaturated oils. We have therefore unwittingly been subject to a chain of events starting with the elimination of animal fats and eventually winding up with aldehydes in our food. Looking ahead, it is little consolation that the FDA is poised to ban trans fats entirely, which will make liquid oils and their oxidation products even more common. Mom-and-pop restaurants, local cafeterias, and corner bakeries will then follow in the footsteps of the large fast-food restaurants in eliminating trans fats but will be less likely to employ rigorous oil-changing and ventilation standards into their operations. Despite the original good intentions behind getting rid of saturated fats, and the subsequent good intentions behind getting rid of trans fats, it seems that the reality, in terms of our health, has been that we've been repeatedly jumping from the frying pan into the fire.

The solution may be to return to stable, solid animal fats, like lard and butter, which don't contain any mystery isomers or clog up cell membranes, as trans fats do, and don't oxidize, as do liquid oils. Saturated fats, which also raise HDL-cholesterol, start to look like a rather good alternative from this perspective. If only saturated fats didn't also raise LDL, the "bad" cholesterol, which remains the key piece of evidence against them. But like so many of the scientific "truths" that we believe but which, upon examination, start to crumble, maybe the LDL-raising effect isn't quite an incontrovertible certainty, either.

10

Why Saturated Fat Is
Good for You

Avoiding saturated fats has come with two unintended consequences: The first, as we've seen, has been the embrace of vegetable oils. The second and probably even more harmful consequence has been the other major dietary shift during the second half of the twentieth century: the replacement of the fats in our diet with carbohydrates. Instead of meat, milk, eggs, and cheese—long central to meals in Western nations—Americans are now eating far more pasta, bread, cereal, and other grains, as well as more fruits and vegetables than ever before. After all, the USDA placed carbohydrates at the base of its food pyramid, as did the Mediterranean Diet, telling the public to eat six to eleven servings of grains a day, plus two to four servings of fruit and three to five of vegetables, altogether 45 percent to 65 percent of all calories as carbohydrates. The AHA advised the same thing. And Americans have duly adopted this guidance. From 1971 to 2000, they increased their consumption of carbohydrates by nearly 25 percent, according to statistics from the Centers for Disease Control and Prevention

(CDC), and they also successfully met the USDA goal of reducing overall fat consumption to 35 percent of total calories or less.

Health authorities consider these accomplishments a step in the right direction, and as the years pass, their official message has remained the same: The USDA's most recent set of *Dietary Guidelines,* in 2010, continued to emphasize that Americans should shift their food intake to a more "plant-based diet that emphasizes vegetables, cooked dry beans and peas, fruits, whole grains, nuts and seeds."

In recent decades, the most famous—one might say infamous voice in the wilderness promoting the opposite point of view was, of course, Robert C. Atkins, a cardiologist in New York City. In 1972, *Dr. Atkins' Diet Revolution* was published and became an overnight best-seller, reprinted twenty-eight times with more than ten million copies sold worldwide. Mainstream nutrition experts consistently disparaged Atkins and his high-fat recommendations, calling him a "fad" diet doctor and accusing him of malpractice, if not worse, but his approach took hold for the simple reason that the "Atkins diet" seemed to work.

Based on his experience treating patients, Atkins believed that meat, eggs, cream, and cheese, exiled to the narrow tip of the food pyramid, were the healthiest of foods. His signature diet plan was more or less the USDA pyramid turned on its head, high in fat and low in carbohydrates. Atkins believed that this diet would not only help people to lose weight but also fight heart disease, diabetes, and possibly other chronic diseases as well.

The Atkins diet has changed somewhat over the years, but its "induction" phase has always been strict, allowing only 5 to 20 grams of carbohydrates daily, or about half a slice of bread at most, although Atkins permitted carbohydrates to tick upward after a patient had stabilized at his or her desired weight. The rest of the diet was protein and fat, with at least twice as much fat as protein. This prescription meant that Atkins's patients ate mainly animal foods—meat, cheese, eggs for the simple reason that these are the only food sources (other than nuts and seeds) where protein and fat are bound together naturally in this proportion.

Atkins started down this path as a young cardiologist struggling with his own expanding girth. He went to a medical library and found a low-carbohydrate diet experiment written up in 1963 by two doctors from the University of Wisconsin Medical School. The diet was a tremendous success for him and then for his patients. Atkins tweaked the Wisconsin paper and expanded it into an article for *Vogue* magazine (his regime was called the "Vogue Diet" for a while). He then published it in a book.

As the low-carbohydrate, high-fat diet became popular, New Yorkers flocked to his Midtown office, and Atkins soon wrote other best-selling books based on his ideas of healthy nutrition. In 1989, he also launched a successful company that sold low-carbohydrate dietary supplements, including Atkins Bars, low-carb pasta, and low-carb, high-fat diet drinks, with millions of dollars in sales annually. Yet even after achieving both fame and fortune, Atkins, to his consternation, could never gain respect from his colleagues or the academic researchers influencing public health policy.

The main reason was that by the time that Atkins arrived on the scene, the diet-heart hypothesis had been firmly fixed at the center of mainstream consciousness for a decade, and Atkins's ideas butted up against this dominant low-fat view. His high-fat, low-carbohydrate diet sounded ludicrously unhealthy to the researchers and clinicians who already believed that saturated fat and fat overall were killers. At the McGovern committee hearings in 1977, the famous Harvard nutrition professor Fredrick J. Stare called

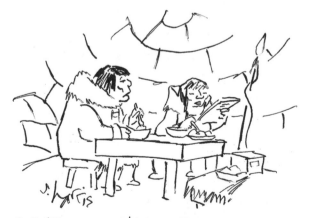

"I DON'T GET IT. WHAT IS THERE BESIDES PROTEIN AND FAT?"

Atkins an "instant money" diet doctor hawking an extremist "fad" regime. The diet was "dangerous," and "the author who makes the suggestion [is] guilty of malpractice," said Stare. The American Dietetic Association referred to Atkins's regime as "a nutritionist's nightmare."

Atkins also confronted America's growing enthusiasm for the polar opposite of his high-fat regime: the very-low-fat, near-vegetarian diet, whose most prominent advocate was the other famous diet doctor of the late twentieth century, Dean Ornish. The two doctors had much in common: they both made millions from their best-selling books; Atkins graced the cover of *Time* while Ornish, *Newsweek*. Atkins had a thriving private practice in Midtown Manhattan and a weekend home in fashionable South Hampton, while Ornish had—and still has—offices in the wealthy waterfront town of Sausalito, across the Golden Gate Bridge from San Francisco. How could they have both been so successful while offering such diametrically opposed solutions for a healthy, disease-free life?

The reality in America from the 1970s onward was that the nation's health was already worsening from the failure of the low-fat diet to prevent heart disease or obesity, and people were scrambling to find an alternative, in one direction or another. Atkins and Ornish shared the view that the AHA diet had been unwise; Atkins coined the term "diabesity" to describe the rising twin scourges of diabetes and obesity in the late twentieth century. These worsening disease rates opened up an opportunity for alternative ideas about healthy nutrition, and both Ornish and Atkins seized that chance. Their solutions just could not have been more different. Like Jack Sprat and his wife, one called for more fat; the other called for less.

In 2000, the two rival diet doctors met in Washington, DC, for a televised debate in a CNN special, "Who Wants to Be a Millionaire Diet Doctor?" On one side, there was Atkins, with his three-egg omelets and two strips of bacon for breakfast. On the other side was Ornish with his fruits and vegetables and his well-honed criticisms of Atkins: "I'd love to tell people that eating pork rinds and bacon and sausage is a healthy way to lose weight, but it isn't," he said, and, "You could go on chemotherapy and lose weight, but I don't recommend it as the optimal way."

Ornish also accused Atkins's diet of causing impotence and bad breath.

Ornish's cleverly polished zingers went straight to the heart and made Atkins apoplectic. "I have treated fifty thousand patients with a high-protein diet," he sputtered, "and all they tell me is that their sex life is better than it ever was."

A crucial problem for Atkins, however, was that he had never performed research to support his dietary claims. While Ornish managed to leverage his one small, ambiguous trial into several publications in the *Journal of the American Medical Association*, as discussed in Chapter 6, the Atkins diet had only been subject to a few small trials, with discouraging results. To defend his regime he had little more than anecdotal evidence: his medical files with tens of thousands of putative success stories. "I would never do a study because I'm a practicing physician. I mean, all I do is treat people," he once told Larry King. Atkins practically begged experts to come in and look at his records, but no one responded to his pleas until he was close to retirement.

It didn't help, either, that in a world where personal politics often seemed capable of steering the entire scientific ship, Atkins clearly lacked the necessary "people skills" to convey his ideas. Whereas Ornish was a smooth cultivator of power, Atkins wore an antagonizing crust, and this curmudgeonly, thin-skinned persona worked against him. "He would be interviewed and would say the American Medical Association is evil, or dieticians are stupid!" said Abby Bloch, a nutrition researcher at Memorial Sloan Kettering Hospital and former director of research at the Robert C. and Veronica Atkins Research Foundation. "And of course he'd alienate the entire audience. So he was a lightning rod." His habit of speaking in hyperbole also irritated his scientific colleagues, according to Bloch. "He'd say, 'I've seen sixty thousand patients, and I've never had a problem.' For doctors, it was like fingernails on a blackboard. And he would say, 'I can cure diabetes!' And doctors, you could see their blood pressure go up."

Perhaps if Atkins had been more patient and politically astute, he might have made inroads, Bloch suggested. Yet even the more judicious and well-respected Pete Ahrens failed to budge his colleagues in the nutrition mainstream. The conventional dietary wisdom was just too entrenched. Ultimately, despite Atkins's wealth of practical knowledge in helping people lose weight and possibly avoid heart disease, he would not get a serious hearing from academic researchers until the twenty-first century.

In April 2003, at the age of seventy-two, Atkins slipped on the ice outside his Manhattan office, hit his head on the pavement, and fell into a coma. He died a week later. Rumors quickly spread about the cause of death; it was said to be a "heart attack," and he was reported to be obese—although he was not.* When Atkins's dietary supplement business declared bankruptcy two years later, apparently done in by both poor management and a flagging interest in the low-carb diet following his death, the experts who had loathed his views portrayed these events as proof of his diet's final death blow. The bankruptcy, especially, was treated as confirmation that the low fat diet had finally trumped low-carb. As Tufts University professor Alice Lichtenstein told me in 2007, "It's over. Atkins just declared bankruptcy. People are already past the low-carbohydrate phase now."

But this was wishful thinking, because while Atkins's fame was such that his name became synonymous with the low-carb diet, his death did not ultimately quash its popularity. The diet's success in helping people to lose weight kept it alive, albeit in a subterranean way. The diet has a surprisingly long history, in fact. The belief that carbohydrates are fattening and high-fat diets healthy predated Atkins and would soon find other, far more mainstream promoters. "Atkins" is merely the name that Americans now most readily associate with this diet, but there were others who developed and nourished this idea long before him, and there would be others after him, as well.

---

*Atkins's death generated controversy much as he had in life. Critics of Atkins publicized a leak from the New York City Medical Examiner's Office, revealing that Atkins suffered from heart disease, but it was not clear whether this condition was due to nutrition or an infection contracted on a trip to the Far East years earlier, as Atkins's cardiologist claimed. Critics also highlighted the fact that Atkins's death certificate listed his weight as 258 lbs, which implied that he was obese; however, at time of admission to the hospital, his weight was recorded as 195 lbs, and his widow plausibly explained that the rapid weight gain had occurred due to fluid retention during his coma (Anon., "Death of a Diet Doctor," 2004).

The Birth of the Low-Carb Diet*

Among the earliest and most famous reports of the low-carbohydrate diet being employed for weight loss was a slim 1863 pamphlet by a retired London undertaker, William Banting. His *Letter on Corpulence, Addressed to the Public* was the *Dr. Atkins' Diet Revolution* phenomenon of its time, selling 63,000 copies in Britain alone, with "large circulations" in France, Germany, and the United States as well. "Of all the parasites that affect humanity," began Banting's little book, "I do not know of, nor can I imagine, any more distressing than that of Obesity." Banting recounts how, at the age of sixty-six and all of 5 feet 5 inches tall, he weighed more than 200 pounds and suffered from failing sight and hearing, an umbilical rupture, weak knees and ankles, acidity, indigestion, and heartburn. To lose weight, his doctors prescribed to him the same two pieces of advice that we are given today: to exercise more, which Banting did by, among other things, rowing for two hours every morning, and to reduce calories. Banting found, however, that the exercise only increased his appetite and that cutting calories left him exhausted.

In 1862, when Banting began losing his hearing, he sought advice from the London ear surgeon William Harvey, who thought that the excessive fat in his ears might be pushing up against the Eustachian tubes. He decided to put Banting on a low-carbohydrate diet. Harvey was aware that farmers sometimes fattened livestock on sugary, starchy diets, and he also correctly guessed that there might be a link between obesity and diabetes, which was then commonly treated in France by a diet free of carbohydrates. Thus, Banting took to eating three meals a day of meat, fish, or game and avoided most foods that might contain sugar or starch, in particular bread, milk (due to its sugar content in the form of lactose), beer, candy, and root vegetables. In a year, Banting lost 46 pounds and claimed to feel marvelous, all his physical ailments having disappeared. In the fourth edition of his book, in 1869, Banting reported that he had lost 50 pounds. He considered his general health "extraordinary." As he wrote,

---

*This history of low-carbohydrate diet practitioners was first compiled in Gary Taubes, *Good Calories, Bad Calories* (2007).

"Indeed, I meet with few men at seventy-two years of age who have so little cause to complain." Banting lived to the age of eighty-one, well beyond the average life expectancy for men in England at the time.

After he died, versions of Banting's diet were taken up by European researchers as well as clinicians to treat their patients. In the United States, Sir William Osler, a worldwide medical authority in the late nineteenth century and one of the founders of Johns Hopkins Hospital, promoted a variation of the diet in his seminal 1892 medical textbook. And a London physician, Nathaniel Yorke-Davis, used a version of the low-carbohydrate diet to treat the obese President William Taft from 1905 on, helping him lose 70 pounds. Although many other doctors during the early years of the twentieth century told their patients to restrict total calories rather than just those from carbohydrates, the low-carbohydrate diet has always endured, "discovered" again and again throughout the twentieth and twenty-first centuries.

In 1919, an internist with a practice on Long Island named Blake Donaldson stumbled on the diet independently. As he recounts in his memoir, *Strong Medicine* (1961), he was frustrated by his inability to help obese patients lose weight simply by cutting back on calories. He discovered the high-fat diet after consulting experts at the American Museum of Natural History in Manhattan, he says, who told him that the Inuit lived mostly disease-free, surviving almost entirely on the "fattest meat they could kill." Donaldson decided to give it a try. Banning all sugar and flour, he prescribed mainly meat to his patients: fatty meat three times a day. There may be an "upper level of meat intake" where people can no longer lose weight, he concluded, "but I've never found it."*

Donaldson insisted that his patients, some seventeen thousand of them over the course of forty years, did remarkably well on this regime, losing

---

*In the mid-1970s, Elliot Danforth at the University of Vermont conducted a series of overeating experiments with different types of food and concluded that eating too much on a meat-centered diet was nearly impossible. His subjects confronted stacks of pork chops that they simply could not consume. "It's very hard to overeat on the Atkins diet, because it sates you," said Danforth. By contrast, he found that people could easily overeat on carbohydrates such as cookies, chips, and cereals (Danforth, interview with author, January 12, 2009).

two to three pounds a week without feeling hunger. The important point, he stressed, was that unlike other "antiobesity treatments" such as calorie restriction, his patients were able to keep the weight off.

In 1944, when Donaldson gave a talk about his diet at a New York hospital, one of the physicians in attendance was Alfred Pennington, an in-house doctor for the E. I. du Pont de Nemours Company. Like many companies in the 1940s, DuPont was concerned about the epidemic of heart disease tearing through the ranks of its middle-aged male executives. Observing that most sufferers were overweight or obese, Pennington and his colleagues assumed that the first step should be a program to slim them down. The executives were put through the paces on various calorie-counting diets as well as an exercise regime, and when these methods failed, Pennington decided to try the approach that he himself had successfully employed after hearing Donaldson's lecture.

Pennington's diet did not restrict total calories. The twenty male executives he selected ate, on average, over 3,000 calories a day, including 6 ounces of meat, 2 ounces of fat, and no more than 80 calories of carbohydrates at each of three daily meals. As Pennington described it, the executives on his diet experienced "a lack of hunger between meals . . . increased physical energy and sense of well-being." And despite eating so much, they lost 7 to 10 pounds a month.

Pennington wrote extensively on the subject of obesity. Rather than being content with seeing his patients lose weight, he sought to understand *why* a low-carb diet might work. Any theory had to take into account that the answer wasn't a reduction in calories, because Pennington's patients didn't seem to be eating fewer calories than normal and in some cases, were eating more. "The explanation, whatever it might be," wrote Pennington, "seemed to lie much deeper." He unearthed a body of research from German and Austrian researchers in the 1920s and thirties who had pinpointed hormones as the driver of obesity. They worked out an entirely new hypothesis about how people got fat—one that had nothing to do with overeating or underexercising, as we commonly believe. These researchers concluded that obesity was a disorder of metabolism in which the fat tissue starts hoarding fat, impeding the way it is normally released and used for energy.

The first step in understanding this metabolic disorder was the realization that our fat tissue is not some inert dead zone but rather a hive of metabolic and hormonal activity. Around the clock, the body continuously stores and withdraws fat as needed, like constant deposits and withdrawals at an ATM. When we eat a meal, we make a deposit, which can then be withdrawn whenever we're not eating, in between meals or during the night while we sleep. Seen from this perspective, fat is just a backstop of energy for the body to use when food is not available in the short term, like having energy bars strapped to one's body. In people with the metabolic disorder, however, while the deposits continue, the withdrawal function ceases to work: the body literally refuses to give up its fat. The fat instead becomes like Godzilla, sucking up energy and converting it into even more fat at the expense of the muscles, the brain, the heart, and all other bodily needs.

The German and Austrian researchers came to believe that hormones were ultimately responsible for this stockpiling of fat. Hormones, after all, could explain why pregnant and postmenopausal women gain weight, why adolescent girls gain fat and adolescent boys gain muscle as they go through puberty. And animal research from the late 1930s onward repeatedly confirmed this idea. Scientists altered hormonal levels in rats by creating lesions to the hypothalamus (the brain's hormone control center), causing their weight to balloon nearly overnight. These rats would not just eat their food; they would "attack" and "devour it," with a "voracious, tigerish appetite." Similar results were found for dogs, cats, and monkeys. And *people* with tumors in the hypothalamus sometimes experienced massive, rapid weight gain, including one case of a fifty-seven-year-old "gardener's wife" who was observed in 1946 to become obese within one year.

The study of hormones, called endocrinology, had revealed by 1921 that insulin, a hormone produced in the pancreas, appeared to trump all others in the deposition of fat. By 1923, doctors were fattening underweight children by injecting them with insulin. Clinicians could get their patients to gain as much as 6 pounds a week by telling them to eat high-carbohydrate meals after receiving insulin injections. The same was found in animal experiments.* And on the other side of that coin, an animal that had been deprived of insulin because its pancreas had been removed could not be induced, no matter how much it ate, to get fat, and it would die from emaciation.

The body secretes insulin whenever carbohydrates are eaten. If carbs are eaten only occasionally, the body has time to recover between the surges of insulin. The fat cells have time to release their stored fat, and the muscles can burn the fat as fuel. If carbohydrates are eaten throughout the day, however, in meals, snacks, and beverages, then insulin stays elevated in the bloodstream, and the fat remains in a state of constant lockdown. Fat accumulates to excess; it is stored, not burned. Pennington described what would theoretically happen on a diet restricted in carbohydrates: the absence of carbohydrates would allow fat to flow out of the fat tissue, no longer held hostage there by the circulating insulin, and this fat could then be used as energy. A person would lose weight, not because they necessarily ate less but because the absence of insulin was allowing the fat cells to release the fat and the muscle cells to burn it.

All these ideas were in the trove of prewar research on hormones and obesity that Pennington was the first to dig up. World War II had scattered these German and Austrian scientists along with their ideas, and because the lingua franca of science shifted after the war from German to English, this early research on an "alternative hypothesis" for obesity had been lost.

In 1953, Pennington reviewed this extensive body of research for the *New England Journal of Medicine* in an article entitled, "A Reorientation on

---

*Animal data supporting this hypothesis includes experiments on rats with surgically induced lesions to the ventromedial hypothalamus. These rats would see dramatic increases in insulin within seconds of surgery and would grow fat in direct proportion to the amount of insulin circulating. How did researchers know that it was the insulin that was making the rats obese? After they'd severed the vagus nerve, which connects the hypothalamus to the pancreas, no insulin could be released, and the rats did not grow fat (Han and Frohman 1970; Hustvedt and Løvø 1972; the theory based on this work that the hypothalamus plays a significant role in hunger is found in Powley 1977).

Obesity."* This was the same year that Ancel Keys had first proposed his idea blaming chronic diseases not on carbohydrates but on fat—a theory that obviously prevailed due to Keys's greater stature in the field, while Pennington's was forgotten until recently. Keys's theory differed from Pennington's in the dietary evil it named, of course, but the two hypotheses were also starkly different in the quality of the scientific research behind them. While Pennington's analysis was based upon a sophisticated understanding of human biological systems, including evidence drawn from endocrinology and biochemistry, Keys's, by contrast, relied almost entirely upon those crude international statistics linking fat and heart disease. His conclusions were based on a statistical correlation, and were not, like Pennington's, grounded in clinical experience with patients or a scholarly understanding of human physiology and biology.

The idea about fat causing obesity, moreover, was founded upon another generality without foundation in human biology: Keys and others thought that because dietary fat contains more calories per gram than do either protein or carbohydrate, fat must make people fat. By this view, people who consume too much fat inadvertently rack up too many calories—a kind of arithmetic error committed when the brain and the stomach fail to communicate with each other. Yet there was no experimental basis for this assumption when Keys wrote about it, and hardly any has accumulated since. The main intellectual advantage to this idea has been its straightforward simplicity. Therefore, in addition to all the other reasons that we've explored for why Keys's ideas traveled so far and wide in the nutrition world, another was probably that nutritionists and cardiologists seeking uncomplicated answers found Keys's mathematical approach easier to imagine than Pennington's complex idea about a hormonal disorder. Yet, as we've seen, a good deal of evidence contradicts the idea that dietary fat causes obesity, just as there was ultimately little evidence for the role

---

*A Hungarian-born obstetrician named Herman Taller, practicing in Brooklyn, read Pennington's articles and began treating his patients with the low-carbohydrate diet in the 1950s. He also wrote a best-selling diet book, *Calories Don't Count* (New York: Simon & Schuster, 1961).

of fat in heart disease. Could the alternative that Pennington identified—carbohydrates—be a biological actor on the heart disease front, as well?

Carbohydrates and Chronic Disease

One of the more startling revelations that Blake Donaldson wrote about lay in his observation that patients on a low-carbohydrate diet not only lost weight but also saw symptoms of *other* health problems disappear. These included heart disease, arteriosclerosis, high blood pressure, osteoarthritis, gallstones, and diabetes—commonly known in the early 1900s as the "obesity sextette," because these six problems were observed to occur more frequently among obese people than among those who were constitutionally lean. (Later, most of these symptoms came to be grouped under the name "syndrome X," also known as metabolic syndrome; see note on page 307.) With patients on his meat-all-the-time diet, Donaldson found himself "less and less likely to resort to drugs" to combat these diseases. Everything seemed to get better when carbohydrates were replaced with fat on his diet. This is, admittedly, exactly the kind of claim that charlatans make about miracle cures, which therefore gave these diets the unfortunate taint of quackery, yet it is a common observation about the high-fat, low-carb diet that it seems to cure a surprising number of health ailments, and this had been true ever since Banting observed it in himself in the early 1860s.

That heart disease, diabetes, and even cancer might be caused by the kinds of carbohydrates consumed in modern diets has also been the conclusion of many doctors and researchers who observed primitive populations as they began to eat these foods. The German doctor Otto Schaefer, for instance, visited some of those famously carnivorous Inuit in the Canadian Arctic in 1951. The population he found on Baffin Island did not import any Western food and was still eating a diet entirely of meat and fat, including such appetizing delicacies as seal intestine, fish eyes, and Arctic char "sewn raw into sealskins and exposed to the sun for two to three days."

In some Arctic regions, the Hudson's Bay Company had begun bringing in annual boatloads of food, mainly flour, biscuits, tea, and molasses. But not all communities got these shipments, giving Schaefer the opportunity to compare communities that received an influx of Western food with those that did not.

Schaefer found that wherever the Inuit ate "in the old native fashion," good health seemed to prevail. After examining four thousand Canadian Inuit, Schaefer reported that he did not see any signs of vitamin or mineral deficiencies, despite the complete absence of fruits or vegetables from their diet. Nor did the lack of light during the winters produce vitamin D deficiency. Anemia for want of iron was also unknown, "so long as a large part of their diet consists of fresh meat and fish, mostly eaten raw and frozen."

From his own observations, as well as from the data he collected at a hospital in Edmonton and at a nearby sanitorium, Schaefer concluded that asthma, ulcers, gout, cancer, cardiovascular disease, diabetes, and ulcerative colitis were nearly nonexistent among the Inuit eating their traditional diet, as were hypertension and psychosomatic diseases. He saw only two cases of blood pressure over 100 mmHg and found arteriosclerosis to be less common in elderly Inuit than in elderly white Canadians. Heart disease, he wrote, "does not appear to exist in Eskimos under 60 years of age."

By contrast, wherever the Inuit ate carbohydrates instead of their traditional food, their health declined. Large numbers of women and children suffered from anemia, and he found his first case of diabetes, previously unreported in the Canadian Arctic, in an Inuit eating these "civilized" foods. He also found chronic ear infections and bad teeth. In some cases, tooth decay was so severe that some Inuit made their own dentures out of walrus tusks.* To Schaefer, it seemed obvious that the Inuit were "unable to cope with starches and sugars" to which they had been introduced.

In a settlement called Iqaluit, where Schaefer found the lowest consumption of traditional foods yet, the health of the Inuit was the worst he had seen anywhere. He observed that the condition of eating large amounts

---

*Tooth decay and a narrowing of facial structure that causes teeth to be crowded in the mouth were among the many health problems seen in societies newly introduced to refined carbohydrates, according to the dentist Weston A. Price, who traveled the world in the early 1900s and documented many populations undergoing such "nutrition transitions" (Price [1939] 2004).

of sugar, which took centuries to develop in Western nations, "has occurred with almost a jolting abruptness in the last twenty years for the Canadian Eskimo." Schaefer witnessed a generation lose their way of life and their health forever. Wherever the Inuit gave up eating meat, they replaced it with carbohydrates. In Iqaluit, where the locals were eating potato chips and drinking soft drinks, he told a local paper that the dietary changes approached a level of "self-inflicted genocide."

Schaefer was not alone in observing this dietary transition and its link to chronic diseases. The British Royal Navy's Surgeon Captain Thomas L. Cleave had seen the same phenomenon in so many remote areas to which he traveled in the early 1900s that he called all chronic illnesses the "saccharine diseases," because so many of these ailments arrived in concert with the introduction of refined carbohydrates—principally sugar and white flour. Boatloads of refined sugar had come to Cleave's own shores when Britain started annexing islands in the West Indies in the 1670s, and the English went from eating 4 pounds of sugar per capita in 1710 to more than 20 pounds per capita in the 1790s, a fivefold increase.*

The latter half of the eighteenth century also saw what appears to be the country's first cases of heart disease. Because this period was also a time when domesticated animals like cows and sheep were being bred to extreme fatness—in pictures they look nearly spherical—a more common explanation for the appearance of heart disease during this time has been the fatty meat, not the sugar.† In the following century, however, average meat consumption stayed constant or even dropped, while rates of heart disease grew. The only element of the diet that kept pace with the increase in heart disease was sugar. By the end of the nineteenth century, the average

---

*The explosion in British sugar consumption coincided exactly with the growing popularity of drinking tea, suggesting that the custom of taking tea functioned as a kind of sugar-delivery vehicle (Walvin 1997, 119–120 and 129–131).

†In addition to sugar, other refined carbohydrates that entered the diet in growing amounts during this time were white flour, which replaced whole wheat with improved milling techniques, and cereals (not all of them refined). Another change in the diet that might have contributed to heart disease was a shift in the animal feed from grass to grains, which would have changed the fatty-acid composition of the meat (Michaels 2001, 50–53).

Briton was eating about 80 pounds per year. (By comparison, the American food industry at the end of the twentieth century was providing more than 150 pounds of sugars per capita, which now included high-fructose corn syrup.)

The other major chronic disease whose appearance seemed to coincide with the coming of refined carbohydrates was cancer. Cancer went from being a rarity in isolated populations such as the Inuits, to a common killer, and the change happened whenever these populations began consuming sugar and white flour. The documentation for this astronomical rise in cancer was not meager, nor was it "restricted to one or two opinions received from a doctor residing in the wilds of Africa or Asia," according to the British journalist and historian J. Ellis Barker. In his book, *Cancer: How It Is Caused; How It Can Be Prevented* (1924), he set out to demonstrate that the evidence included a vast literature of reports and studies from throughout the world, many of which were originally published in the *British Journal of Medicine* or the *Lancet*, both highly respected journals, or in such local publications as the *East African Medical Journal*. Virtually all of the accounts he collected supported the contention that cancer, in addition to other chronic diseases, were indeed absent in isolated populations and only appeared with the coming of western carbohydrates.

George Prentice, a physician who spent time with isolated peoples in Southern Central Africa in the early twentieth century, observed a long list of diseases that tended to appear in these isolated populations almost simultaneously (some of which Donaldson would later include in his "obesity sextette"): cardiovascular disease, hypertension and stroke, cancer, obesity, diabetes mellitus, cavities, periodontal disease, appendicitis, peptic ulcers, diverticulitis, gallstones, hemorrhoids, constipation, and varicose veins.

These diseases clustered. When they came, they came together. And they would inevitably appear when remote populations had their first sustained exposure to Western foods. What did the West introduce to these remote populations? The story that nutrition experts have historically told us is that the industrialized world brought "high-fat, energy-dense diets with a substantial content of animal-based foods." That's a quote from a 2002 World Health Organization report, which reflects the mainstream view. Yet it seems clear from historical accounts such as Schaefer's and others that what Westerners exported to poorer countries from the earliest days onward was limited to what could be easily packaged and preserved. That meant no meat or dairy, since these foods would have spoiled too easily, although lard was an occasional exception. No, what traveled to these populations in every corner a Western trader could reach were four highly portable and popular items: sugar, molasses, white flour, and white rice. In other words: refined carbohydrates. With these western foods came diseases, and so these illnesses came to be called "Western diseases," or the "diseases of civilization."

The Atkins Diet Finally Gets Scientifically Tested

In light of these observations, it makes sense that a diet *without* these carbohydrates would make these diseases go away. This was basically Atkins's idea, which has been dismissed by nutrition authorities, who have been accustomed to thinking of dietary fat, not carbohydrates, as the problem. But practitioners from Banting to Atkins saw broad improvements in health when flour, sugar, and other carbohydrates were removed from the diet. The problem is that once carbohydrates are removed, a high-fat diet is what results, and that's what is supposed to cause heart disease. In the course of this book, we've explored the historical evidence suggesting that a high-fat diet is consistent with good health, but the only way for modern-day medical researchers to find out for sure is to do clinical trials—experiments that could establish if diets loaded in fat and saturated fat might extend life, as Atkins and his predecessors thought, or would kill prematurely, as Keys and his colleagues insisted.

It wasn't until the late 1990s that the diet popularized by Robert Atkins finally attracted a small band of researchers who began to conduct exactly the kinds of experiments that might set the record straight on this issue. These researchers had encountered the low-carb diet in different ways—while practicing medicine or reading the scientific literature. The doctor and researcher Eric Westman at Duke University, for example, had a patient who came to him, saying, "Hey doctor, all I'm eating is steak and eggs!" and boasting about his improved cholesterol markers. Westman was the first physician researcher to take Atkins up on that offer to go through all those medical files. He visited Atkins's office in New York City in the late 1990s and was impressed by his success in helping patients to lose weight and improve health. But he decided that the files weren't good enough. "I need science," he told Atkins. Westman knew that the only way to make sense of various anecdotal accounts was to do randomized controlled trials, the gold standard of medical evidence. So he, along with a few colleagues around the country, started conducting those trials.

This new group of researchers entering the field were young and relatively ignorant about the professional sandpit into which they'd be sinking. Gary Foster, for instance, a professor of psychology at Temple University who took part in a landmark trial comparing different diets in 2003, says he had no idea that including the Atkins regime in his study would be so contentious. "I remember one prominent scientist who stood up in a public meeting and said, 'I am absolutely disgusted that the NIH would waste my money on a study of the Atkins diet,'" he recounted to me. Others in the room piled on, applauding. Given the NIH's antagonism toward high-fat diets, Foster says, it was remarkable he and his colleagues got funding at all, and, in fact, they had needed to apply through an agency "side door," the alternative medicine division, which is the same one that looks at acupuncture.*

By contrast, the NIH never opened even a side door to Stephen Phinney, a doctor and nutritional biochemist. Phinney had started experimenting with high-fat, low-carb diets in the early 1980s and became obsessed with the subject. Unlike Foster, Phinney fully embraced this line of research, although his interest made him what he calls "a heretic" in the field. For more than twenty years, Phinney said, he submitted study proposals that the NIH repeatedly turned down for "reasons that were not serious."

Phinney's closest colleague in this research has been Jeff Volek at the University of Connecticut, who, like Phinney, is a fitness buff. Volek, a kinesiologist, was the Indiana state power-lifting champion at the age of thirty-two, and Phinney has always loved to ski, hike, and bike. Together, they brought a fresh approach to studying nutrition. Rather than seeing

---

*Foster later chose to be more professionally cautious and downplayed any of the positive health outcomes he discovered among the Atkins group in his study.

high-fat diets as a way to lose weight or perhaps prevent heart disease, they were more interested in diet as a means of obtaining peak physical performance. It helped, too, that they hadn't come up through the ranks of academic nutrition departments, since this meant they weren't schooled in the diet-heart hypothesis—which may have allowed them to entertain alternative ideas more easily.

Volek knew that athletes and weight lifters commonly eat a diet high in fat and protein and low in carbohydrates to maximize muscle development and reduce body fat. But for peak performance during long-distance efforts such as marathons, the common wisdom has been that athletes should eat a lot of carbohydrates the night before. This was the first idea that Phinney wanted to test. "We were pretty sure we'd prove that the carb-loading concept was *correct*," Phinney told me. To his surprise, he found just the opposite: athletes in his experiments could perform at their best on nearly zero carbohydrates. In the absence of glycogen (the form of glucose that is stored in muscles and the liver), the body simply switched its fuel source to molecules derived from the fatty acids in the blood, called ketone bodies.

As Phinney and Volek discovered, our bodies can be viewed as the physiological equivalent of hybrid automobiles, switching back and forth between fuel sources: when we can't burn energy from carbohydrates, we burn our fat stores instead.* Phinney was therefore able to refute one of the main criticisms of the Atkins diet: namely that people had to eat at least 100 grams of glucose a day for the body's basic functioning.† Indeed, it's been known for more than half a century, although forgotten or ignored,

---

*When the body shifts over to fatty acids in the form of ketones for its fuel, it enters a state that is called "nutritional ketosis." An enduring fear of the Atkins diet has been that these ketones are toxic, because they have been found to circulate at dangerously high levels in people with uncontrolled diabetes (a condition called "diabetic ketoacidosis.") However, the ketones found among low-carb dieters are at levels five to ten times less than those in diabetics and at this level have been shown to cause no harm.

†An international group in 1999 set the minimum amount of glucose needed at 150 grams per day. This number is derived from the longtime assumed daily minimum of 100 grams, with an arbitrary extra 50 grams added as a safety margin (Bier et al. 1999, S177–S178).

that our bodies have no requirement for carbohydrates and can sustain themselves perfectly well, if not better, on ketones. The small amount of glucose necessary for certain bodily tissue—the lens of the eye and red blood cells, for example—can be created by the liver from the amino acids in the protein we consume.

Phinney was also able to refute other concerns about the Atkins regime that had arisen from a few small trials of the diet in the 1970s and eighties. These studies found that the diet caused headaches, as Ornish mentioned, as well as dizziness, water loss, constipation, and loss of energy, together commonly known as the "Atkins flu." Phinney successfully demonstrated that all these effects were related to the transition period that occurred when people switched from their regular diets over to one low in carbohydrates. This changeover period can last from two to three weeks, during which time big metabolic shifts take place while bodily tissues are adapting to ketones as their new fuel source. Among other things, the kidneys expel water and salt, and Phinney showed that this phenomenon is what causes the light-headedness and constipation experienced by some Atkins dieters.* Phinney's solution to these transition problems was to prescribe several cups of bouillon a day.

This initial loss of water also led critics to the erroneous view that any weight reduction on the diet was due entirely to loss of water rather than fat.† Yet the work of Phinney, Volek, and others demonstrated that the pounds lost on the diet over a longer period of time came from the

---

*The loss of salt and potassium was the Achilles' heel of one of those early studies on the Atkins diet that appeared to condemn it. Researchers at Yale University in 1980 fed participants mostly turkey, which unfortunately had lost much of its salt and potassium content during preparation by boiling. Without an adequate supply of these essential nutrients, subjects experienced a range of unpleasant symptoms, and the study authors concluded that the Atkins diet itself was fundamentally flawed. A more likely explanation was that this boiled-turkey version of the diet lacked essential nutrients (DeHaven et al. 1980).

†The study most commonly cited as "proof" of this point turns out to have lasted only ten days; it was mistakenly assumed that the water loss during this initial period was the only type of weight loss experienced on the Atkins diet (Yang and Van Itallie 1976).

fat stores, not from water loss. By the early 2000s, these researchers were therefore able to discredit many of the misimpressions created by the few early scientific trials of the diet, which were simply too short to get past these transition problems. These researchers also confirmed that the diet's original promise of weight loss held true. In trials comparing the Atkins diet to the standard, calorie-restricted AHA-recommended diet, people lost considerably more weight on the low-carbohydrate diet, and more of that weight was fat rather than muscle.

In addition, they were finally able to demonstrate that cardiovascular health was not impaired by the Atkins diet—quite the reverse actually. In trial after trial and by virtually every indicator that they could measure, the high-fat diet was shown to lower the risk for heart disease and diabetes compared to the one low in fat and saturated fat that the AHA had proposed for Americans for so long. In more than fifteen well-controlled trials that Volek has conducted since the year 2000, he has found that the Atkins diet caused HDL-cholesterol to rise, while triglycerides, blood pressure, and inflammation markers dropped. And the ability of blood vessels to dilate (known as "endothelial function," which many experts believe to be an indicator of heart attack risk) has also been shown to improve on the low-carbohydrate diet, compared to people on one low in fat. Surprised and skeptical, Volek wondered if all these gains could simply be due to weight loss, since his subjects inevitably slimmed down on the Atkins diet. So he did further experiments keeping his subjects' weight constant and found that the low-carb diet yielded the same improvements, even so.

Another dozen or so clinical trials during this time were undertaken by Westman, the Duke University physician who had looked through Atkins's files. Westman was particularly interested in the diet's effect on type 2 diabetes (the kind that is associated with overweight and obesity). Carbohydrate restriction as a "cure" for diabetes had been reported by physicians as far back as the late nineteenth century, but Westman's trials were among the first to give solid scientific backing to the treatment.* Westman

---

*Banting's doctor, Harvey, derived his idea for a low-carbohydrate diet partly from news that French doctors were using this treatment for diabetes. The first recorded instance of the treatment in the United States appears to be work by Elliott Proctor

found that reducing carbohydrates and replacing them with dietary fat was extremely effective in managing diabetes; for some subjects, the disease would go into remission entirely, and their blood-glucose levels and insulin fluctuations would normalize to the point where they could even stop taking their diabetes medication. Based on this work, Westman and his colleagues have argued strenuously that the official low-fat diet, which usually relies on the addition of drugs to "work," should be jettisoned in favor of a low-carb regime as a recommended treatment for this condition. However, the American Diabetes Association (ADA) has stood by its low-fat advice, based on the fact that diabetics have a very high risk of heart disease, and since authorities advise a low-fat diet to fight that disease, that is what the ADA recommends to prevent diabetes, too.

These pioneering researchers of the Atkins diet continued to expand their work throughout the 2000s, conducting trials on a range of subjects: men and women, athletes, and those suffering from obesity, diabetes, and metabolic syndrome.*† And while the gains have varied, they have consis-

---

Joslin, a Harvard- and Yale-educated physician, who put his diabetic patients from 1893 to 1916 on a 10 percent carbohydrate diet. More recently, this approach has been rediscovered and developed by Mary Vernon, a family doctor in Lawrence, Kansas, and Richard K. Bernstein, a doctor in Mamaroneck, New York, who is also the author of *The Diabetes Diet: Dr. Bernstein's Low-Carbohydrate Solution* (New York: Little, Brown, 2005) (Joslin 1919; Joslin's work is also described in Westman, Yancy, and Humphreys 2006, 80–81).

*A portion of this work was funded by the Robert C. and Veronica Atkins Foundation, which was set up in 2003 with a $40 million grant from Atkins to finance research following his death. Although these low-carb researchers were understandably reluctant to accept financing from a foundation with a clear agenda, there were no alternatives, since the NHLBI and AHA have long considered a high-fat diet too unhealthy even to be studied and have therefore funded no trials on it. ("About the Foundation," Robert C. and Veronica Atkins Foundation, accessed October 11, 2013, http://www.atkinsfoundation.org/about.asp.)

†Metabolic syndrome is a name for a group of medical disorders occurring simultaneously in an individual. These include: "central" obesity (around the abdomen), raised triglycerides, low HDL-cholesterol, high fasting plasma glucose, and high blood pressure. A combination of some or all of these problems indicates a sharp increase in risk for coronary artery disease, stroke, and type 2 diabetes. The syndrome was first described by the endocrinologist Gerald Reaven and so is also sometimes

tently pointed in the right direction. One of the more extraordinary experiments involved 146 men suffering from high blood pressure who went on the Atkins diet for almost a year. The group saw their blood pressure drop significantly more than did a group of low-fat dieters—who were *also* taking a blood-pressure medication.

In most of these experiments, the diet with the best results contained more than 60 percent of calories as fat.* This proportion of fat was similar to what the Inuit and the Masai ate but was startlingly high compared to the official recommendations of 30 percent or less. Yet no other well-controlled trials of any other diet had ever shown such clear-cut advantages in the fight against obesity, diabetes, and heart disease, and for so many different kinds of populations.

Despite the consistency of these results, Westman and his colleagues have remained outsiders in the world of nutrition. Their work has perhaps predictably been met with silence, scorn, or both. Getting their research published in prestigious journals has been difficult, and invitations to major conferences are rare. Volek says that even when he's been invited to present his findings at meetings, displaying research that confronts the very foundation of the conventional wisdom on diet, the reception is incurious: "people are just quiet." And despite the substantial body of evidence now supporting the high-fat, low-carbohydrate regime as the healthiest option, his colleagues still routinely refer to the diet as "quackery" and a "fad." Persevering in this field can be dispiriting, Volek told me. "You do deal with bias. . . . It's very difficult to find grant money or journals that want to publish our studies."

Westman has written poignantly about the predicament of working

------

called the "Reaven syndrome." It is also known as "cardiometabolic syndrome," "syndrome X" and "insulin resistance syndrome." The defining symptoms also vary somewhat by authority (NIH, WHO, etc.).

*Only a handful of high-fat diet trials on humans to date have attempted to isolate the effects of saturated fat, because diets high in saturated fats have been considered especially dangerous for study. In the handful of small trials that have been conducted so far, no adverse effects of these diets have been found (Rivellese et al. 2008; Hays et al. 2003; Forsythe 2010; Cassady 2007).

toward paradigm change when the existing bias is so strong: "When an unscientific fear of dietary fat pervades the culture so much that researchers who are on study sections that provide funding will not allow research into high-fat diets for fear of 'harming people,' " as we've seen at the NIH and AHA, "this situation will not allow science to 'self-correct.' A sort of scientific taboo is created because of the low likelihood of funding, and the funding agencies are off the hook because they say that researchers are not submitting requests for grants."

While Volek and his colleagues have long urged the nutrition mainstream to take a "more unbiased, balanced" approach to the low-carbohydrate diet, they remained reluctant to recommend the regime to the entire American population, because it had not yet been subject to a long-term clinical trial.* Only a trial of at least two years or more could answer enduring health concerns about a diet so high in fat, to counter the widespread speculation by researchers and clinicians that the negative effects of eating so much fat and protein might occur only after a prolonged period of time on the diet.†

In 2008, results from a two-year trial were finally published. This was the study in Israel, discussed in the Mediterranean diet chapter, on 322

---

*By the late 2000s, the longest trial had lasted only one year. This was the "A to Z" study, conducted at Stanford University, which showed that premenopausal women on the Atkins diet had better outcomes in every way, compared to women on the Zone diet (moderately low in carbohydrates), the LEARN diet (moderately low in fat, moderately high in carbohydrate), and the Ornish diet (very low in fat and very high in carbohydrates) (Gardner et al. 2007).

†The effects of too much protein was one concern, and this is justified—but is problematic only when a diet lacks fat. When protein is eaten, the kidneys and liver remove the nitrogen and excrete it through the urine. Dietary fat is essential to this process. When overly lean meat is eaten, nitrogen cannot be properly processed and builds up to potentially toxic levels. This condition is a common danger to dieters nowadays, eager to cut back on carbohydrates but, given longtime biases, reluctant to eat more fat. The Inuit considered overly lean meat to be an inadequate source of nourishment. Stefansson dubbed the problem "rabbit-starvation" and suffered from the condition himself when he went through a period of eating lean meat but not enough fat during his yearlong meat-only experiment in 1928 (Stefansson 1956, 31).

overweight men and women. The trial was exceptionally well controlled by the standards of nutrition research, with lunch, the principal meal of the day in Israel, provided at a company cafeteria.

The study separated subjects into three groups: one eating the AHA's prescribed low-fat diet, another on the Mediterranean diet, and a third on the Atkins diet. Iris Shai, the Israeli clinical-trial specialist who directed the study alongside Harvard nutrition professor Meir Stampfer, said that she had initially planned to include only the first two arms. After hearing Eric Westman give a talk at Harvard in 2004 and reading some of the recent low-carbohydrate trials, however, she decided to include the Atkins regime as well.*

Shai found that for nearly every marker of heart disease that could be measured during the two years of the study, Atkins dieters looked the healthiest—and they lost the most weight. For the small subset of diabetics in the study, the results looked about equal for the Atkins and Mediterranean diets. And in every case, the low-fat diet performed the worst.

From the results of this study, plus two other recent trials on the Atkins diet that both lasted two years,† it appeared that concerns about the

---

*For this reason, the study was funded in part by the Atkins Foundation.

†The other two studies did not show such clear advantages for the Atkins diet and are not covered in the text here, because they were less well controlled than the one in Israel. Whereas Shai's team served lunch, the main meal of the day, to participants (which also served as a powerful educational experience in how to follow the assigned diet and was supplemented by counseling sessions), the other two studies merely gave subjects a diet book or other informational materials and weekly advice sessions. The Shai results therefore ought to be considered more reliable. One of the other two studies was by the team that had included Temple's Gary Foster. This trial, on 307 adults, pitted a low-fat, calorie-controlled diet against an Atkins diet that was unlimited in calories, and investigators found almost no difference in the health or weight loss of the subjects on the two diets—except, notably, that HDL-cholesterol improved by 23 percent on the Atkins diet, whereas no such advantage was seen in the low-fat dieting group (Foster et al. 2010). The second study was conducted by Harvard professor Frank M. Sacks, comparing four diets with varying proportions of carbohydrates, protein, and fat. Sacks started with 811 overweight adults and, after two years of study, found little difference in outcomes (Sacks et al. 2009).

regime's potentially harmful long-term effects could finally be put to rest. Kidney function and bone density, two primary concerns, were found to be perfectly fine, if not improved, on the Atkins diet. Yet these crucially important long-term findings have not, on the whole, been discussed by mainstream nutrition experts, nor have they translated into greater support for a higher-fat diet. For the low-carb band of researchers, however, these trials were the last piece of evidence they had been waiting for. Westman, Volek, and Phinney came to the reasonable conclusion that the high-fat, low-carbohydrate diet could now be recommended to the public more broadly.*

Gary Taubes and "The Big Fat Lie"

While these researchers have been ignored by most mainstream medical and nutrition communities, the one person who has successfully redirected the nutrition conversation over the past decade toward the idea that carbohydrates, not fat, are the drivers of obesity and other chronic diseases is the science journalist Gary Taubes. In 2001, he wrote a critical history of the diet-heart hypothesis for *Science* magazine, which was the first time a major scientific journal had published a thorough analysis of the low-fat dogma's scientific weaknesses—at least since Pete Ahrens had ceded the battle against Ancel Keys in the mid-1980s. Taubes also reviewed all the science, from those prewar German and Austrian obesity researchers on through Pennington, and concluded that obesity was indeed a hormonal defect and not the result of gluttony and sloth. In his *Science* piece, Taubes described how the hormone causing obesity is most likely insulin, which spikes when one eats carbohydrates. One of his primary conclusions, in fact, was that dietary fat itself is the nutrient *least* likely to make you fat, because it's the one macronutrient that doesn't stimulate the production of insulin.

---

*In 2010, Phinney, together with Volek and Westman, wrote a new Atkins diet book called *The New Atkins for a New You: The Ultimate Diet for Shedding Weight and Feeling Great* (New York: Touchstone, 2010), which sold more than half a million copies in two years. Phinney and Volek also self-published two books on the low-carbohydrate diet.

The New York Times Magazine Cover, July 7, 2002

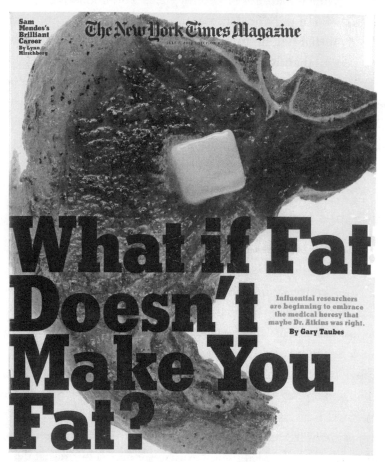

Science journalist Gary Taubes wrote a landmark article, publicly challenging the idea that dietary fat of any kind causes heart disease or obesity.

From *The New York Times*, July 7, 2002 © 2002 *The New York Times*. Used by permission and protected by the Copyright Laws of the United States. The printing, copying, redistribution, or retransmission of this Content without express written permission is prohibited.

Other researchers and scientists had published critiques of the diet-heart hypothesis, but Taubes was the first to put together all the various ideas on the topic into one comprehensive narrative. And Taubes could reach a national audience. He followed up with a second foray in the *New York Times Magazine*, under the headline, "What if It's All Been a Big Fat Lie?" In 2007, he published a book on the subject, *Good Calories, Bad Calories*, a densely annotated and meticulously researched work that made a comprehensive and original case for an "alternative" hypothesis on obesity and chronic disease. It argued that the refined carbohydrates and sugars in our diet are what cause obesity, diabetes, and related diseases, and not the dietary fat or the "excess calories" that are thought to come from eating more than we should.

Taubes has been the most influential recent challenger to the diet-heart hypothesis. Even Michael Pollan, the popular food writer who says we should eat "mostly plants," praised Taubes for exposing the pseudoscience in the low-fat dogma and dubbed him the Alexander Solzhenitsyn of the nutrition world.

Taubes's work shattered dogma to such an extent that most nutrition experts have been unable to respond except by simply dismissing him, as the field has managed to do with challengers so many times before. When Taubes's book came out, Gina Kolata, medical writer for the *New York Times*, called Taubes "a brave and bold science journalist" but ended her review with an airy, "I'm sorry, I'm not convinced." * The chill in the nutrition community toward Taubes was so palpable in the mid-2000s, when I started my own research for this book, that although many diet-and-heart experts had apparently read Taubes, I found that no one was willing to talk about him. Taubes's work as a science journalist had won him many awards, including three science-in-society awards from the National Association of Science Writers, the most that the group allows for any single science reporter. Yet roughly two thirds of my interviews with nutrition experts began with something like: "If you are taking the Gary Taubes line, then I'd rather not talk to you."

Taubes, in turn, was a provocative critic of nutrition science and its practitioners. After one talk at a research institute, a senior faculty member asked, "Mr. Taubes, is it fair to say that one subtext of your talk is that you think we're all idiots?" "A surprisingly good question," Taubes wrote later

---

*Kolata did not address any of the thousands of scientific studies that Taubes covered. Instead, her apparent coup de grâce was several "definitive studies" she found, conducted by researchers in New York City, in which hospitalized subjects were fed diets that varied from zero to 85 percent in their carbohydrate and fat contents, with no observable difference in health outcomes or weight. Taubes replied, accurately, that there was really only one such study on only sixteen people (Taubes, October 28, 2007).

on his blog. He explained that generations of researchers weren't unintelligent; they had simply been educated into a biased way of thinking. Yet if the pursuit of science is about getting the right answer, wrote Taubes, then "getting the wrong answer on such a huge and tragic scale borders on inexcusable." In the last line of his 2002 *New York Times Magazine* article, he quotes a researcher asking the not-so-rhetorical question: "Can we get the low-fat proponents to apologize?"

Despite the no-love-lost nature of the relationship between Taubes and mainstream nutrition experts, much of what he wrote seemed so eminently believable that it was almost immediately adopted. Of course sugar and white flour were bad! Nutrition experts spoke as if this had always been known. A 2010 headline in the *Los Angeles Times* declared, "Fat Was Once the Devil. Now More Nutritionists Are Pointing Accusingly at Sugar and Refined Grains." Researchers around the country who had read and digested Taubes's work were suddenly studying sucrose, fructose, and glucose, comparing them to each other and looking at their insulin effects. Some investigators have made the case recently that the fructose found in fruits, honey, table sugar, and high-fructose corn syrup may be worse than glucose in provoking the inflammation markers linked to heart disease.* The glucose found in sugar and starchy vegetables, meanwhile, seems to work more closely with insulin to cause obesity. The science on these different types of refined carbohydrates is still in its infancy, so we don't really know if all carbohydrates play a role in obesity, diabetes, and heart disease, or if some types are worse than others.

The one statement that seems safe to make is that the refined carbohydrates and sugars that we were recommended to eat by the AHA as part of a healthy, fat-avoiding diet, are not merely indifferent, "empty calories," as we've long been told, but are actively bad for health in a variety of ways.†

---

*Both table sugar (sucrose) and high-fructose corn syrup are comprised of the same roughly fifty-fifty mix of fructose and glucose.

†In 2011, a group of top nutrition experts published the first high-level, formal consensus paper stating that refined carbohydrates were worse than saturated fats in provoking heart disease and obesity (Astrup et al. 2011).

Moreover, the clinical trials in recent years imply that any kind of carbohydrate, including those in whole grains, fruits, and starchy vegetables, are also unhealthy in large amounts. Remember that the Shai study in Israel found that the Mediterranean diet group, eating a high proportion of calories as these "complex" carbohydrates, turned out to be less healthy and fatter than the group on the Atkins diet, although they were healthier than the low-fat alternative. The Women's Health Initiative, too, in which some 49,000 women were tested on a diet high in complex carbohydrates for nearly a decade, showed no reduction in disease risk or weight. This big-picture message about how even too many *unrefined* carbohydrates might be bad for health is alienating for Americans, however, since we are now used to viewing these foods as healthy. And no doubt it would be difficult for nutrition experts to contradict their own half-century's worth of high-carbohydrate advice.

Even so, whatever scientific progress has been made toward our greater understanding of carbohydrates generally in recent years has clearly been due to Taubes's work. "This has been his most important contribution to the field," said Ronald M. Krauss, an influential nutrition expert and the director of research at the Children's Hospital Oakland Research Institute. For a journalist, it was an astonishing coup in the world of science. In 2013, Taubes became one of the rare journalists to write a peer-reviewed article for the highly respected scientific publication, the *British Medical Journal.* Yet given the stranglehold that Keys's ideas have held on nutrition researchers for so many decades, it is perhaps inevitable that an alternative hypothesis had to come from an outsider.*

---

*In 2012, Taubes and the doctor Peter Attia founded a not-for-profit group called the Nutrition Science Initiative (NuSI) with a $40 million grant from the Laura and John Arnold Foundation. It aims to conduct high-quality scientific research on issues that the NIH and AHA have been reluctant to fund. In 2013, NuSI began a pilot experiment to test the hypothesis that carbohydrates, compared to protein and fat, are a uniquely fattening type of calorie. Five centers, including ones at Columbia University and the NIH, are participating in the experiment, and the oversight board includes top nutrition experts. A description of the study protocol can be found in an article in *Scientific American* (Taubes 2013).

The Paradigm Shift on Cholesterol

While Taubes's work pushed to reorient the nutrition conversation away from fat as a dietary evil, and the low-carb band of researchers performed their clinical trials showing that diets without refined carbohydrates had a lot to recommend them, there was a third crucial factor over the past fifteen years that has solidified the evidence behind the idea that a higher fat diet is healthier. This factor has to do with the new science on how to predict heart disease, which has turned everything we originally thought we knew about cholesterol, heart disease, and diet on its head.

Among the most influential researchers in this field is Ronald Krauss. He is indisputably one of the nutrition world's aristocrats, routinely called upon by the AHA and NIH to serve on expert panels, and he has conducted a great deal of NIH-funded research. Krauss is also a rarity among his elite academic colleagues in that he regularly sees patients. While nutritional epidemiologists spend their days poring over questionnaire data, and nutritional biochemists are experimenting under idealized conditions in the lab, Krauss is one of the few nutrition researchers who, like Donaldson and Pennington before him, has the experience of seeing actual people struggling with their weight and health.

Krauss has made several important contributions toward unsettling the case against saturated fat, but the most crucial in scientific terms was his discovery of a new biomarker for heart disease. In the 1990s, Krauss found a way to predict heart disease that both surpassed and undermined the methods upon which the diet-heart hypothesis had been built. The ability to measure some marker in the blood that could reliably indicate heart attack risk is, of course, the holy grail for cardiovascular research. Sixty years ago Keys first proposed total serum cholesterol as this marker, condemning saturated fat entirely on the basis of its capacity to raise it. Then, in the 1970s and eighties, when scientists began to understand the complexities of this "total cholesterol" number—that it wasn't actually a good predictor for heart-attack risk and that it masked the more subtle measures of HDL- and LDL-cholesterol—it seemed that saturated fat might be redeemed. Saturated animal fats *do* raise HDL-cholesterol, after all, which is one of their often-overlooked virtues. Yet saturated fat also raises the "bad" LDL-cholesterol. These conflicting effects have been fatal to saturated fat, because official scientific opinion, for political and other reasons, has favored LDL-cholesterol over HDL-cholesterol as the biomarker of choice for the last few decades.

Krauss was one of the few researchers who was unconvinced that LDL-cholesterol was necessarily the best and most reliable biomarker for heart disease.* In his own practice, he had seen patients who lowered their LDL-cholesterol or already had LDL-cholesterol in the "healthy" zone to begin with, yet suffered heart attacks anyway. The ability of LDL-cholesterol to predict heart disease, Krauss pointed out, is confined mainly to those people with very high LDL-cholesterol levels—160 mg/dL and above. For the garden-variety heart disease patient whose LDL-cholesterol is only borderline high, LDL-cholesterol is relatively meaningless. Indeed, in more than a few major studies, LDL-cholesterol levels were found to be completely uncorrelated with whether people had heart attacks or not.†

Put simply, LDL-cholesterol, despite all the hoopla, is a largely unreliable predictor of heart disease risk. Indeed, many researchers today argue that "high LDL-cholesterol" is no longer especially meaningful. "There is no scientific basis for treating LDL targets," wrote a Yale cardiologist and his colleague in a 2012 open letter to the NIH published in the AHA journal *Circulation*. Or, as Allan Sniderman, a professor of medicine and cardiology at McGill University, described it to me, "LDL is a historical leftover."

---

*One of the problems is very basic: the test to measure LDL cholesterol has always been unreliable. The standard methodology measures total cholesterol and then subtracts HDL-cholesterol, plus the other portion of total cholesterol, which is called very low-density lipoprotein (VLDL). But VLDL itself is not directly measured; it is estimated from measurements of triglycerides, and this confounds results, particularly when triglycerides are high. "The error is very substantial," Allan Sniderman, a biomarker expert at McGill University, told me. He explained, "If your LDL-cholesterol comes back as 130 mg/dL, it could really be anywhere from 115 to 165 or more" (Sniderman interview).

†Moreover, in a study on 304 healthy women that directly measured calcification of the arteries using electron beam tomography, no correlation whatsoever could be found between the degree of calcified plaque and levels of total LDL-cholesterol (Hecht and Superko 2001).

Krauss mined the scientific research literature for clues about better predictors. He found a long line of research, going back to other biomarkers that had long been ignored, one of which had its origins at his own university. In the 1950s, the medical physicist John W. Gofman found that in the same way that total cholesterol can be separated out into LDL and HDL, he could analyze LDL particles as the sum of a number of "LDL subfractions." Krauss confirmed their existence for himself in the mid-1980s, using a technology similar to Gofman's. He found that some LDL particles were large, light, and buoyant, while others were small and dense. The small, dense ones turned out to be very closely associated with heart disease risk, whereas the large, light, buoyant LDL particles were not linked to high risk at all. The upshot, Krauss found, was that "total LDL" masked a more complex reality: a person could have "high total LDL," which by conventional standards sounded bad, yet if the LDL were mainly the light, buoyant kind, it wasn't a problem. Conversely, a person could have relatively low LDL, which seemed like a good thing, but if the LDL-cholesterol were the small, dense kind, it signaled a high degree of risk.

In this one discovery, Krauss revealed why "high LDL-cholesterol," though beloved by mainstream experts and endorsed by the AHA, the NIH, and Nobel Prize–winning scientists, was not living up to its promises for predicting heart attacks. Like total cholesterol in the 1980s, a trusted biomarker turned out to be more complex and to contain more fractions than originally thought. Although public health recommendations had been issued and statin drugs prescribed to millions of Americans based on the idea that these drugs worked by lowering the amount of LDL-cholesterol in the blood, the science of predicting heart disease was still unfolding.

Krauss also tested what happened to LDL subfractions when subjects were fed different kinds of diets. He found that when people ate more total and saturated fats instead of carbohydrates, there was an increase in the large "good" type of LDL, while the small, dense LDL, the kind that was associated with heart disease, went down. If Krauss was right, the case against saturated fat as the main dietary culprit had now been considerably weakened; if saturated fat raised only this relatively innocuous kind of LDL, then its effect on the human body was relatively benign. And combined with saturated fat's ability to raise HDL-cholesterol, then it looked not just benign, but maybe even healthy, and certainly far better than the carbohydrates we've been told to eat in its place.*

Krauss did not push his LDL-subfraction findings too hard with his colleagues, however. He understood that even after it had been successfully replicated, this discovery was something to peddle lightly to fellow nutrition experts, who might take umbrage at the implication that they had been wrong about LDL-cholesterol all along. Indeed, most of his peers found it convenient simply to ignore Krauss's findings. In 2006, for example, when I asked Robert Eckel, then president of the AHA, about them, he told me that although he respected Krauss's work, he did not see why it might be considered particularly important (a view he continued to hold when I checked in with him in 2013). As Penn State's Penny Kris-Etherton, one of the most powerful people in the field, explained to me in 2007, "Academic scientists believe that saturated fat is bad for you, and there is a good deal of reluctance toward accepting evidence suggesting the contrary."

Still, bolstered by his own reading of the evidence, Krauss attempted to take on the AHA's dietary guidelines on fat. Krauss had long been involved in the AHA at the highest levels and thought that if he could move the group toward loosening up its fat reduction advice on both total and saturated fat, he might well have a significant impact on American health. And in 1995, when Krauss assumed the committee chairmanship, he got his chance, ultimately overseeing two iterations of the AHA dietary guidelines, in 1996 and 2000. The person most opposed to saturated fat on the committee was Tufts University's Alice Lichtenstein, another influential member of the nutrition elite. While Krauss argued that the allowable amount of saturated fat should remain as is, Lichtenstein countered that the limit should be ratcheted down even lower than its existing 8 percent level, to 6 or 7 percent. Krauss tried to fend her off by stressing the lack of scientific

---

*Other promising new biomarkers have been discovered and promoted in recent years, such as apolipoprotein B (ApoB) and non-HDL-cholesterol. But only Krauss's LDL subfractions can explain the problematic findings from several large studies that LDL-cholesterol cannot reliably be linked to heart disease outcomes. For this reason, Krauss's subfractions are uniquely significant and important.

evidence for such an extreme recommendation. Even Keys's Cretans, whose saturated-fat intake had been undercounted due to the "Lent problem," had evidently eaten more animal fat than that.

Krauss did manage to make meaningful shifts in the AHA guidelines: In the 1996 version, Krauss made the point, for the first time in any AHA dietary report, that the saturated fatty acids in dairy, meat, and palm oil were of different kinds and did not all have the same effect on blood lipids; in fact, some of these saturated fats had never been found to have any negative effects on cholesterol at all.* But this level of specificity could not be translated into the guidelines distributed to the public, Krauss told me, because "it was too complicated." Even so, Krauss considered it a success that in the next set of guidelines, four years later, he was able to move the advice to reduce saturated fat down the list of priorities, burying it under several subheads.

In the end, however, Krauss lost the battle to the traditionalists, who counterattacked. When Lichtenstein took over the nutrition committee chair, in 2006, she swung the AHA guidelines back in the other direction, dropping the allowable amount of saturated fat from Krauss's 10 percent, past the previous 8 percent, down to 7 percent of calories or less. This was the same tiny amount of saturated fat allowed in the NIH's most aggressive diet, Step 2, which was designed for the highest-risk, post-heart-attack patients. Now it was being recommended to men, women, and children alike. When I asked Lichtenstein whether her committee had considered Krauss's work on LDL subfractions and their implication for saturated fat, she replied that his work was "complicated" and that she "didn't have the time" to review it.

---

*It took another ten years for other guidelines to incorporate these fine points about different kinds of saturated fats, and then only in France. That government's 2010 official dietary advice made the distinction, for the first time, that only those saturated fats found predominantly in palm and coconut oil and to a lesser extent meat and salmon (called lauric, myristic, and palmitic acids) could possibly be linked to heart disease, due to their effect on LDL-cholesterol. Another type of saturated fat (stearic acid), found mainly in meat, dairy, and eggs, was completely exonerated. (In fact, it has been known since the 1950s that stearic acid does not negatively affect cholesterol.)

In 2013, Lichtenstein teamed up with Bob Eckel on a joint task force of the AHA and the American College of Cardiology (ACC) aimed at updating heart disease treatment recommendations for doctors nationwide. Now their advice became even more draconian: all "at-risk" adults, including some 45 million healthy people, were told as a precautionary measure to cut the level of saturated fat back further, to an unprecedented 5 percent to 6 percent of calories.* This was a shockingly low level. To meet that target, a person would need to eat nearly a vegan diet. The Eckel task force justified this recommendation by citing just two clinical trials: the DASH and OmniHeart studies. These experiments fed subjects diets containing 5 percent to 6 percent saturated fat, and their LDL-cholesterol levels dropped significantly. This could be interpreted as a positive finding, but only if Krauss's work were ignored, along with the large trials that negated LDL-cholesterol as a meaningful predictor of risk for most people. The committee also had to disregard the fact that the subjects in these two trials saw their HDL-cholesterol fall significantly, an important indicator of worsening cardiac health. And the subjects saw no improvements in their markers for diabetes, nor did they lose any weight.

In making its very low saturated fat recommendation, the AHA-ACC expert panel stated that it did not consider the impact of its proposed diet on diabetes or metabolic syndrome. And why not? This was a truly startling decision, given that all these conditions have long been established as being tied to each other; the very term "metabolic syndrome" was coined

---

*This AHA-ACC task force is different from the notorious AHA nutrition committee, responsible for dietary guidelines since 1961. By contrast, the AHA-ACC task force was established in 2013 to create treatment guidelines on both diet and drugs for doctors to follow in treating adult patients. These guidelines for doctors have historically been written by the NIH's National Cholesterol Education Program (NCEP) ever since that division was founded in 1986. NCEP wrote three sets of these guidelines, each called "ATP" and numbered 1 to 3. However, the panel convened to write the latest set, ATP4, got so bogged down in rules about reviewing data that NHLBI administrators announced in June 2013, after nearly a decade of unproductive work, that they were handing the job over to the AHA and ACC. This means, effectively, that the government has yielded leadership on its most important diet and disease guidelines to private groups (Gibbons et al. 2013).

to describe a group of risk factors that occur simultaneously, and together increase the risk for coronary artery disease, stroke, and type 2 diabetes. It therefore seems clear that the effect of any treatment, including diet, should be evaluated for all of these conditions jointly.

The reality for mainstream nutrition experts today, however, is that their long-standing loyalty to LDL-cholesterol has backed them into a corner. A great deal of scientific evidence must be ignored to sustain their views; indeed, the AHA-ACC treatment guidelines did not cite any of the several decades' worth of large NIH trials, including MRFIT and the Women's Health Initiative, which collectively tested more than 61,000 men and women for more than seven years, and ultimately failed to show any benefits of a diet low in saturated fats. By contrast, the two trials cited by Eckel's task force tested a total of only 590 people over eight weeks.*

Furthermore, Eckel, Lichtenstein, and their colleagues continued to make the logical leap, as did the LRC trial leaders at the NHLBI in 1984, that LDL-cholesterol-lowering through diet had the same biological effects as LDL-cholesterol-lowering through statins. There is still no data to support this assumption. If anything, the evidence has only gotten weaker in recent years, since a number of studies have now tested an LDL-cholesterol-lowering diet and found that biomarker to be only weakly linked to heart attack risk. Yet despite all this, the AHA-ACC task force's advice to eat a diet limited to between 5 percent and 6 percent saturated fat is now the new norm for people who need to lower their LDL-cholesterol (a group for which no definition is given), and this advice has a good chance of being widely applied to most adult Americans. This guideline is also likely to be enshrined by the USDA, because Alice Lichtenstein is also the chair of the committee writing the 2015 *Dietary Guidelines*.

By ignoring all the evidence on diet and LDL-cholesterol, including the work of Krauss and others on LDL subfractions, the NIH and AHA

---

*It could be argued that these two trials were more rigorously controlled and therefore more likely to yield reliable results than either MRFIT or the Women's Health Initiative. However, the Israeli trial, which came out in favor of the Atkins diet, on 322 people and lasting two *years*, was also very well controlled.

have therefore been able to preserve LDL-cholesterol as their favored bio-marker, as though the last twenty years of science had never happened. And like so much of the advice that we've received on heart disease prevention, the rationale for these changes remains more political and financial than scientific: LDL-cholesterol has a following and a long history; doctors everywhere understand it; the government has an entire bureaucracy, the National Cholesterol Education Program, committed to lowering it; academics have invested their careers in it; pharmaceutical companies, with their profitable LDL-cholesterol-lowering drugs, have promoted it. And LDL-cholesterol has long been the biomarker most widely used to condemn saturated fat, which, in a community of diet and disease researchers biased against that fat, made it especially appealing.

In a highly controversial move, the AHA-ACC task force did appear to downgrade LDL-cholesterol *slightly* in its 2013 guidelines by eliminating the specific numerical treatment targets for them —which had been in place since 1986. The task force also promoted "non-HDL-cholesterol" as a relatively new additional biomarker because it was thought to be a more accurate predictor of cardiovascular risk.* These changes appear to be a step in the right direction for understanding heart disease, yet forces separate from science were probably at work here, too. A cynical observer might point out that in 2013, the patents on statin drugs were expiring and that incentives for pharmaceutical companies to continue favoring LDL-cholesterol would therefore be reduced.

Many diet and disease experts, including Krauss, are disappointed by the continued focus on LDL-cholesterol. Back in 2006, after Lichtenstein's AHA guidelines undid all of Krauss's work on saturated fat, he "became disenchanted with the dietary guideline process," he told me, and ramped down his active work with the AHA. In 2011, he also gave up a coveted spot on that NCEP expert panel led by Eckel and Lichtenstein when he could not endorse the direction in which it was heading.

---

*"Non-HDL-cholesterol" is calculated by subtracting HDL-cholesterol from total cholesterol. Like LDL-cholesterol, however, its accuracy drops significantly when triglycerides are high (van Deventer et al. 2011).

Krauss still had another intellectual contribution to make, however, which would serve to further undermine the foundation of the diet-heart hypothesis and its health claims against saturated fats. This contribution would have a broader and more lasting impact on the nutrition community.

Krauss Lifts the Death Sentence on Saturated Fat, Part 2

Krauss continued to follow the implications of his research on LDL-cholesterol and in 2000, decided to undertake a review of all the scientific evidence against saturated fat. Were those early clinical trials and epidemiological findings that his colleagues cited so frequently to support the diet-heart hypothesis as rock-solid as expert opinion had portrayed them to be? Krauss wasn't the first person to attempt such a review; Taubes himself had recently examined them for his 2007 book, as had others before him, but Krauss was the most influential researcher within the nutrition establishment to undertake such an effort.

In 2009, Krauss told me that he knew it was "going to be a long row to hoe," yet he had no idea just how hard the process would be. Clinical trials such as the Los Angeles Veterans, the Oslo study, and the Finnish Mental Hospital studies (see Chapter 3) were sacred ground. Over the years, Krauss has managed, by couching his arguments carefully and adopting the language of his opponents, to insert many of his ideas into the dialogue. Yet even he met with fierce resistance this time. Krauss told me he had never experienced so much frustration and delay in getting a paper into print as the one he wrote on saturated fat. He confronted an "agonizing series of reviews," he said, first by the *Journal of the American Medical Association*, which ultimately turned his paper down, and then the *American Journal of Clinical Nutrition* (AJCN). The research write-up went through five "major permutations" over three years and finally came out in 2010.

Ultimately Krauss published two papers on what he and his colleagues had learned: one looking at *all* the data from epidemiological studies linking diet and disease and the second looking at *all* the other evidence, including the clinical trials. For the first paper, Krauss and his colleagues concluded that "saturated fat was not associated with an increased risk" for heart disease or stroke. This was the first time a researcher had analyzed all the epidemiological studies together, and Krauss found that they amounted to an absence of incriminating evidence.

In the second paper, Krauss couched his findings with a more judicious set of caveats. One conclusion of the paper was that, judged by the traditional LDL-cholesterol biomarker, saturated fat looked not quite as healthy as polyunsaturated fats. But here Krauss was just toeing the company line. He would not say in print what he would in person: that he didn't believe LDL-cholesterol to be a meaningful biomarker for heart disease, except for people whose levels were abnormally high. Based on the biomarkers that he *did* trust—triglycerides and small, dense LDL-cholesterol—he came to a conclusion that he *did*, unequivocally, believe, namely that eating saturated fat is healthier than eating carbohydrates. In other words: cheese is probably healthier than bread. And eggs and bacon better than oatmeal.

The AJCN editors, recognizing that Krauss's paper would appall the greater portion of their readers, published it alongside an editorial by the diet-heart proponent Jeremiah Stamler, who, at ninety-one years old, was still a zealous defender of that hypothesis. In his lengthy editorial, entitled "Diet Heart: A Problematic Revisit," Stamler made many points, among them the fact that Krauss's conclusions were contrary to pretty much every national and international dietary recommendation on the planet and that therefore they must be wrong. This argument begged the question of how science could ever correct itself if researchers who disagreed with the conventional wisdom must be considered wrong because, well, the conventional wisdom disagreed with them.

Once Krauss's two papers were published, however, they marked a turning point in the nutrition discussion. Linked to Krauss's prestige, the papers allowed subterranean conversations to emerge and the formerly forbidden to be openly spoken.

The Academy of Nutrition and Dietetics (formerly the American Dietetic Association), for example, hosted a meeting in 2010 called "The Great Fat Debate," an event unprecedented for even considering the healthfulness of saturated fat a worthy topic of debate. And one of the four speakers, the rising star of Harvard epidemiologists Dariush Mozaffarian, announced in front of several thousand nutritionists that, based on the current reading of the evidence on heart disease and obesity, experts should be focusing on carbohydrates; "it's not really useful anymore to focus on saturated fats," he said.

More generally, in the United States and around the world, a growing number of researchers in recent years are now willing to criticize the science supporting the diet-heart hypothesis. And more scientists are pursuing investigations based on Taubes's alternative hypothesis. Yet, in what can be seen as a tragic irony, the official nutrition recommendations, under the guardianship of Eckel and Lichtenstein, are simultaneously pushing in the opposite direction, toward an ever more saturated-fat-restricted version.

The sum of the evidence against saturated fat over the past half-century amounts to this: the early trials condemning saturated fat were unsound; the epidemiological data showed no negative association; saturated fat's effect on LDL-cholesterol (when properly measured in subfractions) is neutral; and a significant body of clinical trials over the past decade has demonstrated the absence of any negative effect of saturated fat on heart disease, obesity, or diabetes. In other words, every plank in the case against saturated fat has, upon rigorous examination, crumbled away. It seems now that what sustains it is not so much science as generations of bias and habit—although, as the latest 2013 AHA-ACC guidelines show, bias and habit present powerful, if not impenetrable, barriers to change.

The State of Affairs Today

Americans have dutifully followed official dietary advice to restrict fat and animal products for more than sixty years now, ever since the AHA first recommended this diet in 1961 as the best way to avoid heart disease and obesity. Nineteen years later, in 1980, the USDA guidelines joined in. Since then, the government's own data shows that Americans have reduced their consumption of saturated fat by 14 percent and overall fat by 5 percent.* Red meat consumption has steadily declined, replaced by chicken.

---

*Women have been especially obedient followers of these guidelines, consuming at the lowest end of the recommended calorie range, yet they are nevertheless the most overweight and obese (Dietary Guidelines Advisory Committee, 2010, 67 and 69).

According to a USDA report, Americans also complied with official advice to lower the dietary cholesterol found abundantly in egg yolks and shellfish, even though the cholesterol in food has long been known to have little impact on serum cholesterol (as discussed in Chapter 2).* The original rationale for cutting back on fat was to lower serum cholesterol, and Americans have successfully done that, too. Since 1978, total cholesterol levels among US adults have fallen from an average of 213 mg/dL down to 203 mg/dL. The portion of Americans with "high" cholesterol (over 240 mg/dL) has dropped from 26 percent to 19 percent. Moreover, most of that drop has been due to declines in LDL-cholesterol, the target most emphasized by officials for the past thirty years. In 1952, when Ancel Keys first started arguing for the reduced-fat diet, he predicted that if "mankind stopped eating eggs, dairy products, meats and all visible fats," heart disease would "become very rare." This has certainly not been the case.

Indeed, during these years, and despite or perhaps because of these efforts, Americans have experienced skyrocketing epidemics of obesity and diabetes, and the CDC estimates that 75 million Americans now have metabolic syndrome, a disorder of fat metabolism that, if anything, is ameliorated by eating more saturated fat to raise HDL-cholesterol. And although deaths from heart disease have gone down since the 1960s, no doubt due to improved medical treatment, it's not clear that the actual *occurrence* of heart disease has declined much during that time.

Authorities are naturally reluctant to take responsibility for this outcome. The same recent USDA report that documents the public's success in adhering to its dietary guidelines nevertheless places the onus of blame for obesity and disease squarely on American children and adults, "very few" of whom "currently follow the US Dietary Guidelines"—an unsubstantiated assertion that is repeated throughout the report.

The dietary recommendations now offered by the USDA and AHA for solving the nation's health problems are basically: stay the course. Both groups have backed off their limits on fat slightly. The most recent set of

---

*Only in 2013 did Eckel's task force on lifestyle quietly acknowledge, for the first time among US authorities, that there was "insufficient" evidence to support the advice to limit dietary cholesterol (Eckel 2013, 18).

AHA dietary guidelines shifts its dietary fat recommendation from a limit of 30 percent of calories to a range of between 25 percent and 35 percent, arguably a meaningless change to most people. And the USDA's latest *Dietary Guidelines,* published in 2010, scrapped any specific percentile targets for the three main macronutrient groups, protein, fat, and carbohydrates, altogether.* Yet the prohibitions against saturated fats remain strong, and the USDA report continues to take the stance that "healthy diets are high in carbohydrates."

Rates of Obesity in the United States, 1971–2006

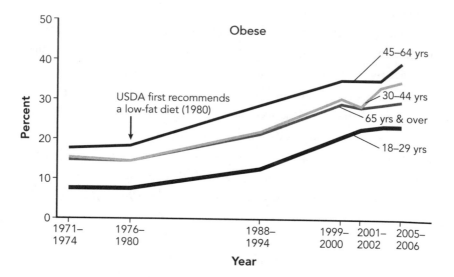

Source: CDC/NCHS, National Health and Nutrition Examination Survey; adapted from "Health, United States, 2008: With Special Feature on the Health of Young Adults," National Center for Health Statistics.

Obesity started rising in America after the USDA first recommended the low-fat, high-carbohydrate diet.

Meanwhile, the same biases that have sustained the diet-heart hypothesis for so many decades remain, and those biases continue to steer the nutrition conversation every step of the way. So, in 2006, when the

---

*The USDA also abandoned its famous food pyramid, opting instead for a simple graphic called "My Plate," which has four sections plus an adjacent white circle, presumably a glass of milk, labeled "dairy." The category of "fats and oils," which used to occupy the tip of the food pyramid, is nowhere to be found.

NINA TEICHOLZ

Women's Health Initiative reported that a low-fat diet made no difference to disease or obesity, the WHI investigators, as well as officials at the AHA and NHLBI, issued press releases stating that this half-a-billion-dollar study had not been conducted well enough to make any conclusions about changing our diets. In 2010, when Krauss's metanalysis came out with good news about saturated fats, the *American Journal of Clinical Nutrition* minimized its impact by publishing the critical editorial by Jerry Stamler as an "introduction" to Krauss's work. And inconvenient findings, such as those by Volek and Westman, continue to be ignored, reasoned away, or misinterpreted by the great majority of nutrition experts.

Moreover, the alliance between the media and the nutrition mainstream endures. Mark Bittman, a food columnist at the *New York Times*, is perhaps the most prominent example of a voice in the media encouraging a diet based on fruits and vegetables while minimizing meat, a mantle he inherited from Jane Brody. Journalists and nutrition authorities also continue to dovetail in amplifying any study finding that appears to condemn either red meat or saturated fat.* And the public gets the message. Americans continue to avoid all fats: the market for "fat replacers," the foodlike substances substituting for fats in processed foods, was, in 2012, still growing at nearly 6 percent per year, with the most common fat replacers being carbohydrate-based.†

---

*A recent example of this emphasis on antimeat studies was the abundance of headlines in 2013 on the finding that a chemical called choline in animal foods might be converted by the liver into the organic compound trimethylamine oxide (TMAO), which appears to cause atherosclerosis in mice. These were small studies, and the media attention given to them seemed disproportionate. *Nature Medicine,* the journal that published the studies, itself appeared to hype them; the cover of the issue in which they were appeared featured a lurid illustration of two dark-skinned, alien-looking restaurant patrons wolfing down steaks. Later, a critic pointed out that the animal foods high in TMAO were not meat and eggs but rather fish and shellfish, and in any case, the evidence connecting TMAO to atherosclerosis in humans was still preliminary. (For studies on TMAO, see Koeth et al. 2013; Wilson Tang et al. 2013. For media coverage, see Kolata April 25, 2013; Kolata April 8, 2013. For "a critic," see Masterjohn April 10, 2013.)

†The low-fat mayonnaise you may buy, for instance, contains a fat replacer to restore the creaminess and rich "mouthfeel" that is lost when fat is removed. The most

If, in recommending that Americans avoid meat, cheese, milk, cream, butter, eggs, and the rest, it turns out that nutrition experts made a mistake, it will have been a monumental one. Measured just by death and disease, and not including the millions of lives derailed by excess weight and obesity, it's very possible that the course of nutrition advice over the past sixty years has taken an unparalleled toll on human history. It now appears that since 1961, the entire American population has, indeed, been subjected to a mass experiment, and the results have clearly been a failure. Every reliable indicator of good health is worsened by a low-fat diet. Whereas diets high in fat have been shown, again and again, in a large body of clinical trials, to lead to improved measures for heart disease, blood pressure, and diabetes, and are better for weight loss. Moreover, it's clear that the original case against saturated fats was based on faulty evidence and has, over the last decade, fallen apart. Despite more than two billion dollars in public money spent trying to prove that lowering saturated fat will prevent heart attacks, the diet-heart hypothesis has not held up.

In the end, what we believe to be true—our conventional wisdom—is really nothing more than sixty years of misconceived nutrition research. Before 1961, there were our ancestors, with their recipes. And before them, there were their ancestors, with their hunting bows or traps or livestock— but like lost languages, lost skills, and lost songs, it takes only a few generations to forget.

---

widely used fat replacers are carbohydrate-based products such as cellulose, malto-dextrins, gums, starches, fiber, and polydextrose.

Conclusion

You may be making yourself miserable three times a day without purpose.
                                    —Edward Pinckney, *The Cholesterol Controversy*, 1973

The advice that comes out of this book is that a higher-fat diet is almost assuredly healthier in every way than one low in fat and high in carbohydrates. The most rigorous science now supports this statement and leads, by simple logic, to the book's other important conclusion, that unless you want to eat like an Italian peasant, drinking bowls of olive oil for breakfast, pretty much the only possible way to consume enough fat for good health is to eat the saturated fats found in animal foods. Practically speaking, this means eating whole fat dairy, eggs, and meat—even fatty meat. In short: all those rich, forbidden foods we've denied ourselves for so long, because these foods are necessarily part of a healthy diet.

Over the past decade, a stack of top-rate scientific studies attesting to the importance of dietary fat has grown to the point where the accumulated body of evidence is nearly undeniable. A high-fat, low-carbohydrate regime has been demonstrated to fight heart disease, obesity, and diabetes; it leads to better health outcomes than does the so-called Mediterranean diet in head-to-head tests; and it performs far better than the standard low-fat approach that has been officially recommended in Western nations for half a century.

That low-fat diet, it turns out, has been terrible for health in every way, as evidenced by skyrocketing rates of obesity and diabetes and the failure to conquer heart disease. Prescribed to the public by the AHA since 1961 to fight heart disease, and then adopted by the USDA in 1980 as the official dietary plan for all men, women, and children, this regime has failed. Rigorous clinical trials, the only kind of science that can demonstrate actual "proof," were a long time in coming after this low-fat advice had already been dispensed to Americans. But over the past decade, a body of these studies has established that a low-fat diet does not fight obesity, heart disease, diabetes, or cancer of any kind. And the low-fat diet tested in these studies wasn't the worst-case version, laden with Snackwell cookies and sugar sodas; it was generally the model of what we are still consistently told to eat today: lots of fruits and vegetables, whole grains, and lean meats.

How is it possible that so many esteemed authorities could have made such an error? The story is long and complex, but it is, like so many other tragic human stories, one of personal ambition and money. This book is full of evidence attesting to these human flaws at work. Yet the misguided nutrition story also has another, more noble element behind it: the passionate desire among high-minded researchers to cure heart disease in America. They wanted to save the nation. It's just that, roughly speaking, they jumped the gun, making official recommendations before proper trials had been conducted* and disregarding those who cautioned that medical interventions should, according to the Hippocratic oath, "first, do no harm."

This original mistake by low-fat diet proponents has been compounded over the years in a number of ways: by billions of dollars spent trying to prove the hypothesis, by vested interests lining up behind it, by research careers coming to depend on it. Biases developed and hardened. Researchers

---

*The low-fat recommendation was instead based on the more impressionistic kind of evidence that comes from epidemiological studies. These kinds of studies have been the source of most of our flip-flopping health advice over the past fifty years, including recommendations for vitamin E supplements, hormone replacement therapy, and yes, the low-fat diet. One of the practical takeaways from this book is therefore that a reader should eye the results from epidemiological studies with a degree of skepticism. The word "association" (often translated in news reports as "linked to") is indicative of this kind of study. A reader might prefer articles with the words "trial," "experiment," or "caused," which are the language of clinical trials.

quoted inadequate studies back and forth to each other, confirming their biases, as if in a hall of mirrors. Critics were sidelined and silenced. And eventually, a universe of nutrition experts came to believe that meat, dairy, and eggs were dangerously unhealthy foods, forgetting that their ancestors had ever milked a cow.

The startling disappointment in 2006 of the largest-ever dietary trial to show any benefits of the low-fat diet has left the nutrition field in a state of near-complete confusion. While authorities now agree that fat overall should not be strictly limited, with the AHA and USDA quietly backing off consumption caps, the most powerful expert panels in the country have nevertheless recently recommended cutting back on the consumption of saturated fats to levels so drastically low as to be nearly unseen in all but the most poverty-stricken chapters of human history.

According to this advice, an ideal diet (low in meat, dairy, and eggs; nearly vegan, in fact) necessarily means obtaining most of one's fat from the only possible alternatives: vegetable and olive oils. Olive oil appears to be fine for health, though it has not successfully been shown to have any particular heart disease–fighting powers, nor does it have the kind of ancient pedigree that has been commonly assumed. However, one of the revelations of this book is that polyunsaturated vegetable oils, when heated to the temperatures required for frying food, create oxidation products that could well be devastating to health. These highly unstable oils are now being used by both fast-food and mom-and-pop restaurants alike to replace trans fats. And this shift might one day be remembered as one of the greatest unintended public health mistakes in the history of manufactured food. Though it would be hard to imagine a greater set of unintended consequences than those resulting from the vast, uncontrolled experiment that the United States and the entire Western world have undergone by adopting a low-fat, high-carbohydrate diet over the past half-century.

The rush to banish animal fats from our diets has exposed us to the health risks of trans fats and oxidizing vegetable oils. If we had not abandoned meat and dairy, we still could still be using lard, suet, tallow, and butter as our principal fats for cooking and eating. These fats are stable, do not oxidize, and have been consumed since the beginning of recorded human history.

Animal fats were originally condemned on the basis of their ability to raise total cholesterol, and later LDL-cholesterol, both biomarkers that turned out to be unreliable predictors of heart attack risk for the great majority of people. The other evidence against saturated fats involved a handful of early, influential clinical trials that were later found not to live up to their original claims. In the end, the case against saturated fat has collapsed.

Moreover, we now know that there are many good reasons to eat animal foods like red meat, cheese, eggs, and whole milk: they are particularly dense in nutrients—far more so than fruits and vegetables. They contain fat and protein in the proportion that humans need. They have been shown to provide the best possible nutrition for healthy growth and reproduction. Saturated fats are also the only foods known to raise HDL-cholesterol, which has shown itself to be a more reliable predictor of heart attacks than LDL-cholesterol. And saturated fats, like all fats, do not make people fat.

Our fear of saturated fats is therefore unsubstantiated. This fear may have seemed reasonable once but persists now only because it fits the preconceptions of researchers, clinicians, and public health authorities; it conforms with their prejudices. Biased researchers writing articles against meat can easily get them into peer-reviewed journals and can count on those findings being promoted by an equally biased media. We've all been living with these biases for so long that it's almost impossible to think otherwise. (I believe it's only been possible for me to write this book, in fact, because I've come to the field of nutrition as an outsider, biased only as much as the average American. And unlike medical or university experts, I'm free from the sorts of pressures they typically confront in order to get their work published, secure research grants, and win promotions.)

We have good reasons for trying to overcome our long-term bias against saturated fats. The science of diet and disease can no longer broker any convincing argument against them. And after all, red meat, cheese, and cream are delicious! Not to mention eggs fried in butter, cream sauces, and the drippings from a pan of roasted meats. The pleasures of these foods are long-forgotten, but they make tasty, deeply satisfying meals. It's recommendable to eat not only the lean meat but the savory fat as well, because it provides the body with much-needed fat and because it also helps offset the

NINA TEICHOLZ

dangers of too much protein, which can lead to nitrogen poisoning if not combined with sufficient fat.

Eat butter; drink milk whole, and feed it to the whole family. Stock up on creamy cheeses, offal, and sausage, and yes, bacon. None of these foods have been demonstrated to cause obesity, diabetes, or heart disease. A large and growing body of recent research now points strongly to the idea that these conditions are caused instead by carbohydrates. Sugar, white flour, and other refined carbohydrates are almost certainly the main drivers of these diseases. Recent scientific research and the historical record all lead to the conclusion that the consumption of refined carbohydrates leads to a higher risk of obesity, heart disease, and diabetes.

These diseases cannot be blamed on genetics: the number of genes associated with them is too large to be meaningful, according to the director of the Human Genome Project, who wrote in 2009 that so many genes were implicated in the development of these chronic diseases that "In pointing at everything, genetics would point at nothing." Nor have any of these diseases been demonstrated in clinical trials to be caused by any other environmental factors. Only carbohydrates have been shown, in clinical experiments, to be the likely principal cause of obesity, heart disease, and diabetes.

I acknowledge that these conclusions seem counterintuitive. They were counterintuitive to me when I started the research for this book. And the implications seem almost impossible to believe, even though they are supported by the best available science: that a beet salad with a fruit smoothie for lunch is ultimately less healthy for your waistline and your heart than a plate of eggs fried in butter. Steak salad is preferable to a plate of hummus and crackers. And a snack of full-fat cheese is better than fruit.

Beyond snacks, we are sorely in need of more foods in the "healthy" column for our main meals, too. Has anyone noticed that a lifetime of dinners comprised merely of vegetables, fish, and pasta is severely limited fare? And fish, since becoming our sole "safe meal," are fast being overfished from the oceans. A broader menu that includes lamb chops, beef stew, and cassoulet would provide some welcome diversity. In sum, the route to higher-fat meals from whole, unprocessed foods is inevitably heaped with animal foods—and that is why humans have taken this path throughout history.

The loss of a historical perspective about our food traditions is perhaps the overriding reason that our nutrition policy has gone so far astray. Authorities tell us that there's "no record" of any long-term "data" on humans eating a diet high in saturated fats, and by this they mean that there are no clinical trials lasting two or more years on a diet high in animal products. But there are four millennia of human history that these experts could have consulted. Cookbooks, histories, diaries, memoirs, novels, food logs, or accounts by missionaries, doctors, explorers, and anthropologists— altogether a virtually limitless number of books, from the Bible to the plays of Shakespeare—which make clear how animal foods made up the core of human meals for thousands of years. During these times, people had shorter life expectancy, true, but they died young of infectious diseases. As adults, their lives and deaths were all but free of the chronic diseases of obesity, diabetes, and heart disease that we die from now; and if they did suffer the latter, it was not at anywhere near the epidemic rates that we do today. From Athena laying down "a fat goat and the chine of a great wild hog rich in lard" for Odysseus, to Isaiah prophesying in the Old Testament that the Lord would "make unto all people a feast of fat things . . . of fat things full of marrow," to Pip's theft of a pork pie in *Great Expectations*, to the historical analyses documenting how Americans in the eighteenth century used to eat three to four times more red meat than they do today, our own written past can tell us a lot. Meat is the central food throughout all of human history, as recorded by humans themselves. We've forgotten our history at our peril.

History tells us that heart disease is interconnected with obesity, diabetes, and other chronic ailments. Known today as metabolic syndrome, this constellation of chronic medical problems used to be called the "obesity sextette," the "Western diseases," the "diseases of civilization," or, in the early 1900s as sugar swept across the English colonies, "the saccharine diseases." As we've seen, conclusions drawn from this history coincide perfectly with results from the best, most careful diet trials of the past decade. The observations line up; there are no paradoxes to explain. And if we can combine the lessons of both science and history, it seems that we may be able to make enlightened decisions about how to start down the path toward curing ourselves of chronic disease.

A Note on Meat and Ethics

In this book, I have not discussed the profound ethical and environmental implications of the conclusions I've drawn from my research. Eating animals gives pause to many people, as it should. Human cultures formerly had elaborate rituals around the act of asking for forgiveness from animals before killing them for food. We no longer have these sacred acts to reconcile us to our biological need for food, and this puts us at a loss. The environmental questions, too, are complicated: cows produce methane, which contributes to greenhouse gases, and they consume a relatively large amount of resources, compared to growing fruits and vegetables, but red meat may be more nutrient-dense per unit of resources consumed and it also provides necessary nutrients not found in plant foods. So it's possible that the greater good health enjoyed by a nation eating more meat might save on health-care costs, thereby evening out the overall ledger. And as a thought experiment: What if we returned to eating tallow and lard again, thereby reducing the demand we place on our land to grow the soybean, rapeseed, cottonseed, safflower, and corn that are expressed into vegetable oils? These questions are all complex and beyond the scope of this book. I have tried to explore here what kinds of dietary fat are good for human health, period. Because America suffers from such a devastating load of chronic disease, the science that relates to this question seemed like a good place to start.

Acknowledgments

This book seized my life for nearly a decade. It sustained me intellectually and fundamentally changed the contours of my thinking, yet it has also been an all-consuming effort that has required enormous support throughout the years from my family. And so it is my husband Gregory, and children, Alexander and Theo, above all, whom I thank. Even as my book intruded on their lives, my boys still embraced it and defended bacon to their teachers. They gave me time for my work ("How many more pages, Mommy?") and fortified me in every way possible. And Gregory, in addition to being a sounding board for my ideas, has been our family's provider, my editor, my cheerleader, my advisor, and my steady love, for which I could not be more grateful. Although he still sneaks gumballs, this book is obviously dedicated to him.

Beyond my family, there are a few people without whom this book never would have been possible. One is my agent and friend Tina Bennett, who has shaped, promoted, and almost single-handedly kept this book alive through the years. Her loyal enthusiasm and abundant kindness are matched by a commanding mastery of every aspect of publishing and a sharp editing eye. She brought wisdom, tact, and the perfect bon mot to every situation, and I could not imagine any aspect of this undertaking without her. Her assistant, Svetlana Katz, has been a warm, resourceful, and astute presence throughout.

Also essential was Emily Loose, who first spotted the book's potential and gave me the confidence that I could write something worthwhile. Then I had the great good fortune to land with my editor Millicent Bennett, who has worked tirelessly to transform my manuscript into a coherent argument. She has been endlessly generous, thoughtful, and tenacious in editing this book. She is a beacon for impeccable standards and logical thinking. My thanks to you, dear Millicent.

The book came out of a story on trans fats assigned by Jocelyn Zuckerman, my smart, effortless editor at *Gourmet*, and then was bravely published by Ruth Reichl. I thank them both for launching me on this journey, which we never could have foreseen. Early on, the people who most opened my eyes to the notion that US nutrition policy might have gone drastically wrong were Mary Enig, Fred Kummerow, and Gary Taubes. Through speaking with them and learning about nutrition science, I began to see the enormous dimensions of this story, which of course appealed to my journalistic instincts. I then entered into what might be called the "complete compulsion" stage of research, during which I felt the need to dig up every last nutrition study from the past sixty years and investigate every lead. For this impulse toward excessive thoroughness, as well as a love of analysis and an independent mind, I thank my parents, Susan and Paul Teicholz. The extent of this compulsion has been wholly my own, however, and is best explained by a desire to get to the bottom of things.

I am deeply thankful to the many officials and researchers in both industry and academia who graciously gave of their time and knowledge to help me along the way. Among those who were especially indefatigable in answering my questions or who offered extraordinary assistance in some way were Tom Applewhite, Christos and Eleni Aravanis, Henry Blackburn, Tanya Blasbalg, Bob Collette, Greg Drescher, Jørn Dyerberg, Ed Emken, Sally Fallon, Anna Ferro-Luzzi, Joe Hibbeln, Stephen Joseph, Ron Krauss, Gil Leveille, Mark Matlock, Gerald McNeill, Michael Mudd, Marion Nestle, Steve Phinney, Uffe Ravnskov, Robert Reeves, Lluís Serra-Majem, Bill Shurtleff, Sara Baer-Sinnott, Allan Sniderman, Jerry Stamler, Steen Stender, Kalyana Sundram, Antonia Trichopoulou, Jeff Volek, Eric Westman, Bob Wainright, Catherine Watkins, Lars Wiedermann, George Wilhite, and Walter Willett. Quite a few of these people will not agree with aspects of this book, but I hope they will recognize my honest endeavor to represent the science fairly, and I thank you all sincerely.

A number of people read all or parts of the book in draft form and offered corrections: Michael Eades, Ron Krauss, George Maniatis, Lydia Maniatis, Stephen Phinney, Chris Ramsden, Jeremy Rosner, David Segal, Christopher Silwood, Gary Taubes, Leslie A. Teicholz, Eric Westman, and Lars Wiedermann. I am extremely grateful to them for their time and for thoughtful attention to the material, as well as the extraordinary efforts that some made to meet deadlines.

I count myself extremely lucky to find a home with Simon & Schuster. Jon Karp has been a warm supporter, Anne Tate is a master of publicity, and Dana Trocker is a spirited marvel of marketing. My superb, hard-working team at S&S also included Alicia Brancato, Mia Crowley-Hald, Gina DiMascia, Suzanne Donahue, Cary Goldstein, Irene Kheradi, Ruth Lee-Mui, and Richard Rhorer. I am deeply grateful to them all, and also to the supremely careful, meticulous team at Dix. My thanks, too, to the ever efficient and lovely Ed Winstead.

My own team of helpers included Linda Sanders, who tracked down hundreds of scientific papers while simultaneously going to medical school, as well as CJ Lotz, Malina Welman, Madeline Blount, and Hannah Bruner. Thank you, also, to Bill and Tia Shuyler for their work on my website and social media.

For their friendship over the years, especially as those years grew longer and friendships more "long-suffering," I am grateful to Ann Banchoff, Cleve Keller, Charlotte Morgan, Sarah Murray, Marge Neuwirth, Lauren Shaffer, David Segal, Jennifer Senior, and Lisa Waltuch. Leaving my writing cave to spend time with you gave me an essential dose of sanity.

Moreover, as any parent of young children knows, it is a luxury to find the time to do work of one's own. I never could have stolen away so many hours with such an easy conscience had it not been for Iulianna Kopanyi and Éva Kobli-Walter, who looked after my boys with devotion and greatly eased my burden in every way.

My deepest thanks go to my family: to my parents, for their endless love and tolerance, to Marc and Leslie for reasons that are too profound to put into words, and again, to Theo, Alexander, and Gregory for being such troupers.

Notes

Introduction

1 *fruits, and vegetables . . . and grains:* Calculated from data in US Department of Agriculture, "Profiling Food Consumption in America," *Agricultural Fact Book 2001–2002* (Washington, DC: US Government Printing Office, 2003), 18–19.

2 *My article received:* Nina Teicholz, "Heart Breaker," *Gourmet,* June 2004, 100–105.

4 *"We were jumped on!":* David Kritchevsky, interview with author, May 31, 2005.

4 *"33 percent of calories or less" . . . "share of those fats that are saturated has also declined":* Centers for Disease Control and Prevention (CDC), "'Trends in Intake of Energy and Macronutrients—United States, 1971–2000," *Morbidity and Mortality Weekly Report* 53, no. 4 (2004): 80–82.

4 *one in seven adult Americans was obese:* US Centers for Disease Control, National Health Examination Survey, 1960–1962, last accessed February 12, 2014, http://www.cdc.gov /nchs/nhanes.htm.

5 *less than 1 percent . . . more than 11 percent:* Maureen I. Harris, "Prevalence of Noninsulin-Dependent Diabetes and Impaired Glucose Tolerance," *Diabetes in America* 6 (1985): 1–31; G. L. Beckles, C. F. Chou, Centers for Disease Control and Prevention, "Diabetes—United States, 2006 and 2010," *Morbidity and Mortality Weekly Report* 62, suppl. 3 (2012): 99–104.

5 *failed to lose weight . . . any major kind of cancer:* Shirley Beresford et al., "Low-Fat Dietary Pattern and Risk of Colorectal Cancer: The Women's Health Initiative Randomized Controlled Dietary Modification Trial," *Journal of the American Medical Association* 295, no. 6 (2006): 643–654. Barbara V. Howard et al., "Low-Fat Dietary Pattern and Weight Change Over 7 Years: The Women's Health Initiative Dietary Modification Trial," *Journal of the American Medical Association* 295, no. 1 (2006): 39–49; Barbara V. Howard et al., "Low-Fat Dietary Pattern and Risk of Cardiovascular Disease: The Women's Health Initiative Randomized Controlled Dietary Modification Trial," *Journal of the American Medical Association* 295, no. 6 (2006): 655–666; Ross L. Prentice et al., "Low-Fat Dietary Pattern and Risk of Invasive Breast Cancer: The Women's Health

Initiative Randomized Controlled Dietary Modification Trial," *Journal of the American Medical Association* 295, no. 6 (2006): 629–642; Ross L. Prentice et al., "Low-Fat Dietary Pattern and Cancer Incidence in the Women's Health Initiative Dietary Modification Randomized Controlled Trial," *Journal of the National Cancer Institute* 99, no. 20 (2007): 1534–1543.

6 *In writing this book:* The author has no conflicts of interest; she has never received any financial or in-kind support, either directly or indirectly, from any party with an interest related to any of the topics covered in this book.

1. The Fat Paradox: Good Health on a High-Fat Diet

9 *Observers estimated that:* Vihjalmur Stefansson, *The Fat of the Land*, enlg. ed. of *Not by Bread Alone* (1946, repr., New York: Macmillan, 1956), 31; calculated by the author from Hugh M. Sinclair, "The Diet of Canadian Indians and Eskimos," *Proceedings of the Nutrition Society* 12, no. 1 (1953): 74.

9 *The fat deposits . . . and the shoulder:* Vihjalmur Stefansson, *The Friendly Arctic: The Story of Five Years in Polar Regions* (New York: Greenwood Press, 1921): 231–232.

9 *The leaner parts:* Vihjalmur Stefansson, *The Fat of the Land*, 25.

9 *"The chief occasion for vegetables . . .":* Ibid., 23.

10 *"no real work":* Stefansson, *The Friendly Arctic*, 24.

10 *"They should have been in a wretched state":* Stefansson, *Fat of the Land*, xvi.

10 *"A storm of protests" . . . "Eating meat raw":* Ibid., 65.

10 *would certainly die:* Ibid., 71.

10 *"The symptoms brought on at Bellevue":* Ibid., 69.

10 *Half a dozen papers published:* Clarence W. Lieb, "The Effects on Human Beings of a Twelve Months' Exclusive Meat Diet Based on Intensive Clinical and Laboratory Studies on Two Arctic Explorers Living under Average Conditions in a New York Climate," *Journal of the American Medical Association* 93, no. 1 (July 6, 1929): 20–22; John C. Torrey, "Influence of an Exclusively Meat Diet on the Human Intestinal Flora," *Proceedings of the Society for Experimental Biology and Medicine* 28, no. 3 (1930): 295–296; Walter S. McClellan, Virgil R. Rupp, and Vincent Toscani, "Prolonged Meat Diets with a Study of the Metabolism of Nitrogen, Calcium, and Phosphorus," *Journal of Biological Chemistry* 87 no. 3 (1930): 669–680; Clarence W. Lieb and Edward Tolstoi, "Effect of an Exclusive Meat Diet on Chemical Constituents of the Blood," *Proceedings of the Society for Experimental Biology and Medicine* 26, no. 4 (1929): 324–325; Edward Tolstoi, "The Effect of an Exclusive Meat Diet Lasting One Year on the Carbohydrate Tolerance of Two Normal Men," *Journal of Biological Chemistry* 83 no. 3 (1929): 747–752; Edward Tolstoi, "The Effect of an Exclusive Meat Diet on the Chemical Constituents of the Blood," *Journal of Biological Chemistry* 83 no. 3 (1929): 753–758.

11 *would drink from 2 to 7 liters of milk each day:* A. Gerald Shaper, "Cardiovascular Studies in the Samburu Tribe of Northern Kenya," *American Heart Journal* 63, no. 4 (1962): 437–442.

11 *Mann found the same with the Masai:* Kurt Biss et al., "Some Unique Biologic Characteristics of the Masai of East Africa," *New England Journal of Medicine* 284, no. 13 (1971): 694–699.

11 *"no vegetable products are taken"*: George V. Mann et al., "Cardiovascular Disease in the Masai," *Journal of Atherosclerosis Research* 4, no. 4 (1964): 289–312.

12 *"These findings hit me very hard"*: A. Gerald Shaper, Interview with Henry Blackburn. In "Preventing Heart Attack and Stroke: A History of Cardiovascular Disease Epidemiology," last accessed February 14, 2014. http://www.epi.umn.edu/cvdepi/interview.asp?id=64.

12 *a review of some twenty-six papers . . . "more or less undisturbed"*: Frank W. Lowenstein, "Blood-Pressure in Relation to Age and Sex in the Tropics and Subtropics: A Review of the Literature and an Investigation in Two Tribes of Brazil Indians," *Lancet* 277, no. 7173 (1961): 389–392. Another study of Bushmen in Kalahari concluded that a "rise in blood pressure is not a characteristic of a normal aging process"; Benjamin Kaminer and W. P. W. Lutz, "Blood Pressure in Bushmen of the Kalahari Desert," *Circulation* 22, no. 2 (1960): 289–295.

12 *subsistence was "easy" . . . "labor light" . . . "seem sedentary"*: Mann, "Cardiovascular Disease in the Masai," 309.

12 *no evidence of a heart attack:* Ibid.

12 *found "possible" signs of heart disease:* A. Gerald Shaper, "Cardiovascular Studies in the Samburu Tribe of Northern Kenya," *American Heart Journal* 63, no. 4 (1962): 439.

12 *on fifty Masai men and found only one:* George V. Mann et al., "Atherosclerosis in the Masai," *American Journal of Epidemiology* 95, no. 1 (1972): 26.

13 *Nor did the Masai suffer from other:* Mann, "Cardiovascular Disease in the Masai, 303–306.

13 *"To eat 'better,' . . . the core of the answer"*: Mark Bittman, "No Meat, No Dairy, No Problem," *New York Times*, December 29, 2011.

13 *The first point on the USDA dietary guidelines:* US Department of Agriculture and US Department of Health and Human Services, *Dietary Guidelines for Americans, 2010*, 7th ed. (Washington, DC. US Government Printing Office, December 2010), viii–ix.

14 *These Indians in the north . . . "in marked contrast"*: Robert McCarrison, *Nutrition and National Health: The Cantor Lectures* (London: Faber and Faber, 1936), 19.

14 *he found that he could reproduce:* Ibid., 24–29.

14 *wrote up his observations in a 460-page report:* Aleš Hrdlička, *Physiological and Medical Observations among the Indians of Southwestern United States and Northern Mexico*, Smithsonian Institution Bureau of American Ethnology Bulletin 34 (Washington, DC: US Government Printing Office, 1908).

14 *were eating a diet predominantly of meat:* Joseph M. Marshall III, *The Day the World Ended at Little Bighorn: A Lakota History* (New York: Penguin Books, 2006).

15 *"no error could account for"*: Hrdlička, *Physiological and Medical Observations*, 40–41.

15 *"not one of these . . . demented or helpless"*: Ibid., 158.

15 *"some seem to assume that it does not exist"*: George Prentice, "Cancer among Negroes," *British Medical Journal* 2, no. 3285 (1923): 1181.

15 *"relative immunity . . . The negroes, when they can get it"*: Ibid.

16 *reported that the meat of the wild animals:* Michael A. Crawford, "Fatty-Acid Ratios in Free-Living and Domestic Animals," *Lancet* 291, no. 7556 (1968): 1329–1333.

17 *"if people had only rabbits . . ."*: John D. Speth, *Bison Kills and Bone Counts: Decision Making by Ancient Hunters* (Chicago: University of Chicago Press, 1983), 151.

17 *half of the fat in a deer kidney:* Sally Fallon Morell and Mary Enig, "Guts and Grease: The Diet of Native Americans," *Wise Traditions in Food, Farming, and the Healing Arts* 2, no. 1 (2001): 43.

17 *a consistent hunting pattern among humans:* Many accounts are collected in Speth, *Bison Kills and Bone Counts,* 146–159: other accounts are in Michael A. Jochim, *Strategies for Survival: Cultural Behavior in an Ecological Context* (New York: Academic Press, 1981), 80–90, and Stefansson, *The Fat of the Land,* 126–131 and 136.

17 *fat was "the determining criteria" when hunting:* Philippe Max Rouja, Éric Dewailly, and Carole Blanchet, "Fat, Fishing Patterns, and Health among the Bardi People of North Western Australia," *Lipids* 38, no. 4 (2003): 399–405.

17 *was considered "rubbish"* . . . *"to be enjoyed":* Ibid., 400.

17 *"tried the meat of horse"* . . . *from five to six pounds* . . . *"continued to grow weak and thin"* . . . *"craving for fat":* Randolph B. Marcy, *The Prairie Traveler: A Handbook for Overland Expeditions* (London: Trubner, 1863): 16.

18 *most of the game "were too lean for use":* Ibid., 152.

2. Why We Think Saturated Fat Is Unhealthy

20 *the prevailing view held that:* Daniel Steinberg, "An Interpretive History of the Cholesterol Controversy: Part 1," *Journal of Lipid Research* 45, no. 9 (2004): 1587.

20 *"defeatist attitude about heart disease":* Ancel Keys, "Atherosclerosis: A Problem in Newer Public Health," *Journal of the Mount Sinai Hospital, New York* 20, no. 2 (1953): 119.

20 *"direct to the point of bluntness":* Henry Blackburn, interview with Ancel Keys, in *Health Revolutionary: The Life and Work of Ancel Keys,* Public Health Leadership Film, Association of Schools of Public Health, last accessed January 5, 2014, http://www.asph.org /document.cfm?page=793.

20 *"to the death"* . . . *"arrogant"* . . . *"ruthless":* Anna Ferro-Luzzi, interview with author, September 18, 2008; George V. Mann, interview with author, October 5, 2005; Michael F. Oliver, interview with author, May 1, 2009.

21 *Keys discovered a passion:* Blackburn, interview with Keys, *Health Revolutionary.*

21 *The K stood for Keys:* Jane Brody, "Dr. Ancel Keys, 100, Promoter of the Mediterranean Diet, Dies," *New York Times,* November 23, 2004.

21 *"biological rust"* . . . *"spread to choke off the flow":* Alton Blakeslee and Jeremiah Stamler, *Your Heart Has Nine Lives: Nine Steps to Heart Health* (New York: Pocket Books, 1966), 24.

21 *One unfortunate girl had a heart attack:* George Lehzen and Karl Knauss, "Über Xanthoma Multiplex Planum, Tuberosum, Mollusciformis," *Archive A, Pathological Anatomy and Histology* 116 (1889): 85–104.

22 *led researchers to believe:* S. J. Thannhauser and Heinz Magendantz, "The Different Clinical Groups of Xanthomatous Diseases: A Clinical Physiological Study of 22 Cases," *Annals of Internal Medicine* 11, no. 9 (1938): 1662–1746.

22 *Anitschkow reported that:* N. Anitschkow, S. Chalatov, C. Müller, and J. B. Duguid, "Über experimentelle Cholesterinsteatose: Ihre Bedeutung für die Enstehung Einiger Pathologischer Prozessen," *Zentralblatt für Allgemeine Pathologie und Pathologische Anatomie* 24 (1913): 1–9.

22 *replicated on all sorts of animals:* Reviewed in Edward H. Ahrens, Jr. et al., "Dietary Control of Serum Lipids in Relation to Atherosclerosis," *Journal of the American Medical Association* 164, no. 17 (1957): 1905–1911.

22 *was widely replicated on all sorts of animals:* On animal models, see, e.g., Edward H. Ahrens Jr. et al., "The Influence of Dietary Fats on Serum-Lipid Levels in Man," *Lancet* 269, no. 6976 (1957): 943–953.

22 *Contemporaries note that rabbits:* Ancel Keys was one of the researchers making this objection; Ancel Keys, "Human Atherosclerosis and the Diet," *Circulation* 5, no. 1 (1952): 115–118.

22 *By contrast, when the experiment:* R. Gordon Gould, "Lipid Metabolism and Athero-sclerosis," *American Journal of Medicine* 11, no. 2 (1951): 209; R. Gordon Gould et al., "Cholesterol Metabolism. I. Effect of Dietary Cholesterol on the Synthesis of Cholesterol in Dog Tissue in Vitro," *Journal of Biological Chemistry* 201, no. 2 (1953), 519.

23 *introduced by two biochemists from Columbia University:* D. Rittenberg and Rudolf Schoenheimer, "Deuterium as an Indicator in the Study of Intermediary Metabolism XI. Further Studies on the Biological Uptake of Deuterium into Organic Substances, with Special Reference to Fat and Cholesterol Formation," *Journal of Biological Chemistry* 121, no. 1 (1937): 235–253.

23 *there was "overwhelming evidence":* Keys, "Human Atherosclerosis and the Diet," 116.

23 *had only a "trivial" effect . . . "requires no further consideration":* Ancel Keys, "Diet and the Epidemiology of Coronary Heart Disease," *Journal of the American Medical Association* 164, no. 17 (1957): 1912–1919. Quote in Ancel Keys et al., "Effects of Diet on Blood Lipids in Man Particularly Cholesterol and Lipoproteins," *Clinical Chemistry* 1, no. 1 (1955): 40.

23 *he later recorded in a book:* Uffe Ravnskov, *The Cholesterol Myths: Exposing the Fallacy that Saturated Fat and Cholesterol Cause Heart Disease* (Washington, DC: New Trends, 2000), 111–112.

23 *has never been shown to have:* Eder Qintão, Scott Grundy, and Edward H. Ahrens, Jr., "Effects of Dietary Cholesterol on the Regulation of Total Body Cholesterol in Man," *Journal of Lipid Research* 12, no. 2 (1971): 233–247; Paul J. Nestel and Andrea Poyser, "Changes in Cholesterol Synthesis and Excretion When Cholesterol Intake Is Increased," *Metabolism* 25, no. 12 (1976): 1591–1599.

23 *one of the most comprehensive analyses:* Paul N. Hopkins, "Effects of Dietary Cholesterol on Serum Cholesterol: A Meta-Analysis and Review," *American Journal of Clinical Nutrition* 55, no. 6 (1992): 1060–1070.

24 *authorities in Britain and most other European nations:* A. Stewart Truswell, "Evolution of Dietary Recommendations, Goals, and Guidelines," *American Journal of Clinical Nutrition* 45, no. 5, suppl. (1987): 1068.

24 *The United States, however, has continued recommending:* Dietary Guidelines Advisory Committee, prepared for the Agricultural Research Service, US Department of Agriculture and US Department of Health and Human Services, *Report of the Dietary Guidelines Advisory Committee on the Dietary Guidelines for Americans, 2010. To the Secretary of Agriculture and the Secretary of Health and Human Services,* 7th ed. (Washington, DC: US Government Printing Office, May 2010), x.

24 *Keys suggested that researchers:* Keys, "Diet and the Epidemiology of Coronary Heart Disease," 1914.

24 *"sleepy old field . . . lipid research" . . . funds . . . each year . . . "lipid research . . . Big Time":* Edward H. Ahrens, Jr., "After 40 Years of Cholesterol-Watching," *Journal of Lipid Research* 25, no. 13 (1984): 1442.

26 *researchers first discovered in 1952:* Lawrence S. Kinsell et al., "Dietary Modification of Serum Cholesterol and Phospholipid Levels," *Journal of Clinical Endocrinology and Metabolism* 12, no. 7 (1952): 909–913.

26 *at Harvard University found:* Mervyn G. Hardinge and Fredrick J. Stare, "Nutritional Studies of Vegetarians: 2. Dietary and Serum Levels of Cholesterol," *Journal of Clinical Nutrition* 2 no. 2 (1954): 82–88.

26 *A Dutch study of vegetarians:* J. Groen, et al., "Influence of Nutrition, Individual, and Some Other Factors, Including Various Forms of Stress, on Serum Cholesterol; Experiment of Nine Months' Duration in 60 Normal Human Volunteers," *Voeding* 13 (1952): 556–587.

26 *found that the saturated fats in butter:* Edward H. Ahrens, Jr., David H. Blankenhorn, and Theodore T. Tsaltas, "Effect on Human Serum Lipids of Substituting Plant for Animal Fat in Diet," *Proceedings for the Society of Experimental Biology and Medicine* 86, no. 4 (1954): 872–878; Ahrens et al., "The Influence of Dietary Fats on Serum-Lipid Levels in Man."

26 *was far more heterogeneity:* Qintão, Grundy, and Ahrens, "Effects of Dietary Cholesterol on the Regulation of Total Body Cholesterol in Man."

26 *one of his most "gratifying contributions":* Ahrens, "After 40 Years of Cholesterol-Watching," 1444.

26 *discovered that the lower-fat diets:* Ancel Keys, Joseph T. Anderson, and Francisco Grande, "Prediction of Serum-Cholesterol Responses of Man to Changes in Fats in the Diet," *Lancet* 273, no. 7003 (1957): 959–966.

26 *"No other variable in the mode of life":* Ancel Keys and Joseph T. Anderson, "The Relationship of the Diet to the Development of Atherosclerosis in Man," *Symposium on Atherosclerosis* (Washington, DC: National Academy of Sciences–National Research Council, 1954), 189.

27 *Keys's graph suggested that:* Keys, "Atherosclerosis: A Problem in Newer Public Health."

29 *Keys thought fat must* make *people fat:* Keys, "Diet and the Epidemiology of Coronary Heart Disease," 1918.

29 *Jerry Seinfeld when he described:* Jerry Seinfeld, *I'm Telling You for the Last Time*, Broadhurst Theatre, New York, 1998.

29 *A lurking fear of fat:* Peter N. Stearns, *Fat History: Beauty in the Modern West* (New York: New York University Press, 1997), 12 and 25–47.

29 *A good portion of his early papers:* Keys, "Diet and the Epidemiology of Coronary Heart Disease," 1913–1914; Ancel Keys and Francisco Grande, "Role of Dietary Fat in Human Nutrition: III. Diet and the Epidemiology of Coronary Heart Disease," *American Journal of Public Health and the Nations Health* 47, no. 12 (1957): 1528–1529.

30 *He and his wife, Margaret . . . the locals' cholesterol:* Keys et al., "Effects of Diet on Blood Lipids in Man," 34–52.

30 *traveled first to Naples then to Madrid:* Ancel Keys et al., "Studies on Serum Cholesterol and Other Characteristics of Clinically Healthy Men in Naples," *A.M.A. Archives of Internal Medicine* 93, no. 3 (March 1954): 328–336; Ancel Keys et al., "Studies on the

Diet, Body Fatness and Serum Cholesterol in Madrid, Spain," *Metabolism Clinical and Experimental* 3, no. 3 (May 1954): 195–212.

30 *It must instead be due to diet:* Keys and Grande, "Role of Dietary Fat in Human Nutrition," 1520–1530.

30 *"only the factor of fat appears":* Keys et al., "Effects of Diet on Blood Lipids in Man," 42.

30 *"dominated by the long-time effects":* Keys, "Diet and the Epidemiology of Coronary Heart Disease," 1912.

30 *"object lesson for the coronary problem":* Ancel Keys, "The Inception and Pilot Surveys," in *The Seven Countries Study: A Scientific Adventure in Cardiovascular Disease Epidemiology,* ed. Daan Kromhout, Alessandro Menotti, and Henry W. Blackburn (Bilthoven, Holland: privately published, 1993): 15–26.

31 *"clearly" a "major factor" . . . of heart disease:* Keys, "Studies on the Diet, Body Fatness and Serum Cholesterol in Madrid, Spain," 209; "major factor" Keys et al., "Studies on the Diet, Body Fatness and Serum Cholesterol in Madrid, Spain," 210.

31 *Keys found further ammunition:* Haqvin Malmros, "The Relation of Nutrition to Health: A Statistical Study of the Effect of the War-Time on Arteriosclerosis, Cardiosclerosis, Tuberculosis and Diabetes," *Acta Medica Scandinavica Supplementum* 138, no. S246 (1950): 137–153. See also, Gotthard Schettler, "Atherosclerosis during Periods of Food Deprivation Following World Wars I and II," *Preventive Medicine* 12, no. 1 (1983): 75–83.

31 *Other scientists noted:* George V. Mann, "Epidemiology of Coronary Heart Disease," *American Journal of Medicine* 23, no. 3 (1957): 463–480.

31 *Keys dismissed them outright:* Ancel Keys, "The Diet and Development of Coronary Heart Disease," *Journal of Chronic Disease* 4, no. 4 (1956): 364–380.

31 *Keys came to this conclusion after conducting:* Keys, Anderson, and Grande, "Prediction of Serum-Cholesterol Responses of Man." Studies are summarized and cited in Ancel Keys, Joseph T. Anderson, and Francisco Grande, "Serum Cholesterol in Man: Diet Fat and Intrinsic Responsiveness," *Circulation* 19, no. 2 (1959): 201.

31 *as Keys announced in a cluster of papers:* Joseph T. Anderson, Ancel Keys, and Francisco Grande, "The Effects of Different Food Fats on Serum Cholesterol Concentration in Man," *Journal of Nutrition* 62, no. 3 (1957); 421–424; Keys, Anderson, and Grande, "Prediction of Serum Cholesterol Responses of Man"; Keys, "Diet and the Epidemiology of Coronary Heart Disease": Ancel Keys, Joseph T. Anderson, and Francisco Grande, "Fats and Disease," *Lancet* 272, no. 6796 (1957): 992–993.

32 *he published a specific mathematical formula:* Keys, Anderson, and Grande, "Serum Cholesterol in Man: Diet Fat and Intrinsic Responsiveness."

32 *"become very rare" . . . "sharp reduction":* E. V. Allen et al., "Atherosclerosis: A Symposium," *Circulation* 5, no. 1 (1952): 99.

32 *he had secured an appointment:* Kromhout, Menotti, and Blackburn, eds., *The Seven Countries Study,* 196.

32 *Keys is the only researcher he mentions by name:* Ibid., 76.

32 *he switched to . . . ate melba toast:* Paul Dudley White, "Heart Ills and Presidency: Dr. White's Views," *New York Times,* October 30, 1955, A1.

32 *"a rich fatty diet" . . . "probable" cause . . . "majority of cases":* Keys, "Diet and the Epidemiology of Coronary Heart Disease," 1912.

34 *Yerushalmy's objection:* Jacob Yerushalmy and Herman E. Hilleboe, "Fat in the Diet and Mortality from Heart Disease: A Methodologic Note," *New York State Journal of Medicine* 57, 14 (1957): 2343–2354.

35 *"I remember the mood in the lab":* Henry Blackburn, interview with author, November 9, 2008.

35 *Mann wrote of his hope:* George V. Mann, "Diet and Coronary Heart Disease," *Archives of Internal Medicine* 104 (1959): 921–929.

35 *national statistics were unreliable:* Ancel Keys, "Epidemiologic Aspects of Coronary Artery Disease," *Journal of Chronic Diseases* 6, no. 4 (1957): 552–559.

35 *an investigation from 1964:* D. D. Reid and G. A. Rose, "Preliminary Communications: Assessing the Comparability of Mortality Statistics," *British Medical Journal* 2, no. 5422 (1964): 1437–1439.

36 *Keys was fully aware:* Keys, *Symposium on Atherosclerosis,* 119.

36 *"negative versus positive":* Ancel Keys, "Epidemiologic Aspects of Coronary Artery Disease," 552.

36 *remembers Blackburn:* Henry W. Blackburn, interview with author, July 22, 2008.

37 *Keys launched the study . . . an annual grant:* "The Fat of the Land," *Time,* January 13, 1961, 48–52.

37 *A number of critics have since pointed out:* Ravnskov, *The Cholesterol Myths,* 18–19; Gary Taubes, *Good Calories, Bad Calories: Fats, Carbs and the Controversial Science of Diet and Health* (New York: Alfred A. Knopf, 2007), 32.

37 *as he wrote, he chose places that he thought:* Alessandro Menotti, email message to author, September 10, 2008.

37 *"where he found enthusiastic help":* Menotti, email message to author, September 10, 2008; Flaminio Fidanza, another original team member on the Seven Countries study, confirmed this assessment: Flaminio Fidanza, email message to author, September 16, 2008.

37 *"Keys just had a personal aversion":* Blackburn, interview.

38 *at least 150,000 Greeks:* George S. Siampos, *Recent Population Change Calling for Policy Action: With Special Reference to Fertility and Migration* (Athens: National Statistical Service of Greece, 1980): 234–257.

38 *monograph published by the AHA:* Ancel Keys, ed., "Coronary Heart Disease in Seven Countries," *Circulation* 61 and 62, suppl. 1, American Heart Association Monograph No. 29 (1970): I-1–I-211.

38 *a book from Harvard University Press:* Ancel Keys, *Seven Countries: A Multivariate Analysis of Death and Coronary Heart Disease* (Cambridge, MA: Harvard University Press, 1980).

38 *according to one tally:* Calculation by John Aravanis, M.D., from personal communication with his father, Christos Aravanis, who directed the Greek portion of the Seven Countries Study.

38 *the number was ridiculously low . . . was 290:* Keys, *Seven Countries: A Multivariate Analysis,* 65.

39 *"heart attacks might be prevented":* Quoted in Jane E. Brody, "Dr. Ancel Keys, 100, Promoter of Mediterranean Diet, Dies," *New York Times,* November 23, 2004.

39 *Saturated fat comprised:* Keys, "Coronary Heart Disease in Seven Countries."

39 *even more paradoxical:* Ancel Keys et al., "The Seven Countries Study: 2,289 Deaths in 15 Years," *Preventive Medicine* 13, no. 2 (1984): 141–154.

40 *"The Greek Orthodox fast is a strict one . . . eggs and butter":* Leland Girard Allbaugh, *Crete: A Case Study of an Underdeveloped Area* (Princeton, NJ: Princeton University Press, 1953), 103.

40 *the expression "pari corajisima":* Vito Teti, "Food and Fatness in Calabria," in *Social Aspects of Obesity,* ed. Igor de Garine and Nancy J. Pollock, trans. Nicolette S. James (Amsterdam: Gordon and Breach, 1995), 13.

40 *A study conducted on Crete:* Katerina Sarri et al., "Greek Orthodox Fasting Rituals: A Hidden Characteristic of the Mediterranean Diet of Crete," *British Journal of Nutrition* 92, no. 2 (2004): 277–284.

40 *"strict adherence [to Lent] did not seem to be common":* Keys, "Coronary Heart Disease in Seven Countries," I-166.

40 *made no mention of the issue at all:* Ancel Keys, Christos Aravanis, and Helen Sdrin, "The Diets of Middle-Aged Men in Two Rural Areas of Greece," *Voeding* 27, no. 11 (1966): 575–586.

40 *"no attempt was made" . . . "a remarkable and troublesome omission":* Katerina Sarri and Anthony Kafatos, letter to the editor, "The Seven Countries Study in Crete: Olive Oil, Mediterranean Diet or Fasting?" *Public Health Nutrition* 8, no. 6 (2005): 666.

41 *"we should not" . . . "the ideal thing all the time":* Daan Kromhout, interview with author, October 4, 2007.

41 *he knew it would go unnoticed:* Keys, Aravanis, and Sdrin, "Diets of Middle-Aged Men in Two Rural Areas of Greece," 577.

42 *category of foods . . . which had a correlation coefficient:* Alessandro Menotti et al., "Food Intake Patterns and 25-Year Mortality from Coronary Heart Disease: Cross-Cultural Correlations in the Seven Countries Study," *European Journal of Epidemiology* 15, no. 6 (1999): 507–515.

42 *"too troublesome" to recode:* Alessandro Menotti, interview with author, July 24, 2008.

42 *"Keys was very opposed to the sugar idea":* Kromhout, interview.

43 *"He was so convinced that fatty acids" . . . "own point of view":* Ibid.

43 *"mountain of nonsense":* Ancel Keys, "Sucrose in the Diet and Coronary Heart Disease," *Atherosclerosis* 14, no. 2 (1971): 200.

43 *"Yudkin and his commercial backers":* Ancel Keys and Margaret Keys, *How to Eat Well and Stay Well the Mediterranean Way* (Garden City, NY: Doubleday, 1975), 58.

43 *Keys published these numbers:* Ancel Keys, "Letter to the Editors," *Atherosclerosis* 18, no. 2 (1973): 352.

43 *"Sugar was never discussed properly":* Menotti, interview.

44 Time *magazine reported:* "Medicine: The Fat of the Land," *Time,* January 13, 1961.

3. The Low-Fat Diet Is Introduced to America

47 *small and underfunded . . . virtually no income:* William W. Moore, *Fighting for Life: A History of the American Heart Association 1911–1975* (Dallas: American Heart Association, 1983): 43.

47   *Procter & Gamble (P&G) designated:* H. M. Marvin, *1924–1964: The 40 Year War on Heart Disease* (New York: American Heart Association, 1964), adapted from an address originally presented before officers of affiliated Heart Associations in 1956.

48   *"suddenly the coffers were filled . . . dreams are made of!":* Ibid., 51.

48   *"bang of big bucks" . . . "launched":* Ibid.

48   *seven chapters . . . $2,650,000:* Ibid., 56.

48   *three hundred chapters . . . $30 million annually:* Moore, *Fighting for Life,* 77; *$30 million:* Marvin, *1924–1964: The 40 Year War on Heart Disease.*

48   *AHA took in 40 percent more:* Moore, *Fighting for Life,* 72.

49   *"People want to know":* Irvine Page et al., "Atherosclerosis and the Fat Content of the Diet," *Circulation* 16, no. 2 (1957): 164.

49   *"uncompromising stands based on evidence":* Ibid.

49   *"the best scientific evidence available":* Irvine Page et al., "Dietary Fat and Its Relation to Heart Attacks and Strokes," *Circulation* 23, no. 1 (1961): 133–136.

50   *"some undue pussy-footing":* "Medicine: The Fat of the Land," *Time,* January 13, 1961.

51   *tucking into scrambled eggs:* Hans H. Hecht, letter to Jeremiah Stamler, February 10, 1969, in author's possession.

51   *"Middle Aged Men Cautioned on Fat":* Murray Illson, "Middle-Aged Men Cautioned on Fat: Heart Attacks Linked to Diet as well as Overweight and High Blood Pressure," *New York Times,* October 24, 1959, 23.

52   *the* New York Times *reported:* "Heart Unit Backs Reduction in Fat," *New York Times,* December 11, 1960, 1.

52   *"whereas people once thought":* Jonathan Probber, "Is Nothing Sacred? Milk's American Appeal Fades," *New York Times,* February 18, 1987.

52   *"mass murder":* Quoted in William Borders, "New Diet Decried by Nutritionists: Dangers Are Seen in Low Carbohydrate Intake," *New York Times,* July 7, 1965.

52   *One article she wrote in 1985:* Jane E. Brody, "America Leans to a Healthier Diet," *New York Times Magazine,* October 13, 1985.

53   *his team identified . . . Zukel could find no difference:* William J. Zukel et al., "A Short-Term Community Study of the Epidemiology of Coronary Heart Disease: A Preliminary Report on the North Dakota Study," *American Journal of Public Health and the Nation's Health* 49, no. 12 (1959): 1630–1639.

54   *In Ireland, researchers analyzed:* Aileen Finegan et al., "Diet and Coronary Heart Disease: Dietary Analysis on 100 Male Patients," *American Journal of Clinical Nutrition* 21, no. 2 (1968): 143–148.

54   *on fifty middle-aged women:* Aileen Finegan et al., "Diet and Coronary Heart Disease: Dietary Analysis on 50 Female Patients," *American Journal of Clinical Nutrition* 21, no. 1 (1969): 8–9.

54   *Malhotra studied the disease:* S. L. Malhotra, "Epidemiology of Ischaemic Heart Disease in Southern India with Special Reference to Causation," *British Heart Journal* 29, no. 6 (1967): 898; S. L. Malhotra, "Geographical Aspects of Acute Myocardial Infarction in India with Special Reference to Patterns of Diet and Eating," *British Heart Journal* 29, no. 3 (1967): 337–344.

55   *"eat more fermented milk products":* S. L. Malhotra, "Dietary Factors and Ischaemic Heart Disease," *American Journal of Clinical Nutrition* 24, no. 10 (1971): 1197.

55 *had a "strikingly low"* . . . *amounts of animal fats:* Clarke Stout et al., "Unusually Low Incidence of Death from Myocardial Infarction: Study of Italian American Community in
Pennsylvania," *Journal of the American Medical Association* 188, no. 10 (1964): 845–849.

55 *The majority of the 179 Roseto men . . . the years of the survey:* Ibid.

55 *"extravagant worldwide publicity":* Ancel Keys, "Arteriosclerotic Heart Disease in Roseto,
Pennsylvania," *Journal of the American Medical Association* 195 no. 2 (1966): 137–139.

55 *Keys concluded that the Roseto data:* Ibid., 139.

56 *collected every study he could find:* Frank W. Lowenstein, "Epidemiologic Investigations
in Relation to Diet in Groups Who Show Little Atherosclerosis and Are Almost Free
of Coronary Ischemic Heart Disease," *American Journal of Clinical Nutrition* 15, no. 3
(1964): 175–186.

56 *The* type *of fat also varied dramatically:* Ibid.

56 *Resisting these "idols of the mind":* Francis Bacon, *Novum Organum Scientiarum*, England, 1620, Book 1: XXXIV.

57 *Karl Popper, described:* Karl Popper, *Objective Knowledge: An Evolutionary Approach*, rev.
ed. (Oxford: Clarendon Press, 1979), 81.

57 *Dozens of trials:* Early clinical trials that did not support the diet-heart hypothesis: A
Research Committee, "Low-Fat Diet in Myocardial Infarction: A Controlled Trial,"
Lancet 2, no. 7411 (1965): 501–504; Research Committee to the Medical Research
Council, "Controlled Trial of Soya-bean Oil in Myocardial Infarction," *Lancet* 2,
no. 7570 (1968): 693–699; J. M. Woodhill et al., "Low Fat, Low Cholesterol Diet in
Secondary Prevention of Coronary Heart Disease," *Advances in Experimental Medicine
and Biology* 109 (1978): 317–330; Marvin L. Bierenbaum et al., "Modified-Fat Dietary
Management of the Young Male with Coronary Disease," *Journal of the American Medi-
cal Association* 202, no. 13 (1967): 59–63.

58 *Ahrens was objecting:* Aherns et al., "Dietary Control of Serum Lipids in Relation to
Atherosclerosis," 1906.

58 *"Silic acid chromatography":* Jules Hirsch and Edward H. Ahrens, Jr., "The Separation of
Complex Lipide Mixtures by Use of Silic Acid Chromatography," *Journal of Biological
Chemistry* 233, no. 2 (1958): 311–320.

58 *consistently revealed that these triglycerides:* Edward H. Ahrens, Jr. et al., "The Influence of
Dietary Fats on Serum-Lipid Levels in Man," *Lancet* 272, no. 6976 (1957): 943–953;
Edward H. Ahrens, Jr. et al., "Carbohydrate-Induced and Fat-Induced Lipemia,"
Transactions of the Association of American Physicians 74 (1961): 134–146; J. L. Knittle
and Edward H. Ahrens, Jr., "Carbohydrate Metabolism in Two Forms of Typerglyceri-
demia," *Journal of Clinical Investigation* 43 (1964): 485–495; Edward H. Aherns, Jr.,
"Carbohydrates, Plasma Triglycerides, and Coronary Heart Disease," *Nutrition Reviews*
44, no. 2 (1986): 60–64.

58 *high triglyceride levels were far more common:* Margaret J. Albrink, "The Significance of
Serum Triglycerides," *Journal of the American Dietetic Association* 42 (1963): 29–31.

58 *a handful of researchers confirmed:* P. T. Kuo et al., "Dietary Carbohydrates in Hyperlipemia (Hyperglyceridemia); Hepatic and Adipose Tissue Lipogenic Activities," *American
Journal of Clinical Nutrition* 20, no. 2 (1967): 116–125; L. E. Bottiger and L. A. Carlson, "Serum Glucoproteins in Men with Myocardial Infarction," *Journal of Atherosclerosis Research* 1 (1961): 184–188.

58 *Ahrens found that triglycerides:* Edward H. Ahrens, Jr. et al., "Carbohydrate-Induced and Fat-Induced Lipemia," *Transactions of the Association of American Physicians* 74 (1961): 136.

58 *whereas a contrasting vial:* Ibid.

59 *"normal chemical process which occurs":* Ibid., 134.

59 *impoverished people in rural Japan . . . were found to have low triglycerides:* Ancel Keys and Noboru Kimora, "Diets of Middle-Aged Farmers in Japan," *American Journal of Clinical Nutrition* 23, no. 2 (1970): 219.

59 *Albrink sketched out a scenario:* Margaret J. Albrink, "Triglycerides, Lipoproteins, and Coronary Artery Disease," *Archives of Internal Medicine* 109, no. 3 (1962): 345–359.

60 *"But let's talk . . . No, we're researching this" . . . "He always opposed any statement":* Jeremiah Stamler, interview with author, April 22, 2009.

61 *"And Yudkin!" . . . "scoundrel":* Ibid.

61 *Raymond Reiser wrote:* Raymond Reiser, "Saturated Fat in the Diet and Serum Cholesterol Concentration: A Critical Examination of the Literature," *American Journal of Clinical Nutrition* 26, no. 5 (1973): 524–555.

61 *a* twenty-four *page reply:* Ancel Keys, Francisco Grande, and Joseph T. Anderson, "Bias and Misrepresentation Revisited: 'Perspective' on Saturated Fat," *American Journal of Clinical Nutrition* 27, no. 2 (1974): "distorting mirrors," 188; "typical distortion," 191; "16-word sentence," 189; "pompously states," 209; "completely ignores," 209; "no comprehension," 209.

61 *he defended the . . . short letter:* Raymond Reiser, "Saturated Fat: A Rebuttal," *American Journal of Clinical Nutrition* 27, no. 3 (1974): 229.

62 *wound up confirming his findings:* Kurt Biss et al., "Some Unique Biologic Characteristics of the Masai of East Africa," *New England Journal of Medicine* 284, no. 13 (1971): 694–699.

62 *cholesterol numbers were fully a quarter higher:* José Day et al., "Anthropometric, Physiological and Biochemical Differences between Urban and Rural Maasai," *Atherosclerosis* 23, no. 2 (1976): 357–361.

62 *"nomads have no relevance":* Ancel Keys, "Coronary Heart Disease—The Global Picture," *Atherosclerosis* 22, no. 2 (1975): 153.

62 *he thought were a better reference point:* Ancel Keys and Margaret Keys, *How to Eat Well and Stay Well the Mediterranean Way* (Garden City, NY: Doubleday, 1975), xi.

63 *"a path of garlands" . . . "And what a fall!":* Vihjalmur Stefansson, *The Fat of the Land,* enlg. ed. of *Not by Bread Alone* (1946, repr., New York: Macmillan, 1956), xxx.

63 *"bizarre manner of life" . . . "on blubber" . . . "no grounds" . . . "demonstrate an exception":* Ancel Keys, "Diet and the Epidemiology of Coronary Heart Disease," *Journal of the American Medical Association* 164, no. 17 (1957): 1913.

63 *"good or bad for you?" . . . " 'choice' cuts":* Fredrick J. Stare, Comment in *The Fat of the Land,* xxxi.

64 *ends by recommending:* Ibid., xii.

64 *announced their first big discovery:* William B. Kannel et al., "Factors of Risk in Development of Coronary Heart Disease—Six-Year Follow-up Experience. The Framingham Study," *Annals of Internal Medicine* 55, no. 1 (1961): 33–50.

65 *"somehow intimately related"*: "Findings of Framingham Diet Study Clarified," *The News*, Framingham-Natick, Friday, October 30, 1970, 36.

65 *total cholesterol was not nearly as strong*: Keaven M. Anderson, William P. Castelli, Daniel Levy, "Cholesterol and Mortality: 30 Years of Follow-up from the Framingham Study," *Journal of the American Medical Association* 257 no. 16 (1987): 2176–2180.

65 *could be found*: Carl C. Seltzer, "The Framingham Heart Study Shows No Increases in Coronary Heart Disease Rates from Cholesterol Values of 205–264 mg/dL," *Giornale Italiano di Cardiologia* (Padua) 21, no. 6 (1991): 683.

65 *In fact, half of the people . . . :* Anderson, Castelli, and Levy, "Cholesterol and Mortality."

66 *"There is an 11% increase":* Ibid., 2176.

66 *many large trials have found similar results:* Among them are M. M. Gertler et al., "Long-Term Follow-up Study of Young Coronary Patients," *American Journal of Medical Sciences* 247, no. 2 (1964): 153; Charles W. Frank, Eve Weinblatt, and Sam Shapiro, "Angina Pectoris in Men," *Circulation* 47, no. 3 (1973): 509–517; Risteard Mulcahy et al., "Factors Influencing Long-Term Prognosis in Male Patients Surviving a First Coronary Attack," *British Heart Journal* 37, no. 2 (1975): 158–165.

66 *study that Mann conducted*: George V. Mann et al., "Diet and Cardiovascular Disease in the Framingham Study I. Measurement of Dietary Intake," *American Journal of Clinical Nutrition* 11, no. 3 (1962): 200–225.

66 *"No relationship found"*: William B. Kannel and Tavia Gordon, "The Framingham Study: an Epidemiological Investigation of Cardiovascular Disease," Section 24, unpublished paper (Washington, DC: National Heart, Lung, and Blood Institute, 1987).

66 *"That went over . . . wanted us to find"*: George V. Mann, interview with author, October 5, 2005.

67 *"a form of cheating"*: George V. Mann, "A Short History of the Diet/Heart Hypothesis," in *Coronary Heart Disease: The Dietary Sense and Nonsense. An Evaluation by Scientists*, ed. George V. Mann for the Veritas Society (London: Janus, 1993), 9.

67 *"the more saturated fat one ate"*: William P. Castelli, "Concerning the Possibility of a Nut . . ." *Archives of Internal Medicine* 152, no. 7 (1992): 1371–1372 (emphasis added).

67 *the problem must have been one of imprecise collection*: William P. Castelli, interview with author, March 16, 2007.

67 *An article he wrote*: George V. Mann, "Diet-Heart: End of an Era," *New England Journal of Medicine* 297, no. 12 (1977): 644–650.

67 *"pretty devastating . . . she was right . . . forceful and persuasive"*: Mann, interview.

68 *they jointly reported "to the nation"*: "National Heart, Lung, & Blood Institute: Important Events in NHLBI History," NIH Almanac 1999, http://www.nih.gov/about/almanac/archive/1999/organization/nhlbi/history.html.

68 *AHA president worked closely*: Moore, *Fighting for Life*, 99 and 271.

69 *the same names continually come up*: "National Heart, Lung, & Blood Institute: Important Events in NHLBI History," *NIH Almanac* 1999, last accessed February 15, 2014, http://www.nih.gov/about/almanac/archive/1999/organization/nhlbi/history.html.

70 AHA presidents *"almost routinely"* directed: Moore, *Fighting for Life*, 98. See also, 271–276.

70 *White helped found:* "The International Society of Cardiology (ISC) and CVD Epidemiology," Division of Epidemiology & Community Health of the School of Public Health, University of Minnesota, http://www.epi.umn.edu/cvdepi/essay.asp?id=186.

70 *$1.5 billion . . . heart disease research:* Henry Blackburn, "Ancel Keys Lecture: The Three Beauties, Bench, Clinical, and Population Research," *Circulation* 86, no. 4 (1992), 1323.

70 *$100 million a year toward original research:* Jan L. Breslow, "Why You Should Support the American Heart Association!" *Circulation* 94, no. 11 (1996): 3016–3022.

70 *"This was a daunting task":* George V. Mann, "A Short History of the Diet/Heart Hypothesis," 12.

71 *"almost embarrassingly high number":* "Coronary Heart Disease and Carbohydrate Metabolism," editorial, *Journal of the American Medical Association* 201, no. 13 (1967): 164–165.

71 *"supported the dogma" . . . "more political than scientific":* George V. Mann, "Coronary Heart Disease—The Doctor's Dilemma," *American Heart Journal* 96, no. 5 (1978), 569.

4. The Flawed Science of Saturated versus Polyunsaturated Fats

72 *"causal relationships are not claimed":* Ancel Keys et al., "The Diet and 15-Year Death Rate in the Seven Countries Study," *American Journal of Epidemiology* 124, no. 6 (1986): 903–915.

73 *Anti-Coronary Club:* Norman Jolliffe, S. H. Rinzler, and M. Archer, "The Anti-Coronary Club: Including a Discussion of the Effects of a Prudent Diet on the Serum Cholesterol Level of Middle-aged Men," *American Journal of Clinical Nutrition* 7, no. 4 (1959): 451–462.

73 *and instructed them to reduce their consumption:* George Christakis et al., "Summary of the Research Activities of the Anti-Coronary Club," *Public Health Reports* 81, no. 1 (1966): 64–70.

74 *reported the* New York Times: Robert K. Plumb, "Diet Linked to Cut in Heart Attacks," *New York Times*, May 17, 1962, 39.

74 *"somewhat unusual" . . . risk factors . . . result was buried:* George Christakis et al., "Effect of the Anti-Coronary Club Program on Coronary Heart Disease Risk-Factor Status," *Journal of the American Medical Association* 198, no. 6 (1966): 597–604.

75 *Los Angeles Veterans Trial:* Seymour Dayton et al., "A Controlled Clinical Trial of a Diet High in Unsaturated Fat in Preventing Complications of Atherosclerosis," *Circulation* 40, no. 1, suppl. 2 (1969): II-1.

75 *died of cancer:* Morton Lee Pearce and Seymour Dayton, "Incidence of Cancer in Men on a Diet High in Polyunsaturated Fat," *Lancet* 297, no. 7697 (1971): 464–467.

75 *"Was it not possible" . . . "that a diet":* Dayton et al., "A Controlled Clinical Trial of a Diet High in Unsaturated Fat," II-2.

75 *In fact, the upward curve of vegetable oil consumption:* Tanya Blasbalg et al., "Changes in Consumption of Omega-3 and Omega-6 Fatty Acids in the United States during the 20th Century," *American Journal of Clinical Nutrition* 93, no. 5 (2011): 950–962.

76 *The* Lancet, *wrote a withering critique:* "Diet and Atherosclerosis," editorial, *Lancet* 294, no. 7627 (1969): 939–940.

76 *defended his study in a letter:* Pearce and Dayton, "Incidence of Cancer in Men on a Diet High in Polyunsaturated Fat," 464–467.

76 *a top nutrition expert:* Barbara V. Howard, interview with author, June 13, 2005.

77 *"exerted a substantial preventive effect":* Osmo Turpeinen et al., "Dietary Prevention of Coronary Heart Disease: The Finnish Mental Hospital Study," *International Journal of Epidemiology* 8, no. 2 (1979): 99–118.

77 *But a closer look reveals:* Matti Miettinen et al., "Effect of Cholesterol-Lowering Diet on Mortality from Coronary Heart-Disease and Other Causes: A Twelve-Year Clinical Trial in Men and Women," *Lancet* 300, no. 7782 (1972): 835–838.

77 *criticize the study in a letter:* M. Halperin, Jerome Cornfield, and S. C. Mitchell, "Letters to the Editor: Effect of Diet on Coronary-Heart-Disease Mortality," *Lancet* 302, no. 7826 (1973): 438–439.

77 *"not ideal" . . . "may perhaps never be performed" . . . "we do not see":* Matti Miettinen et al., "Effect of Diet on Coronary-Heart-Disease Mortality," *Lancet* 302, no. 7840 (1973): 1266–1267.

78 *divided his subjects into two groups:* Paul Leren, "The Effect of Plasma Cholesterol Lowering Diet in Male Survivors of Myocardial Infarction: A Controlled Clinical Trial," *Acta Medica Scandinavica Supplementum* 466 (1966): 1–92.

78 *a traditional Norwegian diet . . . 40 percent fat:* Ibid., 35.

78 *"cholesterol-lowering" diet:* Ibid., 27.

78 *the diets contained about the same amount of fat:* Ibid., 82.

78 *"not with enthusiasm":* Ibid., 30.

78 *Leren published his findings:* Ibid.

78 *eating a great deal of hard margarine and hydrogenated fish oils:* Ibid., 35.

81 *Swift & Co. would make custom margarines:* National Diet-Heart Study Research Group, "The National Diet Heart Study Final Report," *American Heart Association Monograph* 18 in *Circulation* 37 and 38, suppl. 1 (1968): Appendix 1b: I-7.

81 *Stamler remembers:* Jeremiah Stamler, interview with author, April 22, 2009.

81 *Hamburger patties and hot dogs . . . two normal eggs:* National Diet-Heart Study Research Group, "The National Diet Heart Study Final Report," I-100–I-116.

81 *various confirmation tests:* Ibid., I-10–I-11.

81 *"A housewife would order . . . done so well":* Stamler, interview, April 22, 2009.

82 *researchers studied the Israelis:* S. H. Blondheim et al., "Unsaturated Fatty Acids in Adipose Tissue of Israeli Jews," *Israel Journal of Medical Sciences* 12, no. 7 (1976): 658.

82 *to promoting a "prudent" diet:* Stamler, interview, April 22, 2009.

82 *according to two scholarly estimates:* Blasbalg et al., "Changes in Consumption of Omega-3 and Omega-6 Fatty Acids," 950–962; Penny M. Kris-Etherton et al., "Polyunsaturated Fatty Acids in the Food Chain in the United States," *American Journal of Clinical Nutrition* 71, no. 1, suppl. (2000). 179S–188S.

83 *AHA currently recommends:* William S. Harris et al., "Omega-6 Fatty Acids and Risk for Cardiovascular Disease: A Science Advisory from the American Heart Association Nutrition Subcommittee of the Council on Nutrition, Physical Activity, and Metabolism; Council on Cardiovascular Nursing; and Council on Epidemiology and Prevention," *Circulation* 199, no. 6 (2009): 902–907.

83 *more than a few experiments:* Studies are listed in Hans Kaunitz and Ruth E. Johnson, "Exacerbation of the Heart and Liver Lesions in Rats by Feeding Various Mildly Oxidized Fats, *Lipids* 8, no. 6 (1973): 329–336. The most well-known experiment was G. A. Rose, W. B. Thompson, and R. T. Williams, "Corn Oil in Treatment of Ischaemic Heart Disease," *British Medical Journal* 1, no. 5449 (1965): 1531–1533.

84 *cottonseed and some sesame oils . . . Thomas Jefferson tried:* David S. Shields, "Prospecting for Oil," *Gastronomica* 10, no. 4 (2010): 25–34.

85 *"has become a stampede":* Karl Robe, "Focus Gets Clearer on Confused Food Oil Picture," *Food Processing* (December 1961): 62.

85 *"higher and higher amounts of polyunsaturated oils":* Ibid.

86 *Stamler reissued his 1963 book . . . "significant" research support:* Alton Blakeslee and Jeremiah Stamler, *Your Heart Has Nine Lives: Nine Steps to Heart Health* (New York: Pocket Books, 1966).

86 *"must make alliances with":* Stamler, interview, April 22, 2009.

88 *massive advertising campaign:* Gary R. List and M. A. Jackson, "Giants of the Past: The Battle over Hydrogenation (1903–1920)," *Inform* 18, no. 6 (2007): 404.

88 *"new" . . . "better" . . . "shock . . . less progressive" . . . modern woman . . . "Grandmother". . . . "spinning wheel":* Procter & Gamble Company, "The Story of Crisco," in *The Story of Crisco: 250 Tested Recipes* by Marion Harris Neil (Cincinnati, OH: Procter & Gamble, 1914), 6 (italics in original).

88 *easier to digest:* Ibid., 5.

88 *"sparkling bright rooms" . . . "metal surfaces":* Ibid., 10.

88 *"lardy" flavor . . . "true taste":* Ibid., 11.

88 *"Kitchen odors":* Ibid., 12.

88 *forty times in merely four years:* F. J. Massiello, "Changing Trends in Consumer Margarines," *Journal of the American Oil Chemists Society* 55, no. 2 (1978): 262–265.

89 *one and a half billion . . . sixty-five plants . . . eighth-ranking . . . always in the lead:* "Focus," *Journal of the American Oil Chemists Society* 61, no. 9 (1984): 1434.

89 *" 'Crisco' written in their place":* Procter & Gamble, in *The Story of Crisco*, 6.

89 *"the ingenuity of depraved human genius":* Quoted in Richard A. Ball and J. Robert Lilly, "The Menace of Margarine: The Rise and Fall of a Social Problem," *Social Problems* 29, no. 5 (1982): 492.

89 *to call margarine manufacturers "swindlers":* Eugene O. Porter, "Oleomargarine: Pattern for State Trade Barriers," *Southwestern Social Science Quarterly* 29 (1948): 38–48.

90 *"In accordance with Title 6":* In S. F. Riepma, *The Story of Margarine* (Washington, DC: Public Affairs Press, 1970): 51.

90 *Mazola margarine advertised itself:* "Mazola Corn Oil (1960)—Classic TV Commercial," YouTube, accessed January 4, 2014, http://www.youtube.com/watch?v=Y7PW0jUqWeA.

90 *early margarines contained far more trans fats:* Walter H. Meyer, letter to Fred A. Kummerow, May 22, 1967, in author's possession.

91 *nearly every major food corporation:* National Diet-Heart Study Research Group, "National Diet Heart Study Final Report," I-312–I-314.

92 *"everything but the kitchen sink":* Jeremiah Stamler, interview with author, May 1, 2009.

93 *The results, announced in September 1982:* Multiple Risk Factor Intervention Trial Research Group, "Multiple Risk Factor Intervention Trial: Risk Factor Changes and

Mortality Results," *Journal of the American Medical Association* 248, no. 12 (1982): 1465–1477.

93 *floated various possible explanations:* Ibid., 1476.

93 *MRFIT triggered widespread comment:* For example, George D. Lundberg, "MRFIT and the Goals of the Journal," *Journal of the American Medical Association* 248, no. 12 (1982): 1501.

93 *the treatment group was found to have:* Barbara J. Shaten et al., "Lung Cancer Mortality after 16 Years in MRFIT Participants in Intervention and Usual-Care Groups: Multiple Risk Factor Intervention Trial," *Annals of Epidemiology* 7, no. 2 (1997): 125–136.

93 *"I don't know!" . . . "Not rationalized!":* Stamler, interview, May 1, 2009.

93 *"frail but on fire":* Ronald M. Krauss, interview with author, July 2, 2012.

94 *One of the things that Stamler told me:* Stamler, interview, April 22, 2009.

94 *found a link between lowering cholesterol:* These included Pearce and Dayton, "Incidence of Cancer in Men on a Diet High in Polyunsaturated Fat," 464–467; Uris E. Nydegger and René E. Butler, "Serum Lipoprotein Levels in Patients with Cancer," *Cancer Research* 32, no. 8 (1972): 1756–1760; Michael Francis Oliver et al., "A Co-operative Trial in the Primary Prevention of Ischaemic Heart Disease Using Clofibrate. Report from the Committee of Principal Investigators," *Heart* 40, no. 10 (1978), 1069–1118; Robert Beaglehole et al., "Cholesterol and Mortality in New Zealand Maoris," *British Medical Journal* 280, no. 6210 (1980): 285–287; J. D. Kark, A. H. Smith, and C. G. Hames, "The Relationship of Serum Cholesterol to the Incidence of Cancer in Evans County, Georgia," *Journal of Chronic Diseases* 33, no. 5 (1980): 311–322; M. R. Garcia-Palmieri et al., "An Apparent Inverse Relationship between Serum Cholesterol and Cancer Mortality in Puerto Rico," *American Journal of Epidemiology* 114, no. 1 (1981): 29–40; Grant N. Stemmerman et al., "Serum Cholesterol and Colon Cancer Incidence in Hawaiian Japanese Men," *Journal of the National Cancer Institute* 67, no. 6 (1981): 1179–1182; Seth R. Miller et al., "Serum Cholesterol and Human Colon Cancer," *Journal of the National Cancer Institute* 67, no. 2 (1981): 297–300; Djordje Kozarevic et al., "Serum Cholesterol and Mortality: The Yugoslavia Cardiovascular Disease Study," *American Journal of Epidemiology* 114, no. 1 (1981): 21–28.

94 *principally for colon cancer:* Geoffrey Rose et al., "Colon Cancer and Blood-Cholesterol," *Lancet* 303, no. 7850 (1974): 181–183.

94 *three times more likely to get colon cancer:* Roger R. Williams et al., "Cancer Incidence by Levels of Cholesterol," *Journal of the American Medical Association* 245, no. 3 (1981): 247–252.

94 *baseline level of concern:* Elias B. Gammal, Kenneth K. Carroll, and Earl R. Plunkett, "Effects of Dietary Fat on the Uptake and Clearance of 7,12-Dimethylbenz(α)anthracene by Rat Mammary Tissue," *Cancer Research* 28, no. 2 (1968): 384–385.

94 *Another early study that raised a health concern about corn oil was:* Arthur J. Patek et al., "Cirrhosis-Enhancing Effect of Corn Oil," *Archives of Pathology* 82, no. 6 (1966): 596–601.

94 *NIH investigators found:* Hirotsuga Ueshima, Minoru Iida, and Yoshio Komachi, "Letter to the Editor: Is It Desirable to Reduce Total Serum Cholesterol Level as Low as Possible?," *Preventive Medicine* 8, no. 1 (1979): 104–105.

94 *evidence on the topic:* Manning Feinleib, "On a Possible Inverse Relationship Between Serum Cholesterol and Cancer Mortality," *American Journal of Epidemiology* 114, no. 1

(1981): 5–10; Manning Feinleib, "Summary of a Workshop on Cholesterol and Non-cardiovascular Disease Mortality," *Preventive Medicine* 11, no. 3 (1982): 360–367.

95   *clearly dismayed . . . "even more puzzling":* Manning Feinleib, interview with author, April 20, 2009.

95   *it looked especially bad for healthy men:* Stephen B. Hulley, Judith M. B. Walsh, and Thomas B. Newman, "Health Policy on Blood Cholesterol. Time to Change Directions," *Circulation* 86, no. 3 (1992): 1026–1029.

95   *When I mentioned all this to Stamler:* Stamler, interview, May 1, 2009.

96   *Conducted by the biochemist Ivan Frantz:* Ivan D. Frantz et al., "Test of Effect of Lipid Lowering by Diet on Cardiovascular Risk," *Arteriosclerosis, Thrombosis, and Vascular Biology* 9, no. 1 (1989): 129–135.

96   *researchers were unable to find:* Ibid.

96   *"disappointed in the way it came out":* Quoted in Gary Taubes, *Good Calories, Bad Calories: Fats, Carbs, and the Controversial Science of Diet and Health* (New York: Alfred A. Knopf, 2007), 38.

97   *But the results . . . "with risk of death":* Richard B. Shekelle et al., "Diet, Serum Cholesterol, and Death from Coronary Heart Disease: The Western Electric Study," *New England Journal of Medicine* 304, no. 2 (1981): 68.

97   *"It had no INDEPENDENT effect":* Stamler, interview, April 22, 2009.

97   *was to worship God:* Jack H. Medalie et al., "Five-Year Myocardial Infarction Incidence—II. Association of Single Variables to Age and Birthplace," *Journal of Chronic Disease* 26, no. 6 (1973): 325–349.

98   *other large epidemiological study . . . near-vegetarian diet:* Noboru Kimura, "Changing Patterns of Coronary Heart Disease, Stroke, and Nutrient Intake in Japan," *Preventive Medicine* 12, no. 1 (1983): 222–227; Hirotsugu Ueshima, Kozo Tatara, and Shintaro Asakura, "Declining Mortality from Ischemic Heart Disease and Changes in Coronary Risk Factors in Japan, 1956–1980," *American Journal of Epidemiology* 125, no. 1 (1987): 62–72. I am indebted to Uffe Ravnskov, *The Cholesterol Myths: Exposing the Fallacy that Saturated Fat and Cholesterol Cause Heart Disease* (Washington, DC: New Trends Publishing, 2000), for digging up these studies on Japan.

98   lower *rates of heart disease than their fellow:* Hiroo Kato et al., "Epidemiologic Studies of Coronary Heart Disease and Stroke in Japanese Men Living in Japan, Hawaii and California," *American Journal of Epidemiology* 97, no. 6 (1973): 372–385; M. G. Marmot et al., "Epidemiologic Studies of Coronary Heart Disease and Stroke in Japanese Men Living in Japan, Hawaii and California: Prevalence of Coronary and Hypertensive Heart Disease and Associated Risk Factors," *American Journal of Epidemiology* 102, no. 6 (1975): 514–525.

99   *"sub-sample of the cohort in San Francisco":* Kato et al., "Epidemiologic Studies of Coronary Heart Disease and Stroke in Japanese Men," 373.

99   *clearly not the "same method":* Jeanne L. Tillotson et al., "Epidemiology of Coronary Heart Disease and Stroke in Japanese Men Living in Japan, Hawaii, and California: Methodology for Comparison of Diet," *American Journal of Clinical Nutrition* 26, no. 2 (1973): 117–184.

99   *higher rates of stroke:* Robert M. Worth et al., "Epidemiologic Studies of Coronary Heart Disease and Stroke in Japanese Men Living in Japan, Hawaii and California: Mortality,"

American Journal of Epidemiology 102, no. 6 (1975): 481–490; Abraham Kagan et al., "Trends in Stroke Incidence and Mortality in Hawaiian Japanese Men," *Stroke* 25, no. 6 (1994): 1170–1175; on the relationship to animal fat, see Y. Takeya, J. S. Popper, Y. Shimizu, H. Kato, G. G. Rhoads, and Abraham Kagan, "Epidemiologic Studies of Coronary Heart Disease and Stroke in Japanese Men Living in Japan, Hawaii and California: Incidence of Stroke in Japan and Hawaii," *Stroke* 15, no. 1 (1994): 15–23.

100 *higher rates of fatal cerebral hemorrhages:* Heizo Tanaka et al., "Risk Factors for Cerebral Hemorrhage and Cerebral Infarction in a Japanese Rural Community," *Stroke* 13, no. 1 (1982): 62–73.

100 *attempted to dismiss these findings:* Hirotsugu Ueshima, Minoru Iida, and Yoshio Komachi, "Letter to the Editor: Is It Desirable to Reduce Total Serum Cholesterol Level as Low as Possible?" *Preventive Medicine* 8, no. 1 (1979): 104–111; for replies, see Henry Blackburn, Ancel Keys, and David R. Jacobs, *Preventive Medicine* 8, no. 1 (1979): 109; William Kannel, *Preventive Medicine* 8, no. 1 (1979): 106–107.

100 *have endured until today in Japan:* T. Tanaka and T. Okamura, "Blood Cholesterol Level and Risk of Stroke in Community-Based or Worksite Cohort Studies: A Review of Japanese Cohort Studies in the Past 20 Years," *Keio Journal of Medicine* (Tokyo) 61, no. 3 (2012): 79–88.

100 The Lancet *took stock:* "Can I Avoid a Heart Attack?," editorial, *Lancet* 303, no. 7858 (1974): 605.

100 *"very big emotional component"* . . . *"lowering cholesterol":* Michael Oliver, interview with author, May 1, 2009.

101 *"it was not scientific":* A. Gerald Shaper, Interview with Henry Blackburn, in "Preventing Heart Attack and Stroke: A History of Cardiovascular Disease Epidemiology," last accessed February 14, 2014, http://www.epi.umn.edu/cvdepi/interview.asp?id=64.

101 *"no proof that such activity offsets":* "Can I Avoid a Heart Attack?," 605.

101 *"cure should not be worse":* Ibid., 607.

101 *In fact, Seymour Dayton was concerned:* Dayton et al., "A Controlled Clinical Trial of a Diet High in Unsaturated Fat," II-57.

101 *Experts now lament:* Martijn B. Katan, Scott M. Grundy, and Walter C. Willett, "Should a Low-Fat, High-Carbohydrate Diet Be Recommended for Everyone? Beyond Low-Fat Diets," *New England Journal of Medicine* 337, no. 8 (1997): 563–566.

102 *"I sincerely believe we should* not*":* Edward H. Ahrens, Jr., "Drugs Spotlight Program: The Management of Hyperlipidemia: Whether, Rather than How," *Annals of Internal Medicine* 85, no. 1 (1976): 92.

102 *such "unmanageable proportions":* Hans Kaunitz, "Importance of Lipids in Arteriosclerosis: An Outdated Theory," in Select Committee on Nutrition and Human Needs of the United States Senate, *Dietary Goals for the United States—Supplemental Views* (Washington, DC: US Government Printing Office, 1977): 42–54.

102 *according to cholesterol expert Daniel Steinberg:* Daniel Steinberg, "An Interpretive History of the Cholesterol Controversy. Part II. The Early Evidence Linking Hypercholesterolemia to Coronary Disease in Humans," *Journal of Lipid Research* 46, no. 2 (2005): 189.

5. The Low-Fat Diet Goes to Washington

104 *previously dealt with issues of hunger:* William J. Broad, "NIH Deals Gingerly with Diet-Disease Link," *Science* 204, no. 4398 (1979): 1175–1178.

105 *Mottern found them objectionable:* Nick Mottern, interview with author, March 25, 2009.

105 *And he believed the meat industry to be wholly corrupt:* Mottern, interview.

105 *In his eyes, the controversy pitched:* Mottern, interview.

105 *"good guy versus bad guy":* Marshall Matz, interview with author, March 29, 2009.

105 *"I admired them":* Mottern, interview.

108 *investigators reported that the Seventh-day Adventist men:* Roland L. Phillips et al., "Coronary Heart Disease Mortality among Seventh-Day Adventists with Differing Dietary Habits: A Preliminary Report," *American Journal of Clinical Nutrition* 31, no. 10 (1978): S191–S198.

108 *Women, by contrast, saw no benefit:* Paul K. Mills et al., "Cancer Incidence among California Seventh-Day Adventists, 1976–1982," *American Journal of Clinical Nutrition* 59, no. 5 (1994): 1136S–1142S.

108 *this variance alone could have explained:* Rekha Garg, Jennifer H. Madans, and Joel C. Kleinman, "Regional Variation in Ischemic Heart Disease Incidence," *Journal of Clinical Epidemiology* 45, no. 2 (1992): 149–156.

108 *Even the study director acknowledged:* Gary E. Fraser, Joan Sabaté, and W. Lawrence Beeson, "The Application of the Results of Some Studies of California Seventh-Day Adventists to the General Population," *Archives of Internal Medicine* 115, no. 4 (1993): 533.

109 *"Risks: More Red Meat, More Mortality":* Nicholas Bakalar, "Risks: More Red Meat, More Mortality," *New York Times*, March 12, 2012.

109 *a research finding that just three:* An Pan et al., "Red Meat Consumption and Mortality: Results from 2 Prospective Cohort Studies," *Archives of Internal Medicine* 172, no. 7 (2012): 555–563.

110 *the increase in the risk of dying:* Calculated by Zoë Harcombe, "Red Meat & Mortality & the Usual Bad Science," Because Everything You Think About Obesity Is Wrong (blog), March 13, 2012, last accessed February 13, 2014, http://www.zoeharcombe .com/2012/03/red-meat-mortality-the-usual-bad-science/#_ednref2.

110 *the top meat eaters were also found:* Pan et al., "Red Meat Consumption and Mortality," 557.

111 *statisticians generally agree:* Described in Gary Taubes, "Do We Really Know What Makes Us Healthy? *New York Times Magazine*, September 16, 2007.

111 *the reported difference:* World Cancer Research Fund and the American Institute for Cancer Research, *Food, Nutrition, Physical Activity, and the Prevention of Cancer: A Global Perspective* (Washington, DC: American Institute for Cancer Research, 2007), 116–128.

111 *"convincing evidence" . . . Cancer Institute itself:* Nancy Nelson, "Epidemiology in a Nutshell," *Benchmarks*, online publication of the National Cancer Institute, July 8, 2002, last accessed February 13, 2014, http://benchmarks.cancer.gov/2002/07/epidemiology -in-a-nutshell; on "convincing evidence," see World Cancer Research Fund and the

American Institute for Cancer Research, *Food, Nutrition, Physical Activity, and the Prevention of Cancer*, 116.

111 *Experts lambasted:* A. Stewart Truswell, "Problems with Red Meat in the WCRF2," *American Journal of Clinical Nutrition* 89, no. 4 (2009): 1274–1275; Hans Konrad Biesalski, "Meat and Cancer: Meat as a Component of a Healthy Diet," *European Journal of Clinical Nutrition* 56, no. 1, suppl. (2002): S2–S11.

112 *"Our diets have changed radically":* Select Committee on Nutrition and Human Needs of the United States Senate, *Dietary Goals for the United States* (Washington, DC: US Government Printing Office, 1977): 1.

112 *"rich in meat"... "linked to heart disease":* Ibid., 2.

112 *"killer diseases":* Ibid., 1.

112 *"Within this century":* Jane E. Brody, *Jane Brody's Good Food Book: Living the High Carbohydrate Way* (New York: W. W. Norton, 1985), 2.

112 *has been echoed:* Geoffrey Cannon, *Food and Health: The Experts Agree* (London: Consumers' Association, 1992).

112 *"indifferent" farmers:* Quoted in Waverley Root and Richard De Rochemont, *Eating in America: A History* (New York: Morrow, 1976), 56.

113 *"treated with equal carelessness":* Ibid., 81.

113 *apparently so fat... now-extinct species:* Ibid., 72.

114 *food included beef... does not mention:* Ibid., 87.

114 *Infants were fed beef:* Ibid., 132.

114 *Americans ate twice as much beef:* Ibid., 192.

114 *precisely why observers regarded:* Thomas Cooper, *Some Information Respecting America* (London: J. Johnson, 1794).

114 *"bottom of the pork barrel":* James Fenimore Cooper, *The Chainbearer* (Oxford: Oxford University, 1845), 82–83.

114 *relished the viscera... "highly esteemed":* Root and De Rochemont, *Eating in America*, 40.

114 *A survey of eight thousand urban Americans:* Roger Horowitz, *Putting Meat on the American Table: Taste, Technology, Transformation* (Baltimore, MD: Johns Hopkins University Press, 2000), 12.

114 *A food budget published:* Cited in Richard Osborn Cummings, *The American and His Food: A History of Food Habits in the United States* (Chicago: University of Chicago Press, 1940): 264.

115 *Even slaves... "These sources do give us some confidence...":* Horowitz, *Putting Meat on the American Table*, 12.

115 *chicken was considered... for their eggs:* Ibid., 103.

116 *A recent USDA report says:* United States Department of Agriculture, *Agricultural Fact Book 2001–2002* (Washington, DC: US Government Printing Office, 2003): 15.

116 *repeated in the media:* For example Dan Charles, "The Making of Meat Eating America," Morning Edition, National Public Radio, June 26, 2012.

117 *one eighteenth-century observer:* Isaac Weld, *Travels through the States of North America, and the Provinces of Upper and Lower Canada, During the Years 1795, 1796, and 1797* (London: printed for John Stockdale, Piccadilly, 1799), 91.

117 *"avoid leafy vegetables":* Cummings, *The American and His Food*, 128.

117 *fruit and salad were avoided:* Root and De Rochemont, *Eating in America,* 130.

117 *"incorrect to describe Americans":* Ibid., 232.

117 *most authoritative expert on heart disease:* Austin Flint, *A Practical Treatise on the Diagnosis, Pathology, and Treatment of Diseases of the Heart* (Philadelphia: Blanchard and Lea, 1859).

118 *Nor did William Osler:* William Osler, *The Principles and Practice of Medicine* (1892; repr. RareBooksClub.com, 2012).

118 *first clinical description:* William G. Rothstein, *Public Health and the Risk Factor: A History of an Uneven Medical Revolution.* Rochester Studies in Medical History 3 (Rochester, NY: University of Rochester Press, 2003).

118 *"plenty of them over 60":* Paul D. White, "Coronary Heart Disease: Then and Now," *Journal of the American Medical Association* 203, no. 9 (1968): 282.

118 *one fifth of the US population:* US Census Office, *Census Reports II: Twelfth Census of the United States, Taken in the Year 1900. Population, Part II* (Washington, DC: US Census Office, 1902), 4–5.

118 *compared the record on chest pain:* Leon Michaels, "Aetiology of Coronary Artery Disease: An Historical Approach," *British Heart Journal* 28, no. 2 (1966): 258–264.

119 *caused meat sales in the United States to fall:* James Harvey Young, "The Long Struggle for the Law," US Food and Drug Administration, last accessed February 13, 2014, http://www.fda.gov/AboutFDA/WhatWeDo/History/CentennialofFDA/TheLongStrugglefortheLaw.

119 *they did not revive for another twenty years:* Root and De Rochemont, *Eating in America,* 211.

119 *Fat intake did rise during those years:* Mohamed A. Antar, Margaret A. Ohlson, and Robert E. Hodges, "Perspectives in Nutrition: Changes in Retail Market Food Supplies in the United States in the Last Seventy Years in Relation to the Incidence of Coronary Heart Disease, with Special Reference to Dietary Carbohydrates and Essential Fatty Acids," *American Journal of Clinical Nutrition* 14 (1964): 169–178.

120 *carved out an exception:* "Panel Stands by Its Dietary Goals but Eases a View on Eating Meat," *New York Times,* January 24, 1978, A22.

120 *the report advised:* Select Committee on Nutrition and Human Needs, *Dietary Goals for the United States,* 6.

120 *"stood the test of time":* Marshall Matz, interview with author, March 30, 2009.

121 *long been ignored:* Janet M. Levine, "Hearts and Minds: The Politics of Diet and Heart Disease," in *Consuming Fears: The Politics of Product Risks,* ed. Henry M. Sapolsky (New York: Basic Books, 1986), 40–79.

121 *thirteen slices of bread:* Marian Burros, "In the Soda Pop Society—Can the American Diet Change for the Better?" *Washington Post,* September 28, 1978, E1.

122 *"taking a big chance":* Mark Hegsted, "Washington—Dietary Guidelines," Preventing Heart Attack and Stroke: A History of Cardiovascular Disease Epidemiology, ed. Henry Blackburn, last accessed January 29, 2014, http://www.epi.umn.edu/cvdepi/pdfs/Hegsted guidelines.pdf.

122 *panel agreed upon:* Edward H. Ahrens, Jr., "Introduction," *American Journal of Clinical Nutrition* 32, no. 12 (1979): 2627–2631.

123 *"The question . . . is . . .":* Broad, "NIH Deals Gingerly with Diet-Disease Link," 1176.

123 *"hedge their bets":* Robert Levy, director of NHLBI, quoted in William J. Broad, "Academy Says Curb on Cholesterol Not Needed," *Science* 208, no. 4450 (1980): 1355.

123 *"benefits could be expected":* Broad, "NIH Deals Gingerly with Diet-Disease Link," 1176.

123 Dietary Guidelines for Americans: USDA and US Department of Health and Human Services, *Nutrition and Your Health: Dietary Guidelines for Americans*, Home and Garden Bulletin No. 228 (Washington, DC: Science and Education Administration, 1980).

124 *The board had actually been solicited by the USDA:* Broad, "NIH Deals Gingerly with Diet-Disease Link," 1175.

124 *"generally unimpressive results":* National Research Council, Food and Nutrition Board, National Academy of Sciences, *Toward Healthful Diets* (Washington, DC: National Academy Press, 1980).

124 *"best in the world":* Broad, "NIH Deals Gingerly with Diet-Disease Link," 1175.

124 *US Surgeon General, who had responded:* US Public Health Service, Office of the Surgeon General, *Healthy People: The Surgeon General's Report on Health Promotion and Disease Prevention*, US Public Health Service (1979).

125 *"academy were at odds!":* Hegsted, "Washington—Dietary Guidelines."

125 *There were front-page stories:* Jane E. Brody, "Panel Reports Healthy Americans Need Not Cut Intake of Cholesterol: Nutrition Board Challenges Notion That Such Dietary Change Could Prevent Coronary Heart Disease," *New York Times*, May 28, 1980, A1; Susan Okie, "Farmers Are Gleeful, Heart Experts Quiver at Fat-Diet Findings," *Washington Post*, May 29, 1980, A2.

125 *fit to editorialize:* "A Confusing Diet of Fact," editorial, *New York Times*, June 3, 1980, A18; "Cholesterol Does Count," editorial, *Washington Post*, June 2, 1980, A18.

125 MacNeil/Lehrer Report: "The Cholesterol Question," *The MacNeil/Lehrer Report*, May 28, 1980.

125 People *magazine:* Barbara K. Mills, "The Nutritionist Who Prepared the Pro-Cholesterol Report Defends It Against Critics," *People*, June 16, 1980, 58–64.

125 *The* New York Times *accused:* "Confusing Diet of Fact," A18.

125 *The* Times *concluded:* Ibid.

125 Times *ran a front-page story:* Jane E. Brody, "Experts Assail Report Declaring Curb on Cholesterol Isn't Needed," *New York Times*, June 1, 1980, A1.

126 *Harper unapologetically in an interview:* Alfred E. Harper, interview with author, April 2, 2009.

126 *Critics called:* Quoted in "A Few Kind Words for Cholesterol," *Time*, June 9, 1980.

126 *held hearings on the report . . . reputation was raked:* Karen De Witt, "Scientists Clash on Academy's Cholesterol Advice," *New York Times*, June 20, 1980, A15; *National Academy of Sciences Report on Healthful Diets: Hearings before the House Subcommittee on Domestic Marketing, Consumer Relations, and Nutrition of the Committee on Agriculture, House of Representatives*, 96th Congress, 2nd Session, 1980; *Dietary Guidelines for Americans: Hearings before the House Subcommittee on Agriculture, Rural Development and Related Agencies, Committee on Appropriations*, 96th Congress, 2nd Session, 1980.

127 *judged* Science *magazine:* Nicholas Wade, "Food Board's Fat Report Hits Fire," *Science* 209, no. 4453 (1980): 248.

127 Washington Post *editorial board:* "Cholesterol Does Count," *Washington Post*, June 2, 1980, 1.

128 *the LRC results:* LRC Study Group, "The Lipid Research Clinics Coronary Primary Prevention Trial Results. I: Reduction in Incidence of Coronary Heart Disease," *Journal of the American Medical Association* 251, no. 3 (1984): 351–364; LRC Study Group, "The Lipid Research Clinics Coronary Primary Prevention Trial Results. II: The Relationship of Reduction in Incidence of Coronary Heart Disease to Cholesterol Lowering," *Journal of the American Medical Association* 251, no. 3 (1984): 365–374.

129 *men whose cholesterol had gone down:* LRC Study Group, "The Lipid Research Clinics Coronary Primary Prevention Trial Results. I," 356.

129 *metanalysis of six cholesterol-lowering trials:* Matthew F. Muldoon, Stephen B. Manuck, and Karen A. Matthews, "Lowering Cholesterol Concentrations and Mortality: A Quantitative Review of Primary Prevention Trials," *British Medical Journal* 301, no. 6747 (1990): 309; on low-cholesterol and depression: Ju Young Shin, Jerry Suls, and René Martin, "Are Cholesterol and Depression Inversely Related? A Meta-Analysis of the Association between Two Cardiac Risk Factors," *Annals of Behavioral Medicine* 36, no. 1 (2008): 33–43; James M. Greenblatt, "Low Cholesterol and Its Psychological Effects: Low Cholesterol Is Linked to Depression, Suicide, and Violence," *Psychology Today*, June 10, 2011.

129 *Researchers have subsequently suggested:* Jess G. Fiedorowicz and William G. Haynes, "Cholesterol, Mood, and Vascular Health: Untangling the Relationship. Does Low Cholesterol Predispose to Depression and Suicide, or Vice Versa?" *Current Psychiatry* 9, no. 7 (2010).

129 *Other cholesterol-lowering studies:* Manning Feinleib, "On a Possible Inverse Relationship between Serum Cholesterol and Cancer Mortality," *American Journal of Epidemiology* 114, no. 1 (1981): 5–10; Manning Feinleib, "Summary of a Workshop on Cholesterol and Noncardiovascular Disease Mortality," *Preventive Medicine* 11, no. 3 (1982): 360–367.

129 *In addition, populations found to have very low cholesterol:* Tanaka et al., "Risk Factors for Cerebral Hemorrhage and Cerebral Infarction in a Japanese Rural Community"; Kagan et al., "Epidemiologic Studies of Coronary Heart Disease and Stroke in Japanese Men Living in Japan, Hawaii and California: Incidence of Stroke in Japan and Hawaii."

129 *"Any statistician would turn in his badge":* Quoted in Gina Kolata, "Heart Panel's Conclusions Questioned," *Science* 227, no. 4682 (1985): 41.

130 *"I can't fully explain it and it worries":* Ibid.

130 *represented a leap of faith:* Edward H. Ahrens, Jr., "The Diet-Heart Question in 1985: Has It Really Been Settled?" *Lancet* 1, no. 8437 (1985): 1086.

130 *Richard A. Kronmal to write:* Richard A. Kronmal, "Commentary on the Published Results of the Lipid Research Clinics Coronary Primary Prevention Trial," *Journal of the American Medical Association* 253, no. 14 (1985): 2091.

130 *pushed the data . . . it seemed more like "advocacy":* Ibid., 2091 and 2093.

130 *Paul Meier commented:* Quoted in Thomas J. Moore, *Heart Failure: A Critical Inquiry into American Medicine and the Revolution in Heart Care* (New York: Simon & Schuster, 1989), 61.

130 *Rifkind told* Time *magazine:* "Sorry, It's True: Cholesterol Really Is a Killer," *Time*, January 23, 1984.

130 *"keystone in the arch":* Kolata, "Heart Panel's Conclusions Questioned," 40.

132 *The conference "consensus" statement:* National Institutes of Health, "Lowering Blood Cholesterol to Prevent Heart Disease," NIH Consensus Statement 5, no. 7 (1984): 1–11.

132 *in March 1984,* Time *magazine ran:* "Sorry It's True: Cholesterol Really Is a Killer."

133 *wrote a skeptical piece:* Kolata, "Heart Panel's Conclusions Questioned," 40–41.

133 *"dissent [which] is always more newsworthy":* Daniel Steinberg, "The Pathogenesis of Atherosclerosis: An Interpretive History of the Cholesterol Controversy, Part IV: The 1984 Coronary Primary Prevention Trial Ends It—Almost," *Journal of Lipid Research* 47, no. 1 (2006): 11.

134 *there was "a price to pay":* Donald J. McNamara, interview with author, September 26, 2005.

134 *"public is being hosed":* Quoted in Moore, *Heart Failure,* 63.

6. How Women and Children Fare on a Low-Fat Diet

135 *the agency has long been influenced:* Marion Nestle, *Food Politics* (Berkeley, CA: University of California Press, 2002).

135 *Americans were questioning accepted norms:* William G. Rothstein, *Public Health and the Risk Factor: A History of an Uneven Medical Revolution,* Rochester Studies in Medical History 3 (Rochester, NY: University of Rochester Press, 2003), 316.

136 *Jerry Stamler expressed in 1972:* Jeremiah Stamler and Frederick H. Epstein, "Coronary Heart Disease: Risk Factors as Guides to Preventive Action," *Preventive Medicine* 1, no. 1 (1972): 46.

136 *"unsalted pretzels, hard candy, gum drops":* American Heart Association, *An Eating Plan for Healthy Americans: Our American Heart Association Diet* (Dallas, TX: American Heart Association, 1995).

137 *view that has been widely aired:* See, e.g., Baum et al. "Fatty Acids in Cardiovascular Health and Disease: A Comprehensive Update," *Journal of Clinical Lipidology* 6, no. 3 (2012): 216–234, 221.

137 *hefty fee . . . chastened into:* Rothstein, *Public Health and the Risk Factor,* 331–332.

137 *"Do we know enough . . .":* Donald S. Fredrickson, "Mutants, Hyperlipoproteinaemia, and Coronary Artery Disease," *British Medical Journal* 2, no. 5755 (1971): 187–192.

138 *two studies had contradictory results:* A. Korányi, "Prophylaxis and Treatment of the Coronary Syndrome," *Therapia Hungarica* 12 (1963): 17; Research Committee, "Low-Fat Diet in Myocardial Infarction: A Controlled Trial," *Lancet* 2, no. 7411 (1965): 501–504.

138 *"decks stacked against it":* Jane E. Brody, "Tending to Obesity, Inbred Tribe Aids Diabetes Study," *New York Times,* February 5, 1980, C1.

138 The Good Food Book: Jane E. Brody, *Jane Brody's Good Food Book: Living the High Carbohydrate Way* (New York: Norton, 1985).

140 *Group Four foods:* "The Proven Lifestyle," Preventive Medicine Research Institute, last accessed April 2009, http://www.pmri.org/lifestyle_program.html.

140 *"tired, depressed, lethargic and impotent":* Dean Ornish, "Healing through Diet," TED Talks, Monterey, CA, October 2008, last accessed February 13, 2014, http://www.ted.com/talks/dean_ornish_on_healing.html.

140 *as Frank Sacks . . . found:* Quoted in Gina Kolata, "Dean Ornish: A Promoter of Programs to Foster Heart Health," *New York Times,* December 29, 1998, F6.

140 *"It's hard to do a lot of things":* Quoted in George Epaminondas, "The Battle of the Diet Gurus," *The Sun Herald* (Sydney, Australia), February 23, 2003.

141 *control group . . . saw their arteries contract:* Dean Ornish et al., "Can Lifestyle Changes Reverse Coronary Heart Disease? The Lifestyle Heart Trial," *Lancet* 336, no. 8708 (1990): 129–133.

141 *a* Newsweek *cover story:* Geoffrey Cowley, "Healer of Hearts: Dean Ornish's Low-Tech Methods Could Transform American Medicine. But the Doctor Is Still Striving to Transform Himself," *Newsweek*, March 16, 1998.

142 *has never been successfully replicated:* Steven G. Aldana et al., "The Effect of an Intensive Lifestyle Modification Program on Carotid Artery Intima-Media Thickness: A Randomized Trial," *American Journal of Health Promotion* 21, no. 6 (2007): 510–516.

142 *Gould's incredulity:* Kay Lance Gould, interview with author, April 22, 2009.

142 *not been shown to extend life:* Demosthenes G. Katritsis and John P. A. Ioannidis, "Percutaneous Coronary Intervention versus Conservative Therapy in Nonacute Coronary Artery Disease: A Meta-Analysis," *Circulation* 111, no. 22 (2005): 2906–2912.

143 *"Why do you want to know? . . . not the best evidence":* Dean Ornish, interview with author, May 12, 2009.

143 *"actually reversed heart disease . . . totally in agreement":* Dean Ornish, interview with author, May 14, 2009.

143 *opinion piece in the* New York Times*:* Dean Ornish, "Eating for Health, Not Weight," *New York Times*, September 22, 2012.

143 *"we also found improvements . . . quibble about that":* Ornish, interview, May 14, 2009.

143 *"in no case" . . . "judged to be convincing":* World Cancer Research Fund and the American Institute for Cancer Research, Food, Nutrition, Physical Activity, and the Prevention of Cancer: A Global Perspective (Washington, DC: American Institute for Cancer Research, 2007), 114.

144 *overall mortality for vegetarians and nonvegetarians:* Timothy J. Key et al., "Mortality in British Vegetarians: Results from the European Prospective Investigation into Cancer and Nutrition (EPIC-Oxford)," *American Journal of Clinical Nutrition* 89, no. 5 (2009): 1613S–1619S.

144 *to compare the Masai to a neighboring tribe:* John B. Orr and John L. Gilks, *Studies of Nutrition: The Physique and Health of Two African Tribes*, Medical Research Council for the Dietetics Committee of the Economic Advisory Council. Special Report Series, No. 155 (London: H. M. Stationery Office, 1931).

144 *"great bulk" of their food . . . "legumes, and green leaves":* Ibid., 21.

144 *to suffer from . . . to contract rheumatoid arthritis:* Ibid., 9.

144 *5 inches taller . . . 23 pounds . . . narrower waists . . . far more muscular . . . manual labor:* Ibid.

145 *Alice Lichtenstein and a colleague reviewed:* Alice H. Lichtenstein and Linda Van Horn, "Very Low Fat Diets," *Circulation* 98, no. 9 (1998): 935–939.

146 *compelling rationale for including children:* Henry C. McGill et al., "Origin of Atherosclerosis in Childhood and Adolescence," *American Journal of Clinical Nutrition* 72, no. 5, suppl. (2000): 1307S–1315S.

146 *cord blood . . . given serious consideration:* "Questions Surround Treatment of Children with High Cholesterol," *Journal of American Medical Association* 214, no. 10 (1970): 1783–1785.

147 *asked Donald S. Fredrickson:* Fredrickson, "Mutants, Hyperlipoproteinaemia, and Coronary Artery Disease," 187–192.

147 *"scientifically unsound" . . . "needs of the young":* Food and Nutrition Board, Division of Biological Sciences, Assembly of Life Sciences, National Research Council, National Academy of Sciences, *Toward Healthful Diets* (Washington, DC: National Academy Press, 1980), 4.

147 *"The nutritional needs . . . inactive octogenarian":* Ibid.

147 *"absolutely* no *evidence that it's safe":* Quoted in Gina Kolata, "Heart Panel's Conclusion Questioned," *Science* 227, no. 4682 (1985): 41.

147 *"made an* unconscionable *exaggeration":* Ibid., 40.

147 *editorial published in the AAP journal:* American Academy of Pediatrics, Committee on Nutrition, "Prudent Life-Style for Children: Dietary Fat and Cholesterol," *Pediatrics* 78, no. 3 (1986): 524.

148 *"The proposed changes would affect":* Ibid., 521–525.

148 *"provide 60 percent of dietary calcium":* Ibid., 523.

148 *The AAP feared that rates of iron deficiency:* Ibid.

148 *McCollum describes the fate of a rat:* Elmer Verner McCollum, *The Newer Knowledge of Nutrition* (New York: MacMillan, 1921), 58.

149 *"nothing in vegetarianism per se":* Ibid., 62.

149 calcium forms insoluble *"soaps":* J. Bruce German et al., "A Reappraisal of the Impact of Dairy Foods and Milk Fat on Cardiovascular Disease Risk," *European Journal of Nutrition* 48, no. 4 (2009): 194.

150 *consumption of whole milk . . . together increased:* Rothstein, *Public Health and the Risk Factor,* 330.

150 *Lloyd Filer, a professor . . . is quoted:* Marian Burros, "Eating Well," *New York Times,* May 18, 1988.

150 *a survey of about a thousand mothers:* Jane B. Morgan et al., "Healthy Eating for Infants—Mothers' Attitudes," *Acta Pediatrica* 84, no. 5 (1995): 512–515.

151 *In 1989, Fima Lifshitz:* Fima Lifshitz and Nancy Moses, "Growth Failure. A Complication of Dietary Treatment of Hypercholesterolemia," *American Journal of Diseases of Children* 143, no. 5 (1989): 537–542.

151 *"overzealous":* Ibid., 537.

152 *"nutritional dwarfing":* Ibid., 540.

152 *NHLBI in the 1980s finally decided:* DISC Collaborative Research Group, "Dietary Intervention Study in Children (DISC) with Elevated Low Density Lipoprotein Cholesterol: Design and Baseline Characteristics," *Annals of Epidemiology* 3, no. 4 (1993): 399.

152 *Dietary Intervention Study in Children:* The Writing Group for the DISC Collaborative Research Group, "Efficacy and Safety of Lowering Dietary Intake of Fat and Cholesterol in Children with Elevated Low-Density Lipoprotein Cholesterol," *Journal of the American Medical Association* 273, no. 18 (1995): 1429.

152 *in the 80th to 98th percentile:* Ibid., 1429.

152 *entirely different from the way that cholesterol is altered:* See, e.g., William E. Stehbens and Elli Wierzbicki, "The Relationship of Hypercholesterolemia to Atherosclerosis with Particular Emphasis on Familial Hypercholesterolemia, Diabetes Mellitus, Obstructive

Jaundice, Myxedema, and the Nephrotic Syndrome," *Progress in Cardiovascular Diseases* 30, no. 4 (1988): 289–306.

152 *their results could not be generalized:* See, e.g., Alvin M. Mauer, "Should There Be Intervention to Alter Serum Lipids in Children?" *Annual Review of Nutrition* 11 (1991): 383.

152 *They also got less magnesium, phosphorous . . . :* Eva Obarzanek et al., "Safety of a Fat-Reduced Diet: The Dietary Intervention Study in Children (DISC), *Pediatrics* 100, no. 1 (1997): 51–59.

153 *a few other small studies of children:* Robert M. Kaplan and Michelle T. Toshima, "Does a Reduced Fat Diet Cause Retardation in Child Growth?" *Preventive Medicine* 21, no. 1 (1992): 33–52; Mauer, "Should There Be Intervention to Alter Serum Lipids in Children?" 375–391.

153 *authors concluded that "lower fat intakes . . .":* Obarzanek et al., "Safety of a Fat-Reduced Diet," 58.

154 *Bogalusa Heart Study:* Theresa A. Nicklas et al., "Nutrient Adequacy of Low Fat Intakes for Children: The Bogalusa Heart Study," *Pediatrics* 89, no. 2 (1992): 221–228.

154 *STRIP was a loosely controlled experiment:* Helena Lapinleimu et al., "Prospective Randomized Trial in 1062 Infants of Diet Low in Saturated Fat and Cholesterol," *Lancet* 345, no. 8948 (1995): 473.

154 *researchers observed no difference:* Lapinleimu et al., "Prospective Randomised Trial in 1062 Infants"; Harri Niinikoski et al., "Regulation of Growth of 7- to 36-Month-Old Children by Energy and Fat Intake in the Prospective, Randomized STRIP Baby Trial," *Pediatrics* 100, no. 5 (1997): 810–816; Harri Niinikoski et al., "Impact of Repeated Dietary Counseling Between Infancy and 14 Years of Age on Dietary Intakes and Serum Lipids and Lipoproteins: the STRIP Study," *Circulation* 116, no. 9 (2007): 1032–1040, 1034.

154 *lower levels of HDL-cholesterol:* Olli Simell et al., "Special Turku Coronary Risk Factor Intervention Project for Babies (STRIP)," *American Journal of Clinical Nutrition* 72, no. 5, suppl. (2000): 1316S–1331S.

154 *investigators found no vitamin deficiencies:* Ibid., 1317S.

155 *coming mainly from a handful:* Lars Werkö, "Risk Factors and Coronary Heart Disease—Facts or Fancy?" *American Heart Journal* 91, no. 1 (1976): 87–98; Gunnar Biörck, *Contrasting Concepts of Ischaemic Heart Disease* (Stockholm, Sweden: Almqvist & Wiksell International, 1975); John McMichael, "Prevention of Coronary Heart Disease," *Lancet* 308, no. 7985 (1976): 569; Michael Oliver, "Dietary Cholesterol, Plasma Cholesterol and Coronary Heart Disease," *British Heart Journal* 38, no. 3 (1976): 214. A. Stewart Truswell, "Diet and Plasma Lipids—A Reappraisal," *American Journal of Clinical Nutrition* 31, no. 6 (1978): 977–989.

155 *AAP officially adopted:* Academy of Pediatrics, Committee on Nutrition, "Cholesterol in Childhood," *Pediatrics* 101, no. 1 (1998): 141–147.

156 *do not become dangerous, fibrous plaques:* Russell Ross, "The Pathogenesis of Atherosclerosis—An Update," *New England Journal of Medicine* 295 (1986): 488–500.

156 *child's diet is completely unrelated:* Canadian Paediatric Society and Health Canada, Joint Working Group, *Nutrition Recommendations Update: Dietary Fat and Children* (Ottawa, Ontario: Health Canada, 1993).

156 *the lipid profile of the mother:* Claudio Napoli et al., "Influence of Maternal Hypercholes-terolaemia during Pregnancy on Progression of Early Atherosclerotic Lesions in Child-hood: Fat of Early Lesions in Children (FELIC) Study," *Lancet* 354, no. 9186 (1999): 1234–1241.

156 *half of children with high total cholesterol:* William R. Clarke et al., "Tracking of Blood Lipids and Blood Pressure in School Age Children: the Muscatine Study," *Circulation* 58, no. 4 (1978): 626–634; Peter Laskarzewski et al., "Lipid and Lipoprotein Tracking in 108 Children over a Four-Year Period," *Pediatrics* 64, no. 5 (1979): 584–591; Trevor J. Or-chard et al., "Cholesterol Screening in Childhood: Does It Predict Adult Hypercholester-olemia? The Beaver County Experience," *Journal of Pediatrics* 103, no. 5 (1983): 687–691; David S. Freedman et al., "Tracking of Serum Lipids and Lipoproteins in Children over an 8-Year Period: The Bogalusa Heart Study," *Preventive Medicine* 14, no. 2 (1985): 203–216.

156 *Cochrane concluded:* Vanessa J. Poustie and Patricia Rutherford, "Dietary Treatment for Familial Hypercholesterolaemia," Cochrane Database of Systematic Reviews 2 (2001): CD001918-CD001918.

156 *rigorous study on this hypothesis:* Benjamin Caballero et al., "Pathways: A School-Based, Randomized Controlled Trial for the Prevention of Obesity in American Indian School-children," *American Journal of Clinical Nutrition* 78, no. 5 (2003): 1030–1038.

157 *"major contributor of growth failure":* Andrew M. Prentice and Alison A. Paul, "Fat and Energy Needs of Children in Developing Countries," *American Journal of Clinical Nu-trition* 72, suppl. (2000): 1253S.

157 *He compared some 140 Gambian infants . . . 8 pounds more than the Gambians . . . :* Ibid., 1259S–1260S.

157 *5 percent of energy as fat:* Ibid., 1261S.

157 *has zero grams of fat:* "Whole Grain Rice," Earth's Best Organic, accessed November 15, 2013. http://www.earthsbest.com/products/product/2392390001.

157 *18 percent fat:* Prentice, "Fat and Energy Needs of Children," 1256S.

157 *Earth's Best Vegetable Turkey:* "Vegetable Turkey Dinner," Earth's Best Organic, accessed November 15, 2013. http://www.earthsbest.com/products/product/2392350048.

158 *children have reduced their intake of fat:* Meghan M. Slining, Kevin C. Mathias, and Barry M. Popkin, "Trends in Food and Beverage Sources among US Children and Adolescents: 1989–2010," *Journal of the Academy of Nutrition and Dietetics* 113, no. 12 (2013): 1683–1694; Richard P. Troiano, Ronette R. Briefel, Margaret D. Carroll, and Karil Bialostosky, "Energy and Fat Intakes of Children and Adolescents in the United States: Data from the National Health and Nutrition Examination Surveys," *American Journal of Clinical Nutrition* 72, no. 5, suppl. (2000): 1343S–1353S.

158 *scary caveat:* Prentice and Paul, "Fat and Energy Needs of Children," 1262S.

158 *children in their countries had been increasing:* Luis A Moreno, Antonio Sarría, Aurora Lázaro, and Manuel Bueno, "Dietary Fat Intake and Body Mass Index in Spanish Chil-dren," *American Journal of Clinical Nutrition* 72, suppl. (2000): 1399S–1403S; Mitsunori Murata, "Secular Trends in Growth and Changes in Eating Patterns of Japanese Chil-dren," *American Journal of Clinical Nutrition* 72, no. 5, suppl. (2000): 1379S–1383S.

158 *Reports from poorer countries:* Ricardo Uauy, Charles E. Mize, and Carlos Castillo-Duran, "Fat Intake during Childhood: Metabolic Responses and Effects on Growth," *American Journal of Clinical Nutrition* 72, no. 5, suppl. (2000): 1345S–1360S.

158 *in the wealthier countries*: Spain: Moreno, Lázaro, and Bueno, "Dietary Fat Intake and Body Mass Index in Spanish Children"; Germany: Berthold Koletzko et al., "Dietary Fat Intakes of Infants and Primary School Children in Germany," *American Journal of Clinical Nutrition* 72, no. 5, suppl. (2000): 1329S–1398S.

158 *symposium summary statement*: Dennis M. Bier, Ronald M. Lauer, and Olli Simell, "Summary," *American Journal of Clinical Nutrition* 72, no. 5, suppl. (2000): 1410S–1413S.

159 *barely been studied*: Jacques E. Rossouw et al., "The Evolution of the Women's Health Initiative: Perspectives from the NIH," *Journal of the American Medical Women's Association* 50, no. 2 (1995): 50–55.

159 *initially affected more men than women*: Rothstein, *Public Health and the Risk Factor*, 202–206.

159 *represented only 20 percent . . . 25 percent thereafter*: Patrick Y. Lee et al., "Representation of Elderly Persons and Women in Published Randomized Trials of Acute Coronary Syndromes," *Journal of the American Medical Association* 286, no. 6 (2001): 708–713.

159 *researchers had been warning*: Reviewed in Robert H. Knopp et al., "Sex Differences in Lipoprotein Metabolism and Dietary Response: Basis in Hormonal Differences and Implications for Cardiovascular Disease," *Current Cardiology Reports* 8, no. 6 (2006): 452–459.

159 *until ten to twenty . . . until after menopause*: C. M. Flavell, "Women and Coronary Heart Disease," *Progress in Cardiovascular Nursing* 9, no. 4 (Fall, 1994): 18–27.

159 *In the Framingham Study*: William B. Kannel et al., "Serum Cholesterol, Lipoproteins, and the Risk of Coronary Heart Disease: The Framingham Study," *Annals of Internal Medicine* 74, no. 1 (1971): 1–12.

159 *NHLBI expert panel reviewed*: David Jacobs et al., "Report of the Conference on Low Blood Cholesterol: Mortality Associations," *Circulation* 86, no. 3 (1992): 1046–1060.

160 *yielded some disturbing results*: Robert H. Knopp, "The Dietary Alternatives Study," *Journal of the American Medical Association* 278, no. 18 (1997): 1509–1515.

160 *results have been confirmed*: See, e.g., Martijn B. Katan, "High-Oil Compared with Low-Fat, High-Carbohydrate Diets in the Prevention of Ischemic Heart Disease," *American Journal of Clinical Nutrition*, 66, no. 4, suppl. (1997): 974S–979S.

162 *"of all the lipoproteins"*: Tavia Gordon et al., "High Density Lipoprotein as a Protective Factor Against Coronary Heart Disease: The Framingham Study," *American Journal of Medicine* 62, no. 5 (1977): 707.

162 *The correlation was "striking"*: Ibid., 707.

162 *"most important finding"*: William P. Castelli et al., "HDL Cholesterol and Other Lipids in Coronary Heart Disease: The Cooperative Lipoprotein Phenotyping Study," *Circulation* 55, no. 5 (1977): 771.

162 *By 2002, the NCEP was calling*: National Cholesterol Education Program, *Third Report of the National Cholesterol Education Program (NCEP). Expert Panel on Detection, Evaluation, and Treatment of High Blood Cholesterol in Adults: (Adult Treatment Panel III) Final Report*. NIH Publication No. 02–5215 (Washington, DC: NIH, 2002), II-1.

162 *number of epidemiological studies*: Castelli et al., "HDL Cholesterol and Other Lipids," 769–770.

162 *Michael Brown and Joseph Goldstein:* Michael S. Brown and Joseph L. Goldstein, "How LDL Receptors Influence Cholesterol and Atherosclerosis," *Scientific American* 251, no. 5 (1984): 58.

163 *earned $956 billion:* Ryan Fuhrmann, "5 Best-Selling Prescription Meds of All Time," Investopedia, September 24, 2012, last accessed February 12, 2014, http://www.investo pedia.com/financial-edge/0912/5-best-selling-prescription-meds-of-all-time.aspx.

163 *open secrets about statins:* LaRosa et al., "Intensive Lipid Lowering Atorvastin"; Ray et al., "Statins and All Cause Mortality in High Risk Primary Prevention."

163 *journal editors were known to:* Robert H. Knopp, interview with author, February 5, 2009.

163 *one oil chemist described it.* Gerald McNeill, interview with author, December 10, 2012.

164 *Meir Stampfer:* Meir Stampfer, email message to Mark Weyland, November 20, 2004.

164 *seven hundred Boeing employees . . . results showed:* Robert H. Knopp et al., "One-year Effects of Increasingly Fat-Restricted Carbohydrate-Enriched Diets on Lipoprotein Levels in Free-living Subjects," *Proceedings for the Society of Experimental Biology and Medicine* 225, no. 3 (2000): 191–199; Carolyn E. Walden et al., "Differential Effect of National Cholesterol Education Program (NCEP) Step II Diet on HDL Cholesterol, Its Subfractions, and Apoprotein A-1 Levels in Hypercholesterolemic Women and Men after 1 Year: The BeFIT Study," *Arteriosclerosis, Thrombosis, and Vascular Biology* 20, no. 6 (2000): 1580–1587.

164 *women also saw their HDL-cholesterol levels drop:* Actually, these numbers reflect the decrease in a subfraction of HDL-cholesterol called HDL2. The average drop was 16.7 percent for women in the "hypercholesterolemic" group, which started out with high cholesterol, and 7.1 percent for the "hyperlipidemic" group, which started off with high triglycerides. Their total HDL-cholesterol levels went down, too: 7.6 percent and 3.5 percent, respectively.

165 *"mute" reaction . . . "what to make of it":* Robert H. Knopp, interview with author, February 5, 2009.

165 *other trials have also found . . . tend to happen less in these women:* Henry N. Ginsberg et al., "Effects of Reducing Saturated Fatty Acids on Plasma Lipids and Lipoproteins in Healthy Subjects: The Delta Study, Protocol 1," *Arteriosclerosis, Thrombosis, and Vascular Biology* 18, no. 3 (1998): 441–449; Zhengling Li et al., "Men and Women Differ in Lipoprotein Response to Dietary Fat and Cholesterol Restriction," *Journal of Nutrition* 133, no. 11 (2003): 3428–3433.

165 *Knopp summed up:* Robert H. Knopp et al., "Gender Differences in Lipoprotein Metabolism and Dietary Response: Basis in Hormonal Differences and Implications for Cardiovascular Disease," *Current Atherosclerosis Reports* 7, no. 6 (2005): 472–479.

165 *"alternative dietary interventions:* Ibid., 477.

165 *reducing calories:* Dietary Guidelines Advisory Committee, prepared for the Agricultural Research Service, US Department of Agriculture and US Department of Health and Human Services, *Report of the Dietary Guidelines Advisory Committee on the Dietary Guidelines for Americans, 2010. To the Secretary of Agriculture and the Secretary of Health and Human Services,* 7th ed. (Washington, DC: US Government Printing Office, May 2010), Table D1.1, 67.

165 *cut back fat and saturated fat:* Nancy D. Ernst et al., "Consistency Between US Dietary Intake and Serum Total Cholesterol Concentrations: The National Health and Nutrition Examination Surveys," *American Journal of Clinical Nutrition* 66, no. 4, suppl. (1997): 969S.

166 *testified that men and women in Japan:* Gio Gori, Statement to the Senate Select Committee on Nutrition, Select Committee on Nutrition and Human Needs, United States Senate, Volume No. II, Diet Related to Killer Diseases (July 28, 1976): 176–182.

166 *"Now I want to emphasize . . . that food causes cancer":* Ibid., 180.

166 *implied in its report that a low-fat diet:* Select Committee on Nutrition and Human Needs, United States Senate, Ninety-Fifth Congress, 1 Session, *Dietary Goals for the United States* (Washington, DC: US Government Printing Office, 1977).

166 *data on rats:* Albert Tannenbaum, "The Genesis and Growth of Tumors. III. Effects of a High-Fat Diet," *Cancer Research* 2, no. 7 (1942): 468–475.

167 *fat consumption not to be positively linked to breast cancer:* Walter C. Willett et al., "Dietary Fat and the Risk of Breast Cancer," *New England Journal of Medicine* 316, no. 1 (1987): 22–28.

167 *"no evidence" that a reduction:* Michelle D. Holmes, et al., "Association of Dietary Intake of Fat and Fatty Acids with Risk of Breast Cancer," *Journal of the American Medical Association* 281, no. 10 (1999): 914–920.

167 *a paper in the* Journal of the American Medical Association*:* Arthur Schatzkin et al., "The Dietary Fat–Breast Cancer Hypothesis is Alive," *Journal of the American Medical Association* 261, no. 22 (1989): 328–427.

167 *had little effect unless supplemented:* Adrienne E. Rogers and Matthew P. Longnecker, "Biology of Disease: Dietary and Nutritional Influences on Cancer—A Review of Epidemiological and Experimental Data," *Laboratory Investigation* 59, no. 6 (1988): 729–759.

168 *researchers have not been able to find:* D. Mazhar and J. Waxman, "Dietary Fat and Breast Cancer," *QJM* 99, no. 7 (2006): 469–473; Walter C. Willett and David J. Hunter, "Prospective Studies of Diet and Breast Cancer," *Cancer* 74, no. S3 (1994): 1085–1089; Sabina Sieri et al., "Dietary Fat and Breast Cancer Risk in the European Prospective Investigation into Cancer and Nutrition," *American Journal of Clinical Nutrition* 88, no. 5 (2008): 1304–1312.

168 *NCI still could not find:* Rowan T. Chlebowski et al., "Dietary Fat Reduction and Breast Cancer Outcome: Interim Efficacy Results from the Women's Intervention Nutrition Study," *Journal of the National Cancer Institute* 98, no. 24 (2006): 1767–1776.

168 *"probable" evidence . . . a fatty diet . . . wrote the authors:* World Cancer Research Fund and the American Institute for Cancer Research, *Food, Nutrition, Physical Activity, and the Prevention of Cancer*, 139.

168 *"My personal view is that":* Arthur Schatzkin, interview with author, May 1, 2009.

168 *"starting anew" . . . "becoming more agnostic":* Robert N. Hoover, interview with author, October 2, 2012.

169 People *magazine quoted:* Bob Meadows, M. Morehouse, and M. Simmons, "The Problem with Low-Fat Diets," *People*, February 27, 2006, 89–90.

169 *the results . . . series of articles in JAMA:* Shirley Beresford, et al., "Low-Fat Dietary Pattern and Risk of Colorectal Cancer," *Journal of the American Medical Association* 295,

no. 6 (2006): 643–654; Barbara V. Howard et al., "Low-Fat Dietary Pattern and Weight Change over 7 Years," *Journal of the American Medical Association* 295, no. 1 (2006): 39–49; Barbara V. Howard et al., "Low-Fat Dietary Pattern and Risk of Cardiovascular Disease," *Journal of the American Medical Association* 295, no. 6 (2006): 655–666; Ross L. Prentice et al., "Low-Fat Dietary Pattern and Risk of Invasive Breast Cancer," *Journal of the American Medical Association* 295, no. 6 (2006): 629–642; Ross L. Prentice et al., "Low-Fat Dietary Pattern and Cancer Incidence in the Women's Health Initiative Dietary Modification Randomized Controlled Trial," *Journal of the National Cancer Institute* 99, no. 20 (2007): 1534–1543.

170 *"completely null":* Quoted in Gina Kolata, "Low-Fat Diet Does Not Cut Health Risks, Study Finds," *New York Times,* February 8, 2006, A1.

170 *"Rolls Royce" . . . "final word":* Ibid.

170 *Robert Knopp told me:* Knopp, interview.

170 *said Tim Byers:* Quoted in Rob Stein, "New Data on Health: Studies in Confusion," *Washington Post,* February 19, 2006, A1.

170 *Jacques Rossouw:* Ibid.

170 *Newspapers had a heyday:* Cited in Agneta Yngve et al., "Invited Commentary: The Women's Health Initiative. What Is on Trial: Nutrition and Chronic Disease? Or Misinterpreted Science, Media Havoc and the Sound of Silence from Peers?" *Public Health Nutrition* 9, no. 2 (2006): 269.

170 *remarked Marcia Stefanick:* Quoted in Tara Parker-Pope, "In Study of Women's Health, Design Flaws Raise Questions," *Wall Street Journal,* February 28, 2006.

171 *"target around the bullet-hole":* Robert L. Wears, Richelle J. Cooper, and David L. Magid, "Subgroups, Reanalyses, and Other Dangerous Things," *Annals of Emergency Medicine* 46, no. 3 (2005): 254.

172 *A review in 2008 of all studies:* Food and Agriculture Organization of the United Nations, "Fats and Fatty Acids in Human Nutrition: Report of an Expert Consultation 10–14 November 2008," *FAO Food and Nutrition Paper* 91 (Rome: Food and Agriculture Organization of the United Nations, 2010), 13.

172 *in 2013 in Sweden:* Anders Hansen, "Swedish Health Advisory Body Says Too Much Carbohydrate, Not Fat, Leads to Obesity," *British Medical Journal,* 347 (November 15, 2013), doi:10.1136/bmj.f6873.

172 *wrote Frank Hu:* Frank B. Hu, JoAnn E. Manson, and Walter C. Willett, "Types of Dietary Fat and Risk of Coronary Heart Disease: A Critical Review," *Journal of American College of Nutrition* 20, no. 1 (2001): 5.

172 *The USDA and AHA have both quietly eliminated:* USDA/USDHHS, *Dietary Guidelines,* 2010, x; Alice H. Lichtenstein et al., "Diet and Lifestyle Recommendations, Revision 2006," *Circulation* 114, no. 1 (2006): 82–96.

7. Selling the Mediterranean Diet: What Is the Science?

174 *It recommends getting . . . Olive oil is . . . and milk, never:* Walter Willett et al., "Mediterranean Diet Pyramid: A Cultural Model for Healthy Eating," *American Journal of Clinical Nutrition* 61, no. 6, suppl. (1995): 1403S.

175 *The idea had a simple origin, she explains . . . Trichopoulou knew:* Antonia Trichopoulou, interview with author, October 1, 2008.

176 *"We had started cutting down olive trees"* . . . *She had an intuitive sense:* Ibid.

176 *"men of 80 to 100":* Ancel Keys et al., *Seven Countries: A Multivariate Analysis of Death and Coronary Heart Disease* (Cambridge, MA: Harvard University Press, 1980), 76.

177 *"We were freezing in our unheated house":* Ancel Keys, "Mediterranean Diet and Public Health," *American Journal of Clinical Nutrition* 61, no. 6, suppl. (1995): 1322S.

177 *"All the way to Switzerland"* . . . *"warm all over":* Ancel Keys and Margaret Keys, *Eat Well and Stay Well the Mediterranean Way* (Garden City, NY: Doubleday, 1975), 2.

177 *Keys recalled their delight in dining:* Ibid., 4.

177 *"that is the Mediterranean to us":* Ibid., 28.

178 *he reissued his 1959 cookbook:* Ancel Keys and Margaret Keys, *Eat Well and Stay Well* (New York: Doubleday, 1959); Keys and Keys, *Eat Well and Stay Well the Mediterranean Way.* All subsequent citations will refer to this later edition.

178 *"We just wanted to raise the issue":* Trichopoulou, interview.

178 *these early conferences gave rise:* Elisabet Helsing and Antonia Trichopoulou, eds., "The Mediterranean Diet and Food Culture—a Symposium," *European Journal of Clinical Nutrition* 43, suppl. 2 (1989): 1–92.

179 *It had been an uphill battle:* Anna Ferro-Luzzi, interview with author, July 22, 2008.

179 *WHO, which had a greater interest in working:* Elisabet Helsing, interview with author, July 30, 2008.

179 *there were "substantial differences"* . . . *"more butter":* Keys and Keys, *Eat Well and Stay Well,* 38–39.

180 *In a meticulous, landmark paper in 1989:* Anna Ferro-Luzzi and Stefania Sette, "The Mediterranean Diet: An Attempt to Define Its Present and Past Composition," *European Journal of Clinical Nutrition* 43, suppl. 2 (1989): 13–29.

180 *"impossible enterprise":* Ibid., 25.

181 *"while very attractive"* . . . *"should not be used":* Ibid., 26.

181 *did not think of themselves as having a "diet":* Ferro-Luzzi, interview with author, July 22, 2008.

181 *"And bureaucrats didn't like the idea":* Ibid.

181 *"healthy" Cretan diet was virtually overflowing:* Ancel Keys, Christos Aravanis, and Helen Sdrin, "The Diets of Middle-Aged Men in Two Rural Areas of Greece," *Voeding* 27, no. 11 (1966): 575–586; Keys and Keys, *Eat Well and Stay Well,* 31.

181 *"swimming in oil":* Keys and Keys, *Eat Well and Stay Well,* 31.

182 *"You can't recommend high-fat diets":* Bonnie Liebman, "Just the Mediterranean Diet Facts," *Nutrition Action Healthletter* 21, no. 10 (1994).

182 *a considerable effort to confirm:* Antonia Trichopoulou and Pagona Lagiou, "Healthy Traditional Mediterranean Diet: An Expression of Culture, History, and Lifestyle," *Nutrition Reviews* 55, no. 11, pt. 1 (1997): 383.

182 *"You cannot advise less fat!":* Trichopoulou, interview.

182 *took a magnifying glass:* Anna Ferro-Luzzi, W. Philip. T. James, and Anthony Kafatos, "The High-Fat Greek Diet: A Recipe for All?" *European Journal of Clinical Nutrition* 56, no. 9 (2002): 796–809.

182 *"few scientific grounds" for the claim:* Ibid., 806. Ferro-Luzzi's paper solicited a scathing reply not from Antonia Trichopoulou, but from her husband, Dimitrios, also a professor of epidemiology, with joint appointments at the Athens Medical School and

Harvard School of Public Health. Dimitrios defended his wife's research on olive oil generally but did not address any of the methodological problems that Ferro-Luzzi had pointed out in the data on Greek fat consumption. And in an example of the kind of derogatory tone sometimes used among nutrition researchers to defeat their opponents, Dimitrios concluded his letter by suggesting that Ferro-Luzzi's paper "would have been much more useful if it were written more carefully, with more attention to scientific evidence and less arrogance." Dimitrios Trichopoulos, "Letter to the Editor: In Defense of the Mediterranean Diet," *European Journal of Clinical Nutrition* 56 (2002): 928–929; Ferro-Luzzi's reply is here: Anna Ferro-Luzzi, W. Philip T. James, and Anthony Kafatos, "Response to the Letter Submitted by D. Trichopoulos Entitled, 'In Defense of the Mediterranean Diet,' " *European Journal of Clinical Nutrition* 56 (2002): 930–931.

183   *W. Philip T. James:* W. Philip T. James, interview with author, October 26, 2008.

184   *took him to a local tavern:* Trichopoulou, interview, and Walter C. Willett, interview with author, February 8, 2006.

184   *grew up in Michigan eating . . . "revelation":* Willett, interview with author, January 8, 2007.

184   *Trichopoulou remembers:* Trichopoulou, interview.

184   *"their jaws dropped":* Greg Drescher, interview with author, August 14, 2008.

184   *"us in the culinary community" . . . "We were depressed about it":* Ibid.

185   *"Willett was the pivotal figure":* Drescher, interview with author, August 14, 2008.

185   *persuaded by Antonia Trichopoulou's:* Walter C. Willett, email message to author, November 29, 2008.

186   *the "Mediterranean Diet Pyramid":* Justification for the pyramid is given in three papers: Walter C. Willett et al., "Mediterranean Diet Pyramid: A Cultural Model for Healthy Eating," *American Journal of Clinical Nutrition* 61, no. 6, suppl. (1995): 1402S; Lawrence H. Kushi, Elizabeth B. Lenart, and Walter C. Willett, "Health Implications of Mediterranean Diets in Light of Contemporary Knowledge. 1. Plant Foods and Dairy Products," *American Journal of Clinical Nutrition* 61, no. 6, suppl. (1995): 1407S; Lawrence H. Kushi, Elizabeth B. Lenart, and Walter C. Willett, "Health Implications of Mediterranean Diets in Light of Contemporary Knowledge. 2. Meat, Wine, Fats and Oils," *American Journal of Clinical Nutrition* 61, no. 6, suppl. (1995): 1416S.

186   *"olive oil poured all over":* Quoted in Sheryl Julian, "Mediterranean Diet: A Healthy Alternative? Against a Backdrop of Promotion, Experts Debate the Benefits of Olive Oil," *Boston Globe*, January 27, 1993.

188   *"The science just seemed to me too impressionistic":* Marion Nestle, interview with author, July 30, 2008.

188   *"correct in that the evidence":* Lawrence H. Kushi, interview with author, September 6, 2008.

188   *they had only one reviewer:* Marion Nestle, email message to author, August 5, 2008.

188   *a special supplement:* Marion Nestle, ed., "Mediterranean Diets," *American Journal of Clinical Nutrition* 61, no. 6, suppl. (1995): ixS–1427S.

188   *funded by the olive-oil industry:* Marion Nestle, "Mediterranean Diets: Science and Policy Implications," *American Journal of Clinical Nutrition* 61, no. 6 (1995): ixS.

189   *Ferro-Luzzi explained to me:* Ferro-Luzzi, interview.

191   American Journal of Cardiology: Henry Blackburn, "The Low Risk Coronary Male," *American Journal of Cardiology* 58, no. 1 (1986): 161.

191 *"feeling very romantic about Crete":* Henry Blackburn, interview with author, July 22, 2008.

192 *In April 1997:* Oldways Preservation & Exchange Trust, "Crete, Greece, and Healthy Mediterranean Diets: Celebrating the 50th Anniversary of the Scientific Studies of Healthy Traditional Mediterranean Diets Originating on Crete in 1947: An International Symposium," Apollonia Beach Hotel, Heraklion, Crete, April 5–11, 1997.

192 *while the Hale-Bopp comet:* Narsai David, email message to author, August 17, 2008.

192 *"died and gone to heaven"... "absolutely amazing":* Marion Nestle, interview with author, July 30, 2008.

193 *remembers Laura Shapiro:* Laura Shapiro, interview with author, August 5, 2008.

193 *"not just a bunch of slides":* Drescher, interview.

193 *says Shapiro:* Shapiro, interview.

194 *IOOC tried to generate:* Fausto Luchetti, interview with author, November 16, 2008.

194 *the IOOC was glad:* Ibid.

194 *tucked into flower arrangements... shopping bags:* Julian, "Mediterranean Diet: A Healthy Alternative?"

194 *"We'd start with the IOOC money":* Drescher, interview.

194 *"aligning the interests":* Ibid.

195 *funding from the Elais Oil Company:* Christos Aravanis and Anastasios S. Dontas, "Studies in the Greek Islands," in *The Seven Countries Study: A Scientific Adventure in Cardiovascular Disease Epidemiology*, ed. Daan Kromhout, Alessandro Menotti, and Henry Blackburn (Utrecht, Holland: Brouwer, 1994), 112.

195 *as Henry Blackburn recounts:* Blackburn, interview.

195 *Keys "helped significantly":* Aravanis and Dontas, "Studies in the Greek Islands," 112.

195 *when he first came out with his study:* Ancel Keys, ed., "Coronary Heart Disease in Seven Countries," *Circulation* 61 and 62, suppl. 1, American Heart Association Monograph No. 29 (1970): I-88.

195 *in a later publication, only one:* Den C. Hartog et al., *Dietary Studies and Epidemiology of Heart Disease* (The Hague, Holland: Stichting tot wetenschappelijke Voorlichting op Voedingsgebied, 1968), 57.

195 *"what was good for commodities":* Ferro-Luzzi, interview with author, July 22, 2008.

195 *Spain and Greece ran... European Union... $215 million:* Arne Astrup, Peter Mardkmann, and John Blundell, "Oiling of Health Messages in Marketing of Food," *Lancet* 356, no. 9244 (2000): 1786.

195 *also targeted European doctors... researchers to complain:* Ibid.

196 *Nestle spelled out:* Nestle, interview with author, July 30, 2008.

196 *"the fact that it was laundered":* Kushi, interview.

196 *"couldn't get with the program"... "couldn't justify my presence":* Shapiro, interview.

196 *"little olive oil ambassadors":* Ibid.

197 *"food world is particularly prey to corruption":* Nancy Harmon Jenkins, interview with author, August 6, 2008.

197 *nearly fifty papers on the Mediterranean Diet:* The figure of fifty studies was arrived at by counting studies listed in PubMed, www.ncbi.nih.gov.

198 *One ecstatic food writer:* Molly O'Neill, "A Dietary Debate: Is the Mediterranean a Nutritional Eden?" *New York Times*, February 3, 1993.

198 next *"nutritional eden"*: Ibid.

198 *"a velvet glove around the steely reality"*: Ibid.

199 *national consumption statistics . . . three times what it was in 1990:* IndexMundi calculation of USDA statistics, accessed January 4, 2014. http://www.indexmundi.com/agriculture /?country=us&commodity=olive-oil&graph=domestic-consumption.

200 Hippocrates *prescribed its leaves:* Hippocrates, *The Genuine Works of Hippocrates,* trans. Charles Darwin Adams (New York: Dover, 1868), part IV.

200 *"became good friends" . . . "tough scientist" . . . "to the death":* Anna Ferro-Luzzi et al., "Changing the Mediterranean Diet: Effects on Blood Lipids," *American Journal of Clinical Nutrition* 40, no. 5 (1984): 1027–1037.

200 *Ferro-Luzzi recorded:* Ibid.

201 *might help prevent . . . evidence so far is very weak:* Lawrence Kushi and Edward Giovannucci, "Dietary Fat and Cancer," *American Journal of Medicine* 113, no. 9, suppl. 2 (2002): 63S–70S.

201 *various studies on this score:* Álvaro Alonso, Valentina Ruiz-Gutierrez, and Miguel Ángel Martínez-González, "Monounsaturated Fatty Acids, Olive Oil and Blood Pressure: Epidemiological, Clinical and Experimental Evidence," *Public Health Nutrition* 9, no. 2 (2005): 251–257; Álvaro Alonso and Miguel Ángel Martínez-González, "Olive Oil Consumption and Reduced Incidence of Hypertension: The SUN Study," *Lipids* 39, no. 12 (2004): 1233–1238.

201 *flavonoids . . . unable to show:* Lee Hooper et al., "Flavonoids, Flavonoid-Rich Foods, and Cardiovascular Risk: A Meta-Analysis of Randomized Controlled Trials," *American Journal of Clinical Nutrition* 88, no. 1 (2008): 38–50.

201 *published a landmark article:* Antonia Trichopoulou et al., "Adherence to a Mediterranean Diet and Survival in a Greek Population," *New England Journal of Medicine* 348, no. 26 (2003): 2600.

202 *"a high intake of olive oil" . . . "significant and substantial":* Ibid., 2607.

202 *never actually measured the olive oil:* Antonia Trichopoulou, email message to author, December 13, 2013.

202 *not an item on the food-frequency questionnaire:* The Greek dietary questionnaire is an appendix of this description of the study protocol: Klea Katsouyanni et al., "Reproducibility and Relative Validity of an Extensive Semi-Quantitative Food Frequency Questionnaire Using Dietary Records and Biochemical Markers among Greek School-teachers," *International Journal of Epidemiology* 26, suppl. 1 (1997): S119.

202 *"estimated" its use:* Katsouyanni, ibid.

202 *one of the paper's tables:* Trichopoulou et al., "Adherence to a Mediterranean Diet," 2602.

202 *gathered all the available evidence:* Bob Bauer, letter responding to the Health Claim Petition (Docket No 2003Q-0559), Office of Nutritional Products, Labeling and Dietary Supplements, US Food and Drug Administration, November 1, 2004.

202 *FDA was not convinced:* Office of Nutritional Products, Labeling and Dietary Supplements, FDA, Letter Responding to Health Claim Petition dated August 28, 2003: Monounsaturated Fatty Acids from Olive Oil and Coronary Heart Disease (Docket No. 2003Q-0559), November 1, 2004.

202 *"low level of comfort":* Ibid.

202 *a few clinical trials on olive oil have been performed:* N. R. Damasceno et al., "Crossover Study of Diets Enriched with Virgin Olive Oil, Walnuts or Almonds. Effects on Lipids and Other Cardiovascular Risk Markers," *Nutrition Metabolism Cardiovascular Disease* 21, suppl. 1 (2011): 14S–20S; Paola Bogani et al., "Postprandial Anti-Inflammatory and Antioxidant Effects of Extra Virgin Olive Oil," *Atherosclerosis* 190, no. 1 (2007): 181–186; M. Fitó et al., "Anti-Inflammatory Effect of Virgin Olive Oil in Stable Coronary Disease Patients: A Randomized, Crossover, Controlled Trial," *European Journal of Clinical Nutrition* 62, no. 4 (2004): 570–574.

203 *moreover, a few recent studies on animals:* Reviewed in Seth J. Baum et al., "Fatty Acids in Cardiovascular Health and Disease: A Comprehensive Update," *Journal of Clinical Lipidology* 6, no. 3 (2012): 221–223.

203 *an article in* Nature: Gary K. Beauchamp et al., "Phytochemistry: Ibuprofen-Like Activity in Extra-Virgin Olive Oil," *Nature* 437, no. 7055 (2005): 45–46.

203 *"led to the only light-bulb":* Gary Beauchamp, "Oleocanthal: A Pungent Anti-Inflammatory Agent in Extra-Virgin Olive Oil," paper presented at the 15th Anniversary Mediterranean Diet Conference, Oldways Preservation and Exchange Trust and Mediterranean Foods Alliance, Cambridge, Boston, November 17, 2008.

203 *as one critic pointed out:* Vincenzo Fogliano and Raffaele Sacchi, "Oleocanthal in Olive Oil: Between Myth and Reality," *Molecular Nutrition & Food Research* 50, no. 1 (2006): 5–6.

203 *"surprisingly" is the word . . . concluding, in 2011:* Miguel Ruiz-Canela and Miguel A. Martínez-González, "Olive Oil in the Primary Prevention of Cardiovascular Disease," *Maturitas* 68, no. 3 (2011): 245.

204 *actual passage in the* Odyssey: Homer, *The Odyssey,* trans. A. T. Murray (Boston: Harvard University Press, 1919), bk. VI, ll. 211–222. (Emphasis added.)

204 *wrote a French historian:* Hamis Forbes, "Ethnoarchaeology and the Place of Olive in the Economy of the Southern Argolid, Greece," in *La Production du Vin et L'huile en Mediterranee* (The Production of Wine and Oil in the Mediterranean), BCH suppl. 26, eds. M. C. Amouretti and J. P. Brun (Paris: Ecole Française d'Athenes, 1993), 213–226.

204 *Hamilakis concludes . . . "no evidence" . . . "for culinary use":* Yannis Hamilakis, "Food Technologies/Technologies of the Today: The Social Context of Wine and Oil Production and Consumption in Bronze Age Crete," *World Archeology* 31, no. 1; reprinted in *Food Technology in Its Social Context* (London and New York: Routledge, 1999), 45–46.

204 *In Spain, too:* Grigg, "Olive Oil, the Mediterranean and the World," 168.

204 *"doubtful" that olive oil "made a contribution":* Marion Nestle, "The Mediterranean Diet and Disease Prevention," in *The Cambridge World History of Food* 2, eds. K. F. Kiple and K. C. Ornelias (Cambridge, UK: Cambridge University Press, 2000), 1196.

205 *lard:* For Italy, see: Massimo Montanari, *The Culture of Food* (Oxford: Blackwell, 1994), 165; Alan Davidson, "Lard," in *The Penguin Companion on Food* (New York: Penguin Books, 2002), 530–531.

205 *as Ancel Keys originally proposed:* Keys, "Coronary Heart Disease in Seven Countries," I-88.

205 *"psychosocial environment":* Trichopoulou and Lagiou, "Healthy Traditional Mediterranean Diet," 383–389.

206 *Anna Ferro-Luzzi attended an international meeting:* Ferro-Luzzi, interview with author, July 22, 2008.

206 *Trichopoulou found, when she combined:* Antonia Trichopoulou et al., "Modified Mediterranean Diet and Survival: EPIC-Elderly Prospective Cohort Study," *British Medical Journal* 330 (2005): 991–998.

207 *she developed the Mediterranean Diet Score:* Antonia Trichopoulou et al., "Diet and Overall Survival in Elderly People," *British Medical Journal* 311, no. 7018 (1995): 1457–1460.

207 *in a comprehensive review of indexes:* Anna Bach et al., "The Use of Indexes Evaluating the Adherence to the Mediterranean Diet in Epidemiological Studies: A Review," *Public Health Nutrition* 9, no. 1A (2006): 144.

208 *Andy R. Ness . . . told me that the indexes . . . "pretty dire":* Andy R. Ness, interview with author, October 13, 2008.

208 *Trichopoulou replies that her efforts:* Antonia Trichopoulou, interview with author, October 1, 2008.

208 *"This is our cry!":* Ibid.

208 *motivated as much by "Mother Greece":* James, interview; Nestle, interview with author, July 30, 2008; Serra-Majem, interview.

208 *"Antonia is perhaps guilty":* Elisabet Helsing, interview with author, July 30, 2008.

208 *Frank B. Hu wrote:* Frank B. Hu, "The Mediterranean Diet and Mortality—Olive Oil and Beyond," *New England Journal of Medicine* 348 (2003): 2595–2596.

209 *Lyon Diet Heart Study:* Michel de Lorgeril et al., "Mediterranean Alpha-Linolenic Acid-Rich Diet."

209 *"hopelessly underpowered" . . . as one researcher commented:* Andy R. Ness et al., "The Long-Term Effect of Dietary Advice in Men with Coronary Disease: Follow-Up of the Diet and Reinfarction Trial (DART)," *European Journal of Clinical Nutrition* 56, no. 6 (2002): 512–518.

209 *changed their diet . . . a tiny amount:* De Lorgeril et al., "Mediterranean Alpha-Linolenic Acid-Rich Diet," 1456.

210 *"containing star gooseberries, grapes":* Ram B. Singh et al., "Randomised Controlled Trial of Cardioprotective Diet in Patients with Recent Acute Myocardinal Infraction: Results of One Year Follow Up," *British Medical Journal* 304, no. 6833 (1992): 1015–1019; Ram B. Singh et al., "An Indian Experiment with Nutritional Modulation in Acute Myocardinal Infarction," *American Journal of Cardiology* 69, no. 9 (1992): 879.

211 *appeared to have been fabricated:* Caroline White, "Suspected Research Fraud: Difficulties Getting at the Truth," *British Medical Journal* 331, no. 7511 (2005): 285.

211 *the serum cholesterol values:* C. R. Soman, "Correspondence: Indo-Mediterranean Diet and Progression of Coronary Artery Disease," *Lancet* 366, no. 9483 (July 30, 2005): 365–366.

211 *"Suspected Research Fraud":* White, "Suspected Research Fraud."

211 *"either fabricated or falsified":* Sanaa Al-Marzouki et al., "Are These Data Real? Statistical Methods for the Detection of Data Fabrication in Clinical Trials," *British Medical Journal* 331, no. 7511 (July 30, 2005): 270.

211 *expressed their serious reservations:* Jane Smith and Fiona Godlee, "Investigating Allegations of Scientific Misconduct," *British Medical Journal* 331, no. 7511 (July 30, 2005): 245–246; Fiona Godlee, email to author, January 27, 2014. On the same day as *British Medical Journal* editors wrote of their reservations, an editor of the *Lancet* wrote an "Ex-

pression of Concern" about that journal's publication of a 2002 paper by Singh, based on the same trial data. Richard Horton, "Expression of Concern: Indo-Mediterranean Diet Heart Study," *Lancet* 366, no. 9483 (July 30, 2005): 354–356.

211 *an influential one by Lluís Serra-Majem:* Lluís Serra-Majem, Blanca Roman, and Ramón Estruch, "Scientific Evidence of Interventions Using the Mediterranean Diet: A Systematic Review," *Nutritional Review* 64, no. 2, pt. 2, suppl. (2006): S27–S47.

212 *"We have to take care":* Lluís Serra-Majem, interview with author, October 1, 2008.

212 *Indeed, in his literature review:* Serra-Majem, Roman, and Estruch, "Scientific Evidence of Interventions Using the Mediterranean Diet."

212 *"I wanted to leave the door open":* Serra-Majem, interview.

212 *GISSI-Prevenzione trial:* GISSI-Prevenzione Investigators (Gruppo Italiano per lo Studio della Sopravvivenza nell'Infarto micardico), "Dietary Supplementation with n-3 Polyunsaturated Fatty Acids and Vitamin E after Myocardial Infarction: Results of the GISSI-Prevenzione Trial," *Lancet* 354, no. 9177 (1999): 447–455.

213 *conducted in Israel:* Iris Shai et al., "Weight Loss with a Low-Carbohydrate, Mediterranean, or Low-Fat Diet," *New England Journal of Medicine* 359, no. 3 (2008): 229–241.

213 *"So my conservative conclusion is":* Stampfer, interview.

214 *a large Spanish study:* Ramón Estruch et al., "Primary Prevention of Cardiovascular Disease with a Mediterranean Diet," *New England Journal of Medicine* 368, no. 14 (2013): 1279–1290.

215 *announced the* New York Times*:* Gina Kolata, "Mediterranean Diet Shown to Ward Off Heart Attack and Stroke," *New York Times*, February 25, 2013, A1.

215 *Previous shorter trials had found:* See, for instance, Alain J. Nordmann et al., "Meta-Analysis Comparing Mediterranean to Low-Fat Diets for Modification of Cardiovascular Risk Factors," *American Journal of Medicine* 124, no. 9 (2011): 841–851.

215 *largest difference between the low-fat and Mediterranean groups:* Estruch et al., "Primary Prevention of Cardiovascular Disease with a Mediterranean Diet," supplementary appendix, 26.

216 *PREDIMED's appendix:* Ibid.

216 *Serra-Majem told me:* Serra-Majem, interview.

217 *"destroyed in processing":* Keys, Aravanis, and Sdrin, "Diets of Middle-Aged Men," 62.

217 *"absorbed into the clay":* Ibid., and Christos Aravanis, letter to author, October 6, 2008.

218 *"If the thirty-three lined up perfectly":* Sander Greenland, email message to author, January 5, 2008.

218 *"Jell-O in a Cretan earthquake":* Sander Greenland, email message to author, October 7, 2008.

218 *Much later, in the 1980s:* A. Ferro-Luzzi et al., "Changing the Mediterranean Diet: Effects on Blood Lipids," *American Journal of Clinical Nutrition* 40, no. 5 (1984): 1027–1037.

218 *Seven Countries study leaders acknowledged:* Daan Kromhout et al., "Food Consumption Patterns in the 1960s in Seven Countries," *American Journal of Clinical Nutrition* 49, no. 5 (1989): 892.

218 *Keys had published a paper:* Ibid.

218 *"high in saturated fatty acids":* Kushi et al., "Health Implications of Mediterranean Diets in Light of Contemporary Knowledge. 1," 1410S.

218 *"In Crete the meat is mostly goat":* Keys, Aravanis, and Sdrin, "Diets of Middle-Aged Men," 575–586.

218 *An earlier survey of the Cretan diet:* Leland Girard Allbaugh, *Crete: A Case Study of an Underdeveloped Area* (Princeton, NJ: Princeton University Press, 1953), 100.

219 *"Patrokles put a big bench in the firelight":* Quoted in John C. Waterlow, "Diet of the Classical Period of Greece and Rome," *European Journal of Clinical Nutrition* 43, suppl. 2 (1989): 6.

219 *"major hallmark" of his pyramid:* Kushi, "Health Implications of the Mediterranean Diets in Light of Contemporary Knowledge. 2," 1416S.

219 *Willett and his colleagues don't cite:* Ibid. Willett, "Health Implications of Mediterranean Diets in Light of Contemporary Knowledge. 2."

219 *Willett told me:* Walter Willett, email message to author, November 29, 2008.

220 *a thorough study of the Cretan diet:* Allbaugh, *Crete: A Case Study of an Underdeveloped Area.*

220 *"consisted chiefly of foods of vegetable origins":* Ibid., 100.

220 *"We are hungry most of the time . . . 72% of the families questioned":* Ibid., 105.

220 *"not very nourishing":* Vito Teti, "Food and Fatness in Calabria," in *Social Aspects of Obesity,* eds., Igor De Garine and Nancy J. Pollock, trans. Nicolette S. James (Amsterdam: Gordon and Breach, 1995).

221 *Teti to conclude:* Ibid., 9.

221 *18 percent of men . . . 5 percent in the north:* Instituto Nazionale di Statistica, "Analisi Statistica sui Giovani Iscritti nelle Liste di Leva" (Statistical Analysis of Young Conscripts), *ISTAT Notiziaro,* Serie 4, Foglio 41 (1993); 14:1–10 (in Italian).

221 *the shortest men in the entire country:* Cited in Teti, "Food and Fatness in Calabria," 9.

221 *"Meat is what . . . who had eaten meat":* Ibid., 15.

221 *ten times more meat . . . biggest change:* Anna Ferro-Luzzi and Francesco Branca, "Mediterranean Diet, Italian-Style: Prototype of a Healthy Diet," *American Journal of Clinical Nutrition* 61, no. 6, suppl. (1995): 1343S.

221 *by almost three inches:* World Health Organization, "Health for All: Statistical Database," Geneva: Regional Office for Europe, 1993.

221 *It was the same in Spain:* Lluís Serra-Majem et al., "How Could Changes in Diet Explain Changes in Coronary Heart Disease Mortality in Spain? The Spanish Paradox," *American Journal of Clinical Nutrition* 61, no. 6 (1995): 1353S.

222 *The Swiss ate:* E. Guberan, "Surprising Decline of Cardiovascular Mortality in Switzerland: 1951–1976," *Journal of Epidemiology and Community Health* 33, no. 2 (1979): 114–120.

222 *he found that the farmers:* Christos Aravanis, "The Classic Risk Factors for Coronary Heart Disease: Experience in Europe," *Preventive Medicine* 12, no. 1 (1983): 19.

222 *heart attack rates remained:* Christos D. Lionis et al., "Mortality Rates in a Cardiovascular 'Low-risk' Population in Rural Crete," *Family Practice* 10, no. 3 (1993): 300–304.

222 *In a 2004 paper:* Lluís Serra-Majem et al., "Does the Definition of the Mediterranean Diet Need to be Updated?" *Public Health Nutrition* 7, no. 7 (2004): 928.

223 *"pie almost never":* Allbaugh, *Crete: A Case Study,* 103.

223 *"hardly any pastries were eaten":* Kromhout et al., "Food Consumption Patterns in the 1960s in Seven Countries," 892.

223 *the intake of sugar and other carbohydrates fell:* Serra-Majem et al., "How Could Changes in Diet Explain Changes?," 1351S–1359S.

223 *Italian sugar consumption:* Paolo Rubba et al., "The Mediterranean Diet in Italy: An Update," *World Review of Nutrition and Dietetics* 97 (2007): 86.

223 *As Serra-Majem told me:* Lluís Serra-Majem, interview with author, August 2, 2008.

8: Exit Saturated Fats, Enter Trans Fats

227 *drop by his office to "ok":* Mark Matlock, interview with author, November 7, 2005.

228 *campaign called "Saturated Fat Attack":* Center for Science in the Public Interest, "Building a Healthier America, 35th Anniversary Report" (Washington, DC: Center for Science in the Public Interest, 2006); Center for Science in the Public Interest, "Saturated Fat Attack," booklet (Washington, DC: Center for Science in the Public Interest, 1988).

228 *Hydrogenated oils were therefore "not a bad bargain":* Michael F. Jacobson and Sarah Fritschner, *The Fast-Food Guide: What's Good, What's Bad, and How to Tell the Difference* (New York: Workman, 1986), 51.

228 *CSPI campaign successfully convinced:* Center for Science in the Public Interest, "Popcorn: Oil in Day's Work," *Nutrition Action Health Letter*, May 1994, last accessed February 12, 2014, http://www.cspinet.org/nah/popcorn.html.

228 *"a great boon":* Jacobson and Fritschner, *The Fast-Food Guide*, 132.

230 *now thought to be minimal:* K. C. Hayes for the Expert Panel, "Fatty Acid Expert Roundtable: Key Statements about Fatty Acids," *Journal of the American College of Nutrition* 29, no. 3, suppl. (2010): 285S–288S.

230 *funded by his own millions:* Ronald J. Adams and Kenneth M. Jennings, "Media Advocacy: A Case Study of Philip Sokolof's Cholesterol Awareness Campaigns," *Journal of Consumer Affairs* 27, no. 1 (1993): 145–165.

230 *"THE POISONING OF AMERICA":* Phil Sokolof, "The Poisoning of America," *New York Times*, November 1, 1988, A29. Identical full-page ads were also placed in the *Wall Street Journal*, *Washington Times*, *New York Post*, and *USA Today*, among other papers.

230 *"thousands of letters" . . . "only a few replies":* "Food Industry Gadfly Still Buzzing," Associated Press, March 5, 2009.

230 *his "greatest triumph":* Quoted in ibid.

232 *"We want to hold this market":* D. G. Wing, Testimony on Behalf of the American Soybean Association, to the US Congress, House Agricultural Committee, Hearings in March, 1948, printed in *Soybean Digest* (April 1948): 22.

232 *"remembers Steven Drake":* Steven Drake, interview with author, November 8, 2012.

232 *only 4 percent to 10 percent of the fats:* Oil World estimate for 1986, cited in "Tropical Fats Labeling: Malaysians Counterattack ASA Drive," *Journal of the American Oil Chemists' Society* 64, no. 12 (1987): 1596–1598; the 4 percent figure refers to 1985 consumption and comes from Youngmee K. Park and Elizabeth A. Yetley, "Trench Changes in Use and Current Intakes of Tropical Oils in the United States," *American Journal of Clinical Nutrition* 51, no. 5 (1990): 738–748.

233 *the name "'tree lard' for it":* Drake, interview.

233 *Part of the ASA's so-called "Fat-Fighter" kits:* Susan J. Duthie, "Soybean Growers Move to Label Palm Oil as Unhealthy, Bringing Rivalry to a Boil," *Wall Street Journal*, August 31, 1987.

233 *the* Wall Street Journal *described it:* Ibid.

233 *demonstrators turned up:* Barbara Crossette, "International Report: Malaysia Opposes Labels on Palm Oil," *New York Times*, October 19, 1987.

233 *"racist picture . . . to tell you the truth":* Drake, interview.

233 *"only 5 percent to 10 percent":* Kalyana Sundram, interview with author, January 8, 2008.

233 *have a chilling effect:* Sundram, interview.

234 *said Tan Sri Augustine Ong:* Tan Sri Augustine Ong, interview with author, March 11, 2008.

234 *protect against blood clots:* On protection against blood clots, see Gerard Hornstra and Anna Vendelmans-Starrenburg, "Induction of Experimental Arterial Occlusive Thrombi in Rats," *Atherosclerosis* 17, no. 3 (1973): 369–382; on rats, see Margaret L. Rand, Adje A. Hennissen, and Gerard Hornstra, "Effects of Dietary Palm Oil on Arterial Thrombosis, Platelet Responses and Platelet Membrane Fluidity in Rats," *Lipids* 23, no. 11 (1988): 1019–1023.

234 Nutrition Reviews *wrote:*"New Findings on Palm Oil," editorial, *Nutrition Reviews* 45, no. 9 (1987): 205–207.

234 *discovered in 1981:* Ian A. Prior et al., "Cholesterol, Coconuts, and Diet on Polynesian Atolls: A Natural Experiment: The Pukapuka and Tokelau Island Studies," *American Journal of Clinical Nutrition* 34, no. 8 (1981): 1552–1561.

234 *In Malaysia and the Philippines:* Pramod Khosla, "Palm Oil: A Nutritional Overview," *Journal of Agricultural and Food Industrial Organization* 17 (2000): 21–23.

234 *"a trade issue under the guise":* Ong, interview.

235 Ronk's testimony . . . *was widely credited:* Crossette, "International Report: Malaysia Opposes Labels on Palm Oil."

235 *told the* New York Times: Douglas C. McGill, "Tropical-Oil Exporters Seek Reprieve in U.S." *New York Times*, February 3, 1989, D1.

235 *Nabisco spokeswoman:* Ibid.

235 *yet some products:* Ibid.

236 *nearly 2 billion pounds:* "Tropical Fats Labeling: Malaysians Counterattack ASA Drive," *Journal of the American Oil Chemists' Society* 64, no. 12 (1987): 1596.

236 *was replaced pound for pound:* Based on multiple interviews, including Walter Farr, February 22, 2008, Frank Orthofer, January 15, 2008, Gil Leveille, February 21, 2008, and Lars Wiedermann, January 16, 2004.

236 *his "nuclear" option:* Ong, interview.

236 *ran full-page ads:* Malaysian Oil Palm Grower's Council, "To the American People—The Facts about Palm Oil," full-page advertisements in the *New York Times, Wall Street Journal, USA Today,* and other papers, January–February 1989; McGill, "Tropical Oils Exporters."

236 *ASA was well-aware:* Drake, interview.

236 *"pretty scary," "really shook us up" . . . "attacking one oil":* Ibid.

236 *"technically unsound . . . bad manners":* Lars Wiedermann, letter to author, March 3, 2008.

237 Wall Street Journal *reported:* Quoted in "US Soybean Group to Stop Depicting Palm Oil as Risk," *Wall Street Journal*, August 10, 1989, 1.

237 *the end of a "bitter, two-year feud":* Ibid.

237 *explained Ron Harris:* Ron Harris, interview with author, August 20, 2007.

237 *a trans-fat expert at USDA:* Gary List, interview with author, February 15, 2008.

237 *Walter Farr . . . "We intentionally upped trans fats":* Farr, interview with author, February 22, 2008.

237 *"Over my career . . . leaps and bounds":* Ibid.

237 *18 billions pounds . . . more than 80 percent:* Robert Reeves, email message to author, February 2, 2004.

238 *In the 1920s and thirties:* Thomas Percy Hilditch and N. L. Vidyarthi, "The Products of Partial Hydrogenation of Higher Monoethylenic Esters," *Proceedings of the Royal Society of London. Series A, Containing Papers of a Mathematical and Physical Character* 122, no. 790 (1929): 552–563.

238 *"in no way objectionable":* A. D. Barbour, "The Deposition and Utilization of Hydrogenation Isoleic Acid in the Animal Body," *Journal of Biological Chemistry* 10, no. 1 (1933): 71.

238 *grew more slowly:* A. K. Pickat, "The Nutritive Value of Margarine and Soy Bean-Oil," *Voprosy Pitaniia* 2, no. 5 (1933): 34–60.

238 *yin-yang of conflicting results:* Kenneth P. McConnel and Robert Gordon Sinclair, "Passage of Elaidic Acid through the Placenta and Also into the Milk of the Rat," *Journal of Biological Chemistry* 118, no. 1 (1937): 118–129; E. Aaes-Jørgensen et al., "The Role of Fat in the Diet of Rats," *British Journal of Nutrition* 10, no. 4 (1956): 292–304.

238 *was a 1944 study:* H. J. Deuel et al., "Studies of the Comparative Nutritive Value of Fats: I. Growth Rate and Efficiency of Conversion of Various Diets to Tissue," *Journal of Nutrition* 27 (1944): 107–121; H. J. Deuel, E. Movitt, and L. F. Hallman, "Studies of the Comparative Nutritive Value of Fats: The Negative Effect of Different Fats on Fertility and Lactation in the Rat," *Journal of Nutrition,* 27, no. 6 (1944): 509–513.

238 *opinion piece:* Harry J. Deuel, "The Butter-Margarine Controversy," *Science* 103, no. 2668 (1946): 183–187.

239 *The only published . . . "almost hopelessly complex" . . . "We are consuming" . . . "indeed fortunate":* Ahmed Fahmy Mabrouk and J. B. Brown, "The Trans Fatty Acids of Margarines and Shortenings," *Journal of the American Oil Chemists Society* 33, no. 3 (1956): 102.

239 *In 1961, Ancel Keys:* Joseph T. Anderson, Francisco Grande, and Ancel Keys, "Hydrogenated Fats in the Diet and Lipids in the Serum of Man," *Journal of Nutrition* 75 (1961): 368–394.

239 *Joseph T. Judd:* Joseph T. Judd, interview with author, October 27, 2005.

240 *a study out of its company lab:* Don E. McOsker et al., "The Influence of Partially Hydrogenated Dietary Fats on Serum Cholesterol Levels," *Journal of the American Medical Association* 180, no. 5 (1962): 380–385.

240 *study in* Science: Patricia V. Johnston, Ogden C. Johnson, and Fred A. Kummerow, "Occurrence of Trans Fatty Acids in Human Tissue," *Science* 126, no. 3276 (1957): 698–699.

241 *"a big wheel":* Fred A. Kummerow, interview with author, November 6, 2005.

241 *for posing in an ad with a bottle of Crisco:* Fred A. Kummerow, letter to Campell Moses, July 11, 1968, in author's possession.

242 *agreed with him about the trans fat language:* Kummerow, interview with author, September 25, 2003.

242 *had 150,000 dietary-guideline pamphlets printed up:* American Heart Association, Committee on Nutrition, "Diet and Heart Disease: This Statement was Developed by the Committee on Nutrition and Authorized for Release by the Central Committee for Medical and Community Program of the American Heart Association," American Heart Association, 1968.

242 *It didn't want anything revealed:* Letter from Malcolm R. Stephens, president of the Institute of Shortening and Edible Oils, to Campbell Moses, July 2, 1968, in author's possession.

242 *new batch of guidelines printed up:* American Heart Association, Committee on Nutrition, "Diet and Heart Disease: Revised Report of the Committee on Nutrition Authorized by the Central Committee for Medical and Community Program of the American Heart Association—1968," American Heart Association, 1968.

242 *"any of the heart association"... giving him money:* Kummerow, interview, September 25, 2003.

243 *confirmed Kummerow's original 1957 study:* Patricia V. Johnston, Ogden C. Johnson, and Fred A. Kummerow, "Deposition in Tissues and Fecal Excretion of Trans Fatty Acids in the Rat," *Journal of Nutrition* 65, no. 1 (1958): 13–23.

243 *are like foreign agents:* Walter J. Decker and Walter Mertz, "Effects of Dietary Elaidic Acid on Membrane Function in Rat Miochondria and Erythrocytes," *Journal of Nutrition* 91, no. 3 (1967): 327; William E. M. Lands et al., "A Comparison of Acyltransferase Activities in Vitro with the Distribution of Fatty Acids in Lecithins and Triglycerides in Vivo," *Lipids* 1, no. 3 (1966): 224; Mohamedain M. Mahfouz, T. L. Smith, and Fred A. Kummerow, "Effect of Dietary Fats on Desaturase Activities and the Biosynthesis of Fatty Acids in Rat-Liver Microsomes," *Lipids* 19, no. 3 (1984): 214–222.

243 *ramped up their uptake of calcium:* Fred A. Kummerow, Sherry Q. Zhou, and Mohamedain M. Mahfouz, "Effects of Trans Fatty Acids on Calcium Influx into Human Arterial Endothelial Cells," *American Journal of Clinical Nutrition* 70, no. 5 (1999): 832–838.

243 *fifty unnatural ones:* Randall Wood, Fred Chumbler, and Rex Wiegand, "Incorporation of Dietary *cis* and *trans* Isomers of Octadecenoate in Lipid Classes of Liver and Hepatoma," *Journal of Biological Chemistry* 252, no. 6 (1977): 1965–1970.

243 *Wood told me:* Randall Wood, interview with author, December 18, 2003.

243 *echoed David Kritchevsky:* David Kritchevsky, interview with author, May 31, 2005.

244 *American Dairy Association would not fund:* Thomas H. Applewhite, interview with author, December 11, 2003.

245 *explained Lars H. Wiedermann:* Wiedermann, interview with author, January 16, 2004.

245 *"the ringleader on trans":* Applewhite, interview.

245 *Wiedermann remembers going after Kummerow:* Wiedermann, interview with author, January 16, 2004.

245 *Kummerow found them intimidating:* Kummerow, interview with author, August 21, 2007.

245 *"their main effect"... "they would blindside you":* Wood, interview with author, December 18, 2003.

246 *a study he had conducted on miniature pigs:* Fred A Kummerow et al., "The Influence of Three Sources of Dietary Fats and Cholesterol on Lipid Composition of Swine Serum Lipids and Aorta Tissue," *Artery* 4 (1978): 360–384.

246 *as a USDA chemist . . . described it to me:* Gary List, interview with author, February 15, 2008.

246 *"We spent lots of time" . . . "nothing either wrong or immoral":* Wiedermann, letter to author, March 19, 2008.

247 *set off "alarm bells":* Wiedermann, interview with author, February 7, 2008.

247 *a paper documenting:* Mary Enig, R. Munn, and M. Keeney, "Dietary Fat and Cancer Trends—A Critique," *Federation Proceedings,* Federation of American Societies for Experimental Biology, 37, no. 9 (1978): 2215.

247 *three highly critical Letters to the Editor:* Thomas H. Applewhite, " 'Statistical Correlations' Relating Trans-Fats to Cancer: A Commentary," *Federation Proceedings,* Federation of American Societies for Experimental Biology 38, no. 11 (1979): 2435; J. C. Bailar, "Dietary Fat and Cancer Trends—A Further Critique," *Federation Proceedings,* Federation of American Societies for Experimental Biology 38, no. 11 (1979): 2435; W. H. Meyer, "Dietary Fat and Cancer Trends—Further Comments," *Federation Proceedings,* Federation of American Societies for Experimental Biology 38, no. 11 (1979): 2436.

247 *Enig recalled . . . those "guys" included:* Applewhite, interview; Mary G. Enig, interview with author, October 15, 2003.

247 *As Enig describes:* Enig, interview with author, December 29, 2004.

247 *"nutso" . . . "off-the-wall" . . . "a zealot":* "nutso," Edward A. Emken, interview with author, October 25, 2007; "paranoid," Robert J. Nicolosi, interview with author, October 27, 2005; "off the wall," Rick Crystal, interview with author, October 27, 2005; "a zealot," Steve Hill, interview with author, February 4, 2008.

248 *said one attendee:* List, interview with author, February 15, 2008.

248 *commented another:* Frank T. Orthoefer, interview with author, January 15, 2008.

248 *review . . . found "no evidence":* Life Sciences Research Center, Federation of American Societies for Experimental Biology, *Evaluation of the Health Aspects of Hydrogenated Soybean Oil as a Food Ingredient,* Prepared for Bureau of Foods, Food and Drug Administration, Department of Health, Education, and Welfare (Bethesda, MD: Life Sciences Research Office, Federation of American Societies for Experimental Biology, 1976), 30.

248 *Kummerow's disturbing finding:* Ibid., 29.

249 *to conclude that trans fats:* Frederic R. Senti, ed., *Health Aspects of Dietary Trans-Fatty Acids,* Prepared for the Center for Food Safety and Applied Nutrition, Food and Drug Administration, Department of Health and Human Services (Bethesda, MD: Life Sciences Research Office, Federation of American Societies for Experimental Biology, 1985).

249 *Enig told the assembled experts:* "FASEB Nutrition Study Using 'Flawed Data,' Researcher Charges," *Food Chemical News,* January 25, 1988, 52–54.

250 *continued to criticize Enig's work:* Thomas H. Applewhite, "Nutritional Effects of Isomeric Fats: Facts and Fallacies," in *Dietary Fats and Health,* eds. Edward George Perkins and W. J. Visek (Chicago: American Oil Chemists' Society, 1983), 421–422.

250 *David Ozonoff . . . once observed:* David Ozonoff, "The Political Economy of Cancer Research," *Science and Nature* 2 (1979): 15.

250 *submitted a paper:* J. Edward Hunter and Thomas H. Applewhite, "Isomeric Fatty Acids in the US Diet: Levels and Health Perspectives," *American Journal of Clinical Nutrition* 44, no. 6 (1986): 707–717.

250 *Enig claimed that Hunter's calculations:* "FASEB Nutrition Study Using 'Flawed Data,' " 52–54.

251 *when the reality was 22 percent:* Mary G. Enig, *Trans Fatty Acids in the Food Supply: A Comprehensive Report Covering 60 Years of Research*, 2nd ed. (Silver Spring, MD: Enig Associates, 1995), 152.

251 *According to her measurements:* Ibid., 108.

251 *says Enig's colleague, Beverly B. Teter:* Beverly B. Teter, interview with author, December 15, 2003.

251 *Enig's best estimate:* Mary G. Enig et al., "Isomeric *Trans* Fatty Acids in the US Diet," *Journal of the American College of Nutrition* 9, no. 5 (1990): 471–486.

251 *set up by FASEB in 1986:* Sue Ann Anderson, "Guidelines for Use of Dietary Intake Data," *Journal of the American Dietetic Association* 88, no. 10 (1988): 1258–1260.

251 *"No one other than Enig":* "Trans Fatty Acids Dispute Rages in Letters to FASEB," editorial, *Food Chemical News*, May 30, 1988, 8.

251 *"unwarranted and unsubstantiated"* . . . *"physiological effects":* Ibid., 6.

251 *"trans fatty acids do not pose any harm":* Ibid.

251 *publicly wondered in a letter:* Ibid.

252 *grumbled Hunter:* J. Edward Hunter, interview with author, December 17, 2003.

252 *read and been troubled . . . to look into it:* Martijn B. Katan, interview with author, September 27, 2005.

252 *Korver explains that:* Onno Korver, interview with author, November 2, 2007.

252 *"It took some persuasion":* Ibid.

252 *Katan conducted a feeding trial:* Ronald P. Mensink and Martijn B. Katan, "Effect of Dietary Trans Fatty Acids on High-Density and Low-Density Lipoprotein Cholesterol Levels in Healthy Subjects," *New England Journal of Medicine* 323, no. 7 (1990): 439–445.

253 *"I thought the HDL-effect must be incorrect":* Katan, interview.

253 *Associated Press headline:* "Margarine's Fatty Acids Raise Concern," Associated Press, August 16, 1990.

253 *a letter to the editor:* Robert M. Reeves, "Letter to the Editor: Effect of Dietary Trans Fatty Acids on Cholesterol Levels," *New England Journal of Medicine* 324, no. 5 (1991): 338–340.

253 *"not totally convincing":* Hunter, interview.

253 *says Katan:* Katan, interview.

253 *number of follow-up studies:* Peter L. Zock and Martijn B. Katan, "Hydrogenation Alternatives: Effects of *Trans* Fatty Acids and Stearic Acid Versus Linoleic Acid on Serum Lipids and Lipoproteins in Humans," *Journal of Lipid Research* 33 (1992): 399–410; Alice H. Lichtenstein et al., "Hydrogenation Impairs the Hypolipidemic Effect of Corn Oil in Humans," *Arteriosclerosis and Thrombosis* 13, no. 2 (1993): 154–161; Randall Wood et al., "Effect of Butter, Mono- and Polyunsaturated Fatty Acid-Enriched Butter, *Trans* Fatty Acid Margarine, and Zero *Trans* Fatty Acid Margarine on Serum Lipids and Lipoproteins in Healthy Men," *Journal of Lipid Research* 34, no. 1 (1993): 1–11; Randall Wood et al., "Effect of Palm Oil, Margarine, Butter and Sunflower Oil on Serum Lipids and Lipoproteins of Normocholesterolemic Middle-Aged Men," *Journal Nutritional Biochemistry* 4, no. 5 (1993): 286–297; Antti Aro et al., "Stearic Acid, *Trans*

Fatty Acids, and Dairy Fat: Effects on Serum and Lipoprotein Lipids, Apolipoproteins, Lipoprotein(a), and Lipid Transfer Proteins in Healthy Subjects," *American Journal of Clinical Nutrition* 65, no. 5 (1997): 1419–1426.

253 *as ISEO experts pointed out:* Thomas H. Applewhite, "Trans-Isomers, Serum Lipids and Cardiovascular Disease: Another Point of View," *Nutrition Reviews* 51, no. 11 (1993): 344–345.

254 *"close all of them":* Korver, interview.

254 *observes Katan:* Katan, interview.

255 *"All of us get industry money":* Robert J. Nicolosi, interview with author, October 27, 2005.

255 *Gerald McNeill . . . spelled this out for me:* Gerald McNeill, interview with author, December 10, 2012 and January 29, 2014.

255 *a number of reviews have shown that industry-funded trials:* See, for instance, Justin E. Bekelman, "Scope and Impact of Financial Conflicts of Interest in Biomedical Research: A Systematic Review," *Journal of the American Medical Association* 289, no. 4 (2003): 454–465.

256 *"therefore neutralize them":* Joseph T. Judd, interview with author, October 27, 2005.

256 *Judd confirmed them:* Joseph T. Judd et al., "Dietary Trans Fatty Acids: Effects on Plasma Lipids and Lipoproteins of Healthy Men and Women," *American Journal of Clinical Nutrition* 59, no. 4 (1994): 861–868.

256 *recalled Judd:* Judd, interview.

256 *relished K. C. Hayes:* K. C. Hayes, interview with author, February 18, 2008.

256 *acknowledged Hunter:* Hunter, interview.

256 *found himself transferred:* George Wilhite, interview with author, February 26, 2008.

256 *said Michael Mudd:* Michael Mudd, interview with author, September 30, 2005.

257 *said Mudd:* Ibid.

257 *yet another review:* Penny M. Kris-Etherton and Robert J. Nicolosi, "Trans Fatty Acids and Coronary Heart Disease Risk," International Life Sciences Institute, Technical Committee on Fatty Acids, ILSI Press, 1995; reprinted in "Trans Fatty Acids and Coronary Heart Disease Risk," *American Journal of Clinical Nutrition* 62, no. 3, suppl. (1995): 655S–708S.

257 *said Penny Kris-Etherton:* Penny Kris-Etherton, interview with author, June 8, 2007.

257 *Katan considered the report:* Katan, interview.

9. Exit Trans Fats, Enter Something Worse?

260 *found that eating trans fats was correlated:* Walter C. Willett et al., "Intake of Trans Fatty Acids and Risk of Coronary Heart Disease among Women," *Lancet* 341, no. 8845 (1993): 581–585.

260 *an opinion piece:* Walter C. Willett and Alberto Ascherio, "Trans Fatty Acids: Are the Effects Only Marginal?," *American Journal of Public Health* 84, no. 5 (1994): 722–724.

260 *"I'll never forget as long as I live":* Michael Mudd, interview with author, September 30, 2005.

261 *"It's a month that will live with me in infamy":* Rick Cristol, interview with author, October 27, 2005.

261 *"The industry went nuclear over it":* Martijn B. Katan, interview with author, September 27, 2005.

262 *July 1994 group:* "Trans Fatty Acids and Risk of Myocardial Infarction," Toxicology Forum Annual Meeting, July 11–15, 1994.

262 *After Willett presented his epidemiological findings:* Ibid., and Samuel Shapiro, interview with author, December 27, 2005.

262 *No one really knows exactly:* Ibid.

263 *"weak" to "very weak":* David J. Hunter et al., "Comparisons of Measures of Fatty Acid Intake by Subcutaneous Fat Aspirate, Food Frequency Questionnaire, and Diet Records in a Free-Living Population of US Men," *American Journal of Epidemiology* 135, no. 4 (1992): 418–427.

263 *National Cancer Institute concluded:* Ernst J. Schaefer et al., "Lack of Efficacy of a Food-Frequency Questionnaire in Assessing Dietary Macronutrient Intakes in Subjects Consuming Diets of Known Composition," *American Journal of Clinical Nutrition* 71, no. 3 (2000): 746–751. Other problems with the food-frequency questionnaire are described in the following papers: Somdat Mahabir et al., "Calorie Intake Misreporting by Diet Record and Food Frequency Questionnaire Compared to Doubly Labeled Water among Postmenopausal Women," *European Journal of Clinical Nutrition* 60, no. 4 (2005): 561–565; Alan R. Kristal, Ulrike Peters, and John D. Potter, "Is It Time to Abandon the Food Frequency Questionnaire?" *Cancer Epidemiology, Biomarkers and Prevention* 14, no. 12 (2005): 2826–2828; Arthur Schatzkin et al., "A Comparison of a Food Frequency Questionnaire with a 24-Hour Recall for Use in an Epidemiological Cohort Study: Results from the Biomarker-Based Observing Protein and Energy Nutrition (OPEN) Study," *International Journal of Epidemiology* 32, no. 6 (2003): 1054–1062.

263 *hardly the full list of concerns:* Sheila A. Bingham, "Limitations of the Various Methods for Collecting Dietary Intake Data," *Annals of Nutrition and Metabolism* 35, no. 3 (1991): 117–127.

263 *thirtyfold increase:* R. Doll et al., "Mortality in Relation to Smoking: 40 Years' Observations on Male British Doctors," *British Medical Journal* 309, no. 6959 (1994): 901–911.

264 *Richard Hall . . . recalled:* Richard Hall, interview with author, December 19, 2007.

264 *Michael Pariza . . . said:* Michael Pariza, interview with author, February 6, 2008.

264 *published multiple articles:* Frank Sacks and Lisa Litlin, "Trans-Fatty-Acid Content of Common Foods," *New England Journal of Medicine* 329, no. 26 (1993): 1969–1970; K. Michels and F. Sacks, "Trans Fatty Acids in European Margarines," *New England Journal of Medicine* 332, no. 8 (1995); 541–542; Tim Byers, "Hardened Fats, Hardened Arteries?" *New England Journal of Medicine* 337, no. 21 (1997), 1544–1545; A. Ascherio et al., "Trans Fatty Acids and Coronary Heart Disease," *New England Journal of Medicine* 340, no. 25 (1999): 1994–1998; S. J. Dyerberg, and A. N. Astrup, "High Levels of Industrially Produced Trans Fat in Popular Fast Foods," *New England Journal of Medicine* 354, no. 15 (2006): 1650–1652; D. Mozaffarian et al., "Trans Fatty Acids and Cardiovascular Disease," *New England Journal of Medicine* 354, no. 15 (2006): 1601–1613.

265 *"multiple testing" . . . said S. Stanley Young:* S. Stanley Young, interview with author, January 2, 2007; S. Stanley Young, "Gaming the System: Chaos from Multiple Testing," *IMS Bulletin* 36, no. 10 (2007): 13.

265 *Looking at the astrological signs:* Peter C. Austin et al., "Testing Multiple Statistical Hypotheses Resulted in Spurious Associations: A Study of Astrological Signs and Health," *Journal of Clinical Epidemiology* 59, no. 9 (2006): 964–969.

265 *said Bob Nicolosi:* Bob Nicolosi, interview with author, October 27, 2005.

265 *"We are really conducting a very large human-scale":* "Trans Fatty Acids and Risk of Myocardial Infarction," Toxicology Forum Annual Meeting.

266 *originally been a major force . . . headlining them as "Trans":* Elaine Blume, "The Truth About Trans: Hydrogenated Oils Aren't Guilty as Charged," *Nutrition Action Healthletter* 15, no. 2 (1988): 8–9; Margo Wootan, Bonnie Liebman, and Wendie Rosofsky, "Trans: The Phantom Fat," *Nutrition Action Healthletter* 23, no. 7 (1996): 10–14.

266 *said Jacobson:* Michael Jacobson, interview with author, October 25, 2005.

267 *FDA issued a "proposed rule":* Food and Drug Administration, Department of Health and Human Services, "Food Labeling: Trans Fatty Acids in Nutrition Labeling, Nutrient Content Claims, and Health Claims," *Federal Register* 68, no. 133 (July 11, 2003), docket no. 94P–0036: 41436.

267 *the IOM expert panel recommended:* Institute of Medicine of the National Academies, Panel on Macronutrients, Panel on the Definition of Dietary Fiber, Subcommittee on Upper Reference Levels of Nutrients, Subcommittee on Interpretation and Uses of Dietary Reference Intakes, and the Standing Committee on the Scientific Evaluation of Dietary Reference Intakes, "Letter Report on Dietary Reference Intakes for Trans Fatty Acids," drawn from the report, *Dietary Reference Intakes for Energy, Carbohydrate, Fiber, Fat, Fatty Acids, Cholesterol, Protein, and Amino Acids*, part 1 (Washington, DC: National Academies Press, 2002), 14.

267 *would have excessively disparaged:* FDA, *Federal Register* 68, 41459.

267 *"scientifically inaccurate and misleading":* Ibid., 41452.

268 *"sufficient" to conclude:* Ibid., 41444.

268 *were deemed secondary:* Ibid., 41448.

268 *it has long suffered:* See, for example, "The F.D.A. in Crisis: It Needs More Money and Talent," editorial, *New York Times*, February 3, 2008, 14.

268 *Mark Matlock . . . described to me:* Mark Matlock, interview with author, November 7, 2005.

269 *said Farr:* Walter Farr, interview with author, February 22, 2008.

269 *"had to confess them":* Bruce Holub, interview with author, September 23, 2007.

269 *in some 42,720 packaged food products:* Food and Drug Administration, Department of HHS, "Food Labeling: Trans Fatty Acids in Nutrition Labeling, Nutrient Content Claims, and Health Claims: Proposed Rule" (1999), 62776–62777.

269 *said ADM's Mark Matlock:* Matlock, interview, October 9, 2005.

270 *said Pat Verduin:* Qutoted in Kim Severson and Melanie Warner, "Fat Substitute Is Pushed Out of the Kitchen," *New York Times*, February 15, 2005, A1.

270 *Said Martijn Katan:* Martijn Katan, interview with author, September 27, 2005.

270 *exclaimed Gil Leveille:* Gil Leveille, interview with author, February 27, 2008.

271 *pointed out Au Bon Pain's Master Baker:* Quoted in P. Cobe et al., "Best Do-Over That We'll All Be Doing Soon," *Restaurant Business*, April 6, 2007.

271 *said Kris Charles:* Quoted in Delroy Alexander, Jeremy Manier, and Patricia Callahan, "For Every Fad, Another Cookie: How Science and Diet Crazes Confuse Consumers,

Reshape Recipes and Rail, Ultimately, to Reform Eating Habits," *Chicago Tribune*, August 23, 2005.

271 *creamy middle melted . . . wafers tended to break:* Ibid.

271 *what he wanted was an injunction:* Stephen L. Joseph, interview with author, November 2003.

272 *"deeply concerned and angry":* BanTransFat.com, Inc., "Citizen Petition Regarding Trans Fats Labeling," Ban Trans Fats, May 22, 2003, http://bantransfats.com/fdapetition .html.

272 *to reformulate the Oreo cookie:* Kantha Shelke, "How Food Processors Removed Trans Fats Ahead of Deadline," *Food Processing*, October 4, 2006, http://www.foodprocessing.com /articles/2006/013/.

273 *"Interesterification is akin to":* Gil Leveille, interview with author, June 24, 2006.

273 *"We just don't know" . . . "another trans lurking":* Ibid.

274 *the "fat replacers":* Mimma Pernetti et al., "Structuring Edible Oil with Lecithin and Sorbitan Tri-Stearate," *Food Hydrocolloids* 21, nos. 5–6 (2007): 855–861.

274 *Danisco:* Keith Seiz, "Formulations: Sourcing Ideal Trans-Free Oils," *Functional Foods & Nutraceuticals*, July 2005, 37.

275 *the oil may actually be beneficial for health:* See the entire supplement, Pramad Khasla and Kalyanan Sundram, eds., "A Supplement on Palm Oils," *Journal of the American College of Nutrition* 29, no. 3, suppl. (2010): 237S–342S. Note that the editors are employed by the palm oil industry.

276 *omega-6s are related to depression:* Joseph R. Hibbeln and Norman Salem Jr., "Dietary Polyunsaturated Fatty Acids and Depression: When Cholesterol Does Not Satisfy," *American Journal of Clinical Nutrition* 62, no. 1 (1995): 1–9; J. R. Hibbeln et al., "Do Plasma Polyunsaturates Predict Hostility and Violence?" in *Nutrition and Fitness: Metabolic and Behavior Aspects in Health and Disease, World Review of Nutrition and Diatetics* 82, eds., A. P. Simopoulos and K. N. Pavlou (Basel, Switzerland: Karger, 1996): 175–186.

276 *AHA most recent dietary review:* William S. Harris et al., "Omega-6 Fatty Acids and Risk for Cardiovascular Disease. A Scientific Advisory from the American Heart Association Nutrition Subcommittee of the Council of Nutrition, Physical Activity, and Metabolism; Council on Cardiovascular Nursing; and Council on Epidemiology and Prevention," *Circulation* 119, no. 6 (2009): 902–907.

276 *Gerald McNeill . . . explained that:* Gerald McNeill, interview with author, December 10, 2012.

277 *"As those oils are heated":* Ibid.

277 *Robert Ryther . . . "It builds up":* Robert Ryther, interview with author, January 11, 2013.

278 *"Anybody that has a fryer has this problem":* Ibid.

278 *higher among chefs and restaurant "workers":* D. Coggon et al., "A Survey of Cancer and Occupation of Young and Middle Aged Men. Cancers of the Respiratory Tract," *British Journal of Industrial Medicine* 43, no. 5 (1986): 332–338; E. Lund and J. K. Borgan, "Cancer Mortality among Cooks," *Tidsskrift for Den Norske Legeforening* 107 (1987): 2635–2637; I. Foppa and C. Minder, "Oral, Pharyngeal and Laryngeal Cancer as a Cause of Death among Swiss Cooks," *Scandinavian Journal of Work, Environment and Health* 18 (1992): 287–292. See, also, She-Ching Wu and Gow-Chin Yen, "Effects of

Cooking Oil Fumes on the Genotoxicity and Oxidative Stress in Human Lung Carcinoma (A-549) Cells," *Toxicology in Vitro* 18, no. 5 (2004): 571–580.

278 *"probably" carcinogenic to humans:* World Health Organization, International Agency for Research on Cancer (IARC), "Household Use of Solid Fuels and High-Temperature Frying," IARC Monographs on the Evaluation of Carcinogenic Risks to Humans, vol. 95 (Lyon, France: IARC, 2006), 392.

279 *piece of fried chicken:* Jian Tang et al., "Isolation and Identification of Volatile Compounds from Fried Chicken," *Journal of Agricultural and Food Chemistry* 31, no. 6 (1983): 1287–1292.

279 *published a large body of work:* Reviewed in E. W. Crampton et al., "Studies to Determine the Nature of the Damage to the Nutritive Value of Some Vegetable Oils from Heat Treatment: IV. Ethyl Esters of Heat Polymerized Linseed, Soybean and Sunflower Seed Oils," *Journal of Nutrition* 60, no. 1 (1956): 13–24. See also John S. Andrews et al., "Toxicity of Air-Oxidized Soybean Oil," *Journal of Nutrition* 70, no. 2 (1960): 199–210; and Samuel M. Greenberg and A. C. Frazer, "Some Factors Affecting the Growth and Development of Rats Fed Rancid Fat," *Journal of Nutrition* 50, no. 4 (1953): 421–440.

279 *"stuck to the wire floor":* Crampton et al., "Studies to Determine the Nature of the Damage to Nutritive Value," 18.

279 *the chemist Denham Harman:* Denham Harman, "Letter to the Editor. Atherosclerosis: Possible Ill-Effects of the Use of Highly Unsaturated Fats to Lower Serum Cholesterol Levels," *Lancet* 275, no. 7005 (1957): 1116–1117.

280 *food chemists from Japan reported:* Takehi Ko Ohfuji and Takashi Kaneda, "Characterization of Toxic Components in Thermally Oxidized Oil," *Lipids* 8, no. 6 (1973): 353–359; Toshimi Akiya, Chuji Araki, and Kiyoko Igarashi, "Novel Methods of Evaluation Deterioration and Nutritive Value of Oxidized Oil," *Lipids* 8, no. 6 (1973): 348–352.

280 *pathologist . . . reported:* Hans Kaunitz and Ruth E. Johnson, "Exacerbation of the Heart and Liver Lesions in Rats by Feeding Various Mildly Oxidized Fats, *Lipids* 8, no. 6 (1973): 329–336.

280 *in 1991, he took stock of the field:* Hermann Esterbauer, Rudolf Jörg Schaur, and Helmward Zollner, "Chemistry and Biochemistry of 4-Hydroxynonenal, Malonaldehyde and Related Aldehydes," *Free Radical Biology & Medicine* 11, no. 1 (1991): 81–128; "rapid cell death": 91, "great diversity of deleterious effects" and "rather likely": 118.

280 *Aldehydes are "very reactive compounds . . . reacting constantly":* A. Saari Csallany, interview with author, February 21, 2013.

280 *one of the reasons that aldehydes were ignored:* Earl G. Hammond, interview with author, October 9, 2007.

280 *Csallany refined the ability to detect:* Song-Suk Kim, Daniel D. Gallaher, and A. Saari Csallany, "Lipophilic Aldehydes and Related Carbonyl Compounds in Rat and Human Urine," *Lipids* 34, no. 5 (1999): 489–495.

281 *showed that they were produced by a range:* C. M. Seppanen and A. Saari Csallany, "Simultaneous Determination of Lipophilic Aldehydes by High-Performance Liquid Chromatography in Vegetable Oil," *Journal of the American Oil Chemists' Society* 78, no. 12 (2001): 1253–1260; C. M. Seppanen and A. Saari Csallany, "Formation of 4-Hydroxynonenal, a Toxic Aldehyde, in Soybean Oil at Frying Temperature," *Journal*

of the American Oil Chemists' Society 79, no. 10 (2002): 1033–1038; In Hwa Han and A. Saari Csallany, "Formation of Toxic a,b-Unsaturated 4-Hydroxy-Aldehydes in Thermally Oxidized Fatty Acid Methyl Esters," *Journal of the American Oil Chemists' Society* 86, no. 3 (2009): 253–260.

281 *not detected by the standard tests:* Csallany, interview; Mark Matlock, interview with author, February 19, 2013; Kathleen Warner, interview with author, November 8, 2013.

281 *One of Csallany's recent projects:* A. Saari Csallany et al., "4-Hydroxynonenal (HNE), a Toxic Aldehyde in French Fries from Fast Food Restaurants," poster presentation at the HNE Symposium of the 16th Bi-Annual Conference of the Free Radical Society and HNE Symposium, London, September 1–9, 2012.

281 *She would like to do more studies:* Csallany, interview

281 *says Giuseppi Poli:* Giuseppi Poli, interview with author, February 12, 2014.

281 *cause LDL-cholesterol to oxidize:* Hermann Esterbauer et al., "Autoxidation of Human Low Density Lipoprotein: Loss of Polyunsaturated Fatty Acids and Vitamin E and Generation of Aldehydes," *Journal of Lipid Research* 28, no. 5 (1987): 495–509.

281 *role in atherosclerosis:* I. Staprans et al., "Oxidized Cholesterol in the Diet Accelerates the Development of Atherosclerosis in LDL Receptor- and Apolipoprotein E-Deficient Mice," *Arteriosclerosis, Thrombosis, and Vascular Biology* 20, no. 3 (2000): 708–714. On all diseases: see major reviews on aldehydes: Giuseppi Poli et al., "4-Hydroxynonenal: A Membrane Lipid Oxidation Product of Medicinal Interest," *Medicinal Research Reviews* 28, no. 4 (2008): 569–631; Anne Negre-Salvayre et al., "Pathological Aspects of Lipid Peroxidation," *Free Radical Research* 44, no. 10 (2010): 1125–1171; Neven Zarkovic, "4-Hydroxynonenal as a Bioactive Marker of Pathophysiological Processes," *Molecular Aspects of Medicine* 24, nos. 4–5 (2003): 285–286; Rachel M. Haywood et al., "Detection of Aldehydes and Their Conjugated Hydroperoxydiene Culinary Oils and Fats: Investigations Using High Resolution Proton NMR Spectroscopy," *Free Radical Research* 22, no. 5 (1995): 441–482; Hermann Esterbauer, "Cytotoxicity and Genotoxicity of Lipid Oxidation Products," *American Journal of Clinical Nutrition* 57, no. 5, suppl. (1993): 779S–786S; Giuseppe Poli and Rudolf Jörg Schaur, eds., "4-Hydroxynonenal: A Lipid Degradation Product Provided with Cell Regulatory Functions," *Molecular Aspects of Medicine* 24, nos. 4–5, suppl. (2003): 147S–313S; V. J. Feron et al., "Aldehydes: Occurrence, Carcinogenic Potential, Mechanism of Action and Risk Assessment," *Mutation Research* 259, nos. 3–4 (1991): 363–385; Quing Zhang et al., "Chemical Alterations Taken Place During Deep-Fat Frying Based on Certain Reaction Products: A Review," *Chemistry and Physics of Lipids* 165, no. 6 (2012): 662–681; Martin Grootveld et al., "Health Effects of Oxidized Heated Oils," *Foodservice Research International* 13, no. 1 (2001): 41–55.

281 *formal marker for the process:* Zarkovic, "4-Hydroxynonenal as a Bioactive Marker," 285–286.

281 *stress was observed in an experiment on mice:* Daniel J. Conklin et al., "Acrolein Consumption Induces Systemic Dyslipidemia and Lipoprotein Modification," *Toxicology and Applied Pharmacology* 243, no. 1 (2010): 1–12; Daniel J. Conklin et al., "Acrolein-Induced Dyslipidemia and Acute-Phase Response Are Independent of HMG-CoA Reductase," *Molecular Nutrition and Food Research* 55 (2011): 1411–1422.

282 *told me he was "stunned" to find:* Daniel J. Conklin, interview with author, November 8, 2013.

282 *a trial in New Zealand:* A. J. Wallace et al., "The Effects of Meals Rich in Thermally Stressed Olive and Safflower Oils on Postprandial Serum Paraoxonase Activity in Patients with Diabetes," *European Journal of Clinical Nutrition* 55, no. 11 (2001): 951–958.

282 *olive oil has consistently been shown:* Andres Fullana, Angel A. Carbonell-Barrachina, and Sukh Sidhu, "Comparison of Volatile Aldehydes Present in the Cooking Fumes of Extra Virgin Olive, Olive, and Canola Oils," *Journal of Agriculture and Food Chemistry* 52, no. 16 (2004): 5207–5214.

282 *fats that produce the fewest oxidation products:* On beef fat and lard, see Andrew W. D. Claxson et al., "Generation of Lipid Peroxidation Products in Culinary Oils and Fats during Episodes of Thermal Stressing: A High Field 'H NMR Study," *FEBS Letters* 355, no. 1 (1994): 88. On butter, see Hwa Han and A. Saari Csallany, "Temperature Dependence of HNE Formation in Vegetable Oils and Butter Oil," *Journal of the American Oil Chemists' Society* (June 2008). On coconut oil, see Claxson et al., "Generation of Lipid Peroxidation Products in Culinary Oils," 88.

282 *"First they were alarmed, then nothing":* Csallany, interview.

282 *a letter to the journal* Food Chemistry: Martin Grootveld, Christopher J. L. Silwood, and Andrew W. D. Claxson, "Letter to the Editor. Warning: Thermally-Stressed Polyunsaturates are Damaging to Health," *Food Chemistry* 67 (1999): 211–213.

282 *followed by a paper directed to alert:* Martin Grootveld et al., "Health Effects of Oxidized Heated Oils," *Foodservice Research International* 13, no. 1 (2001): 41–55.

282 *"Since I am not a food chemist":* Rudolf Jörg Schaur, email message to author, February 10, 2014.

282 *In 2006, the European Union formed a group:* Tilman Grune, Neven Zarkovic, and Kostelidou Kalliopi, "Lipid Peroxidation Research in Europe and the COST B35 Action 'Lipid Peroxidation Associated Disorders,'" *Free Radical Research* 44, no. 10 (2010): 1095–1097.

283 *simply to "hope":* Warner, interview with author, November 8, 2013.

283 *Large fast-food chains also employ sophisticated:* Bob Wainright, email message to author, February 9, 2014.

283 *he couldn't understand . . . so preoccupied:* Poli, interview.

283 *"how deadly used frying oils are":* Lars Wiedermann, email message to author, November 9, 2013.

283 *Mark Matlock at ADM:* Mark Matlock, interview with author, February 19, 2013.

283 *FDA press office finally responded:* Shelly Burgess, email message to author, April 11, 2013.

284 *European Food and Safety Authority:* European Food and Safety Authority, "Analysis of Occurrence of 3-monochloropropane-1,2-diol (3-MCPD) in Food in Europe in the Years 2009–2011 and Preliminary Exposure Assessment," *EFSA Journal* 11, no. 9 (2013): 3381. doi:10.29303/j.efsa.2013.3381.

284 *schools of medicine and public health:* See, for instance, Beatrice Trum Hunter, *Consumer Beware* (New York: Simon & Schuster, 1971): 30–50.

10. Why Saturated Fat Is Good for You

286 *according to statistics from the Centers for Disease Control:* Centers for Disease Control and Prevention (CDC), "Trends in Intake of Energy and Macronutrients—United States, 1971–2000," *Morbidity and Mortality Weekly Report* 53, no. 4 (2004): 80–82.

287 *"plant-based diet that"*: Dietary Guidelines Advisory Committee, prepared for the Agricultural Research Service, US Department of Agriculture and US Department of Health and Human Services, *Report of the Dietary Guidelines Advisory Committee on the Dietary Guidelines for Americans, 2010. To the Secretary of Agriculture and the Secretary of Health and Human Services,* 7th ed. (Washington, DC: US Government Printing Office, May 2010), 2.

287 Dr. Atkins' Diet Revolution: Robert C. Atkins, *Dr. Atkins' Diet Revolution: The High Calorie Way to Stay Thin Forever* (New York: David McKay, 1972).

288 *experiment written up in 1963:* Edgar S. Gordon, Marshall Goldberg, and Grace J. Chosy, "A New Concept in the Treatment of Obesity," *Journal of the American Medical Association* 186, no. 1 (1963): 156–166.

288 *"Vogue Diet" for a while:* "Beauty: *Vogue's* Take It Off, Keep It Off Super Diet . . . Devised with the Guidance of Dr. Robert Atkins," *Vogue* 155, no. 10 (1970): 84–85.

289 *"guilty of malpractice":* Select Committee on Nutrition and Human Needs of the United States Senate, "Obesity and Fad Diets," Ninety-Third Congress (Washington, DC: US Government Printing Office, April 12, 1973).

289 *"a nutritionist's nightmare":* Quoted in "The Battle of Pork Rind Hill," *Newsweek,* March 5, 2000.

289 *cover of* Time: Joel Stein, "The Low-Carb Diet Craze," *Time,* November 1, 1999.

289 *Ornish,* Newsweek: Geoffrey Cowley, "Healer of Hearts: Dean Ornish's Low-Tech Methods Could Transform American Medicine. But the Doctor Is Still Striving to Transform Himself," *Newsweek,* March 16, 1998.

289 *coined the term "diabesity":* Robert C. Atkins, *Larry King Live,* CNN, January 6, 2003.

289 *a CNN special:* "What's the Healthiest Way to Lose Weight?" *Crossfire,* CNN, May 30, 2000.

290 *once told Larry King:* Atkins, *Larry King Live.*

290 *said Abby Bloch:* Abby Bloch, interview with author, August 24, 2005.

291 *done in by both poor management and a flagging interest:* Pallavi Gogoi, "Atkins Gets Itself in a Stew," *Bloomberg Businessweek,* August 1, 2005.

291 *Alice Lichtenstein told me:* Alice C. Lichtenstein, interview with author, October 11, 2005.

292 *1863 pamphlet:* William Banting, "Letter on Corpulence: Addressed to the Public," in *Letter on Corpulence* (New York: Cosimo Classics, 2005).

292 *began Banting's little book:* Ibid., 6–7.

292 *was then commonly treated in France:* Alfred W. Pennington, "Treatment of Obesity: Developments of the Past 150 Years," *American Journal of Digestive Diseases* 21, no. 3 (1954): 65.

292 *Banting took to eating three meals a day:* Ibid., 65–69.

293 *average life expectancy:* Paul Clayton and Judith Rowbotham, "How the Mid-Victorians Worked, Ate and Died," *International Journal of Environmental Research and Public Health* 6, no. 3 (2009): 1239.

293 *European . . . clinicians:* Per Hanssen, "Treatment of Obesity by a Diet Relatively Poor in Carbohydrates," *Acta Medica Scandinavica* 88, no. 1 (1936): 97–106; Robert Kemp, "Carbohydrate Addiction," *Practitioner* 190 (1963): 358–364; H. R. Rony, *Obesity and Leanness* (Philadelphia: Lea and Febiger, 1940).

293 *Yorke-Davies, used a version . . . lose 70 pounds:* Deborah Levine, "Corpulence and Correspondence: President William H. Taft and the Medical Management of Obesity," *Annals of Internal Medicine* 159, no. 8 (2013): 565–570.

293 *his memoir,* Strong Medicine*:* Blake F. Donaldson, *Strong Medicine* (London: Cassell, 1961).

293 *"fattest meat they could kill":* Ibid., 34.

293 *"upper level" . . . "never found it:* Ibid., 35.

294 *"antiobesity treatments":* Ibid.

294 *"a lack of hunger between meals":* Alfred W. Pennington, "Obesity in Industry: The Problem and Its Solution," *Industrial Medicine & Surgery* 18, no. 6 (1949): 259.

294 *7 to 10 pounds a month:* Alfred W. Pennington, "Symposium on Obesity: A Reorientation on Obesity," *New England Journal of Medicine* 248, no. 23 (1953): 963.

294 *Pennington wrote extensively:* Ibid., 959–964.

294 *"seemed to lie much deeper":* Pennington, "Treatment of Obesity," 67.

295 *a hive of metabolic and hormonal activity:* E. Wertheimer and B. Shapiro, "The Physiology of Adipose Tissue," *Physiology Reviews* 28, no. 4 (1948): 451–464.

295 *altered hormonal levels in rats:* John R. Brobeck, "Mechanism of the Development of Obesity in Animals with Hypothalamic Lesions," *Physiological Reviews* 26, no. 4 (1946): 544.

295 *"attack" and "devour it" . . . "tigerish appetite":* Ibid., 549.

295 *Similar results were found:* Ibid., 541–559. Also see A. W. Hetherington and S. W. Ranson, "The Spontaneous Activity and Food Intake of Rats with Hypothalamic Lesions," *American Journal of Physiology—Legacy Content* 136, no. 4 (1942): 609.

295 *people with tumors in the hypothalamus:* Brobeck, "Mechanism of the Development of Obesity," 541.

295 *insulin . . . appeared to trump all others:* C. Von Noorden, *Clinical Treatises on Pathology and Therapy of Disorders of Metabolism and Nutrition, Part VIII. Diabetes Mellitus* (New York: E. B. Treat, 1907), 60.

295 *doctors were fattening underweight children:* Louis Fischer and Julian Rogatz, "Insulin in Malnutrition," *Archives of Pediatrics & Adolescent Medicine* 31, no. 3 (1926): 363.

296 *an animal that had been deprived of insulin:* Wilhelm Falta, *Endocrine Diseases: Including Their Diagnosis and Treatment* (Philadelphia: P. Blakiston's Son, 1923), 584.

296 *Pennington described:* A. W. Pennington, "Obesity: Overnutrition or Disease of Metabolism?" *American Journal of Digestive Diseases* 20, no. 9 (1953): 268–274.

296 *Pennington reviewed this extensive body:* Alfred W. Pennington, "Obesity," *Medical Times* 80, no. 7 (1952): 390; Alfred W. Pennington, "A Reorientation on Obesity," *New England Journal of Medicine* 248, no. 23 (1953): 959–964.

298 *One of the more startling revelations . . . "obesity sextette":* Donaldson, *Strong Medicine*, 2.

298 *"less and less likely to resort to drugs":* Ibid., 3.

298 *The population he found on Baffin Island:* Otto Schaefer, "Medical Observations and Problems in the Canadian Arctic: Part II," *Canadian Medical Association Journal* 81, no. 5 (1959): 387

298 *boatloads of food:* David Damas, *Arctic Migrants/Arctic Villagers: The Transformation of Inuit Settlement in the Central Arctic* (Quebec: McGill-Queen's Press, 2002), 29–30.

299 *"consists of fresh meat"*: Schaefer, "Medical Observations and Problems in the Canadian Arctic: Part II," 386.

299 *Heart disease . . . "does not appear to exist"*: Ibid., 387.

299 *"unable to cope"*: Otto Schaefer, "Glycosuria and Diabetes Mellitus in Canadian Eskimos: A Preliminary Report and Hypothesis," *Canadian Medical Association Journal* 99, no. 6 (1968): 252–262.

300 *"a jolting abruptness"*: Otto Schaefer, "When the Eskimo Comes to Town," *Nutrition Today* 6, no. 6 (1971): 11.

300 *"self-inflicted genocide"*: Quoted in *Yukon News* (June 4, 1975), 19: in Gerald W. Hankins, *Sunrise Over Pangnirtung: The Story of Otto Schaefer, M.D.* (Calgary, Canada: Arctic Institute of North America of the University of Calgary, 2000), 168.

300 *called all chronic illnesses the "saccharine diseases"*: Thomas L. Cleave and George Duncan Campbell, *Diabetes, Coronary Thrombosis, and the Saccharine Disease* (Bristol: John Wright & Sons, 1966).

300 *a fivefold increase*: James Walvin, *Fruits of Empire: Exotic Produce and British Taste, 1660–1800* (New York: New York University Press, 1997), 119.

300 *first cases of heart disease*: Leon Michaels, *The Eighteenth-Century Origins of Angina Pectoris: Predisposing Causes, Recognition and Aftermath*, Medical History, suppl. 21 (London: The Wellcome Trust Centre for the History of Medicine at UCL, 2001), 9.

301 *150 pounds of sugars*: US Department of Agriculture, "Profiling Food Consumption in America," *Agricultural Fact Book 2001–2002* (Washington, DC: US Government Printing Office, 2003), 20.

301 *George Prentice, a physician who spent time*: H. C. Trowell and D. P. Burkitt, eds., *Western Diseases: Their Emergence and Prevention* (London: Edward Arnold, 1981).

301 *quote from a 2002 World Health Organization report*: Joint WHO/FAO Expert Consultation, "Diet, Nutrition, and the Prevention of Chronic Diseases," *World Health Organization Technical Report Series* 916 (2003): 6.

302 *four highly portable and popular items*: There are many stories in Cleave and Campbell, *Diabetes, Coronary Thrombosis, and the Saccharine Disease*; Weston A. Price, *Nutrition and Physical Degeneration* (1936, repr., La Mesa, CA: The Price-Pottenger Nutrition Foundation, 2004); Vilhjalmur Stefansson, *The Fat of the Land*, enlarg. ed. of *Not By Bread Alone* (1946, repr., New York: Macmillan, 1956).

302 *"Hey doctor, all I'm eating is steak and eggs!"*: Eric C. Westman, interview with author, September 12, 2004.

303 *landmark trial*: Gary Foster et al., "Weight and Metabolic Outcomes after 2 Years on a Low-Carbohydrate versus Low-Fat Diet: A Randomized Trial," *Annals of Internal Medicine* 153, no. 3 (2010): 147–157.

303 *he recounted to me*: Gary Foster, interview with author, August 18, 2005.

303 *"heretic" in the field . . . "reasons that were not serious"*: Stephen D. Phinney, email message to author, August 28, 2012.

304 *"We were pretty sure we'd prove" . . . "concept was correct"*: Ibid.

304 *he found just the opposite*: Stephen D. Phinney et al., "Capacity for Moderate Exercise in Obese Subjects after Adaptation to a Hypocaloric, Ketogenic Diet," *Journal of Clinical Investigation* 66, no. 5 (1980): 1152.

305　*perfectly well, if not better, on ketones:* Robert S. Gordon, Jr. and Amelia Cherkes, "Un-esterified Fatty Acids in Human Blood Plasma," *Journal of Clinical Investigation* 35, no. 2 (1956): 206–212.

305　*can be created by the liver:* Combined Staff Clinic, "Obesity," *American Journal of Medicine* 19, no. 1 (1955): 117

305　*related to the transition period:* Stephen D. Phinney et al., "The Human Metabolic Response to Chronic Ketosis without Caloric Restriction: Physical and Biochemical Adaption," *Metabolism* 32, no. 8 (1983): 757–768; P. C. Kelleher et al., "Effects of Carbohydrate-Containing and Carbohydrate-Restricted Hypocaloric and Eucaloric Diets on Serum Concentrations of Retinol-Binding Protein, Thyroxine-Binding Prealbumin and Transferrin," *Metabolism* 32, no. 1 (1983): 95–101; G. L. Blackburn, "Mechanisms of Nitrogen Sparing with Severe Calorie Restricted Diets," *International Journal of Obesity* 5, no. 3 (1981): 215–216.

305　*Phinney showed that this phenomenon:* Phinney et al., "The Human Metabolic Response to Chronic Ketosis."

306　*In trials comparing the Atkins diet to the standard:* Jeff S. Volek et al., "Comparison of Energy-Restricted Very Low-Carbohydrate and Low-Fat Diets on Weight Loss and Body Composition in Overweight Men and Women," *Nutrition & Metabolism* 1, no. 13 (2004): 1–32; J. W. Krieger et al., "Effects of Variation in Protein and Carbohydrate Intake on Body Mass and Composition During Energy Restriction: A Meta-Regression," *American Journal of Clinical Nutrition* 83, no. 2 (2006): 260–274.

306　*"endothelial function" . . . has also been shown:* Jeff S. Volek et al., "Effects of Dietary Carbohydrate Restriction versus Low-Fat Diet on Flow-Mediated Dilation," *Metabolism* 58, no. 12 (2009): 1769–1777.

306　*further experiments keeping his subjects' weight constant:* Eric C. Westman, Jeff S. Volek, and Richard D. Feinman, "Carbohydrate Restriction Is Effective in Improving Atherogenic Dyslipidemia even in the Absence of Weight Loss," *American Journal of Clinical Nutrition* 84, no. 6 (2006): 1549–1549.

306　*solid scientific backing to the treatment:* One study that predated Westman's is Bruce R. Bistrian et al., "Nitrogen Metabolism and Insulin Requirements in Obese Diabetic Adults on a Protein-Sparing Modified Fast," *Diabetes* 25, no. 6 (1976): 494–504.

307　*could even stop taking their diabetes medication:* Mary C. Vernon et al., "Clinical Experience of a Carbohydrate-Restricted Diet: Effect on Diabetes Mellitus," *Metabolic Syndrome and Related Disorders* 1, no. 3 (2003): 234.

307　*Westman and his colleagues have argued:* Anthony Accurso et al., "Dietary Carbohydrate Restriction in Type 2 Diabetes Mellitus and Metabolic Syndrome: Time for a Critical Appraisal," *Nutrition & Metabolism* 5, no. 1 (2008): 1–8.

307　*since authorities . . . ADA:* American Diabetes Association, position statement, "Nutrition Recommendations and Interventions for Diabetes," *Diabetes Care* 31, suppl. 1 (2008): S66.

307　*conducting trials on a range of subjects:* Eric C. Westman et al., "Low-Carbohydrate Nutrition and Metabolism," *American Journal of Clinical Nutrition* 86, no. 2 (2007): 276–284; Volek et al., "Comparison of Energy-Restricted Very Low-Carbohydrate and Low-Fat Diets," 1–32; Jeff S. Volek et al., "Comparison of a Very Low-Carbohydrate and Low-Fat Diet on Fasting Lipids, LDL Subclasses, Insulin Resistance, and Postprandial Lipemic

Responses in Overweight Women," *Journal of the American College of Nutrition* 23, no. 2 (2004); 177–184; Matthew J. Sharman et al., *Human Nutrition and Metabolism* 134, no. 4 (2004): 880–885; Frederick F. Samaha et al., "A Low-Carbohydrate as Compared with a Low-Fat Diet in Severe Obesity," *New England Journal of Medicine* 348, no. 21 (2003): 2074–2081; Linda Stern et al., "The Effects of Low-Carbohydrate versus Conventional Weight Loss Diets in Severely Obese Adults: One-Year Follow-up of a Randomized Trial," *Annals of Internal Medicine* 140, no. 10 (2004): 778–786; William S. Yancy et al., "A Low-Carbohydrate, Ketogenic Diet versus a Low-Fat Diet to Treat Obesity and Hyperlipidemia: A Randomized, Controlled Trial," *Annals of Internal Medicine* 140, no. 10 (2004): 769–777; James H. Hays et al., "Effect of a High Saturated Fat and No-Starch Diet on Serum Lipid Subfractions in Patients with Documented Atherosclerotic Cardiovascular Disease," *Mayo Clinic Proceedings* 78, no. 11 (2003): 1331–1336; Kelly A. Meckling, Caitriona O'Sullivan, and Dayna Saari, "Comparison of a Low-Fat Diet to a Low-Carbohydrate Diet on Weight Loss, Body Composition, and Risk Factors for Diabetes and Cardiovascular Disease in Free-Living, Overweight Men and Women," *Journal of Clinical Endocrinology & Metabolism* 89, no. 6 (2004): 2717–2723; Eric C. Westman, "A Review of Low-Carbohydrate Ketogenic Diets," *Current Atherosclerosis Reports* 5 (2003): 476–483.

308 *One of the more extraordinary experiments:* Yancy, et al., "A Low-Carbohydrate, Ketogenic Diet versus a Low-Fat Diet."

308 *Volek says . . . "people are just quiet":* Jeff Volek, interview with author, April 18, 2006.

308 *Westman has written poignantly:* Eric C. Westman, "Rethinking Dietary Saturated Fat," *Food Technology* 63, no. 2 (2009): 30.

309 *"more unbiased, balanced":* Jeff S. Volek, Matthew J. Sharman, and Cassandra E. Forsythe, "Modification of Lipoproteins by Very Low-Carbohydrate Diets," *Journal of Nutrition* 135, no. 6 (2005): 1339–1342.

309 *results from a two-year trial:* Iris Shai et al., "Weight Loss with a Low-Carbohydrate, Mediterranean, or Low-Fat Diet," *New England Journal of Medicine* 359, no. 3 (2008): 229–241.

312 *Other researchers and scientists had published:* Russell L. Smith and Edward R. Pinckney, *Diet, Blood Cholesterol and Coronary Heart Disease: A Critical Review of the Literature* (Santa Monica, CA: privately published, 1988); Thomas J. Moore, *Heart Failure: A Critical Inquiry into American Medicine and the Revolution in Heart Care* (New York: Random House, 1989); George V. Mann, "A Short History of the Diet/Heart Hypothesis," in *Coronary Heart Disease: The Dietary Sense and Nonsense. An Evaluation by Scientists,* ed. George V. Mann for the Veritas Society (London: Janus, 1993), 1–17; Uffe Ravnskov, *The Cholesterol Myths: Exposing the Fallacy that Saturated Fat and Cholesterol Cause Heart Disease* (Washington, DC: New Trends, 2000).

312 *"What if It's All Been a Big Fat Lie?":* Gary Taubes, "What if It's All Been a Big Fat Lie?" *New York Times Magazine,* July 7, 2002.

312 *In 2007, he published a book:* Gary Taubes, *Good Calories, Bad Calories: Challenging the Conventional Wisdom on Diet, Weight Control, and Disease* (New York: Alfred A. Knopf, 2007).

313 *Gina Kolata . . . called:* Gina Kolata, "Carbophobia," *New York Times,* October 7, 2007.

313 *Taubes wrote later on his blog:* Gary Taubes, "Catching Up on Lost Time: The Ancestral Health Symposium, Food Reward, Palatability, Insulin Signaling and Carbohydrates, Ket-

tles, Pots and Other Odds and Ends (with Some Philosophy of Science as a Special Added Attraction). Part I," *Gary Taubes* (blog), September 2, 2011, accessed February 12, 2014 http://garytaubes.com/2011/09/catching-up-on-lost-time-ancestral-health-symposium -food-reward-palatability-insulin-signaling-carbohydrates-kettles-pots-other-odds-ends -part-i/.

314 *"borders on inexcusable":* Ibid.

314 Los Angeles Times *declared:* Marni Jameson, "A Reversal on Carbs: Fat Was Once the Devil. Now More Nutritionists Are Pointing Accusingly at Sugar and Refined Grains," *Los Angeles Times,* December 20, 2010.

314 *made the case recently that the fructose found in fruit:* Richard J. Johnson, *The Fat Switch* (Mercola.com, 2012).

315 *said Ronald M. Krauss:* Ronald M. Krauss, interview with author, August 21, 2013.

315 British Medical Journal*:* Gary Taubes, "The Science of Obesity: What Do We Really Know About What Makes Us Fat? An Essay by Gary Taubes," *British Medical Journal* 346 (2013), doi: 10.1136/bmj.f1050.

317 *more than a few major studies:* Michel de Lorgeril et al., "Mediterranean Alpha-Linolenic Acid-Rich Diet in Secondary Prevention of Coronary Heart Disease," *Lancet* 343, no. 8911 (1994): 1454–1459; Jean-Pierre Després, "Bringing Jupiter Down to Earth," *Lancet* 373, no. 9670 (2009): 1147–1148; J. C. LaRosa et al., "Intensive Lipid Lowering with Atorvastatin in Patients with Stable Coronary Disease," *New England Journal of Medicine* 352 (2005): 1425–1435; K. K. Ray et al., "Statins and All-Cause Mortality in High-Risk Primary Prevention: A Meta-Analysis of 11 Randomized Controlled Trials Involving 65,229 Participants," *Archives of Internal Medicine* 170 (2010): 1024–1031; Castelli et al., "HDL Cholesterol and Other Lipids," in "Coronary Heart Disease: The Cooperative Lipoprotein Phenotyping Study," *Circulation* 55, no. 5 (1977): 771.

317 *the AHA journal* Circulation*:* Rodney A. Hayward and Harlan M. Krumholz, "Three Reasons to Abandon Low-Density Lipoprotein Targets: An Open Letter to the Adult Treatment Panel IV of the National Institute of Health," *Circulation* 5 (2012): 2–5. See also Harlan M. Krumholz, "Editorial: Target Cardiovascular Risk Rather than Cholesterol Concentration," *British Medical Journal* 347 (2013): doi:10.1136/bmj.f7110.

317 *"historical leftover":* Allan Sniderman, interview with author, September 6, 2012.

318 John W. Gofman *found:* John W. Gofman et al., "The Role of Lipids and Lipoproteins in Atherosclerosis," *Science* 111, no. 2877 (1950): 166–186.

318 *Krauss confirmed their existence:* Darlene M. Dreon et al., "A Very-Low-Fat Diet Is Not Associated with Improved Lipoprotein Profiles in Men with a Predominance of Large, Low-Density Lipoproteins," *American Journal of Clinical Nutrition* 69, no. 3 (1999): 411–418; Ron M. Krauss and Darlene M. Dreon, "Low-Density-Lipoprotein Subclasses and Response to a Low-Fat Diet in Healthy Men," *American Journal of Clinical Nutrition* 62, no. 2 (1995): 478S–487S.

318 *He found that . . . total and saturated fats:* Krauss and Dreon, "Low-Density-Lipoprotein Subclasses and Response to a Low-Fat Diet"; Dreon et al., "A Very-Low-Fat Diet Is Not Associated with Improved Lipoprotein Profiles"; Ronald M. Krauss, "Dietary and Genetic Probes of Atherogenic Dyslipidemia," *Arteriosclerosis, Thrombosis, and Vascular Biology* 25, no. 11 (2005): 2265–2272; Ronald M. Krauss et al. "Separate Effects of Re-

duced Carbohydrate Intake and Weight Loss on Atherogenic Dyslipidemia," *American Journal of Clinical Nutrition* 83, no. 5 (2006): 1025–1031.

319 *He understood that even after:* Krauss, interview with author, June 12, 2006.

319 *it had been successfully replicated:* Benoît Lamarche et al., "Small, Dense Low-Density Lipoprotein Particles as a Predictor of the Risk of Ischemic Heart Disease in Men," *Circulation* 95, no. 1 (1997): 69–75.

319 *I asked Robert Eckel . . . I checked in with him:* Robert H. Eckel, interviews with author, May 1, 2006, and November 19, 2013.

319 *Penny Kris-Etherton . . . told me:* Penny Kris-Etherton, interview with author, June 7, 2007.

319 *Lichtenstein countered:* Krauss, interview; Eric B. Rimm, interview with author, January 7, 2008; Lichtenstein, interview.

320 *Krauss made the point:* Ronald M. Krauss et al., "AHA Dietary Guidelines Revision 2000: A Statement for Healthcare Professionals from the Nutrition Committee of the American Heart Association," *Circulation* 102, no. 18 (2000): 2284–2299.

320 *"it was too complicated":* Krauss, interview, August 20, 2012.

320 *Krauss was able to move:* Ibid.

320 *swung the AHA guidelines back in the other direction:* Alice H. Lichtenstein et al., "Diet and Lifestyle Recommendations Revision 2006: A Scientific Statement from the American Heart Association Nutrition Committee," *Circulation* 114, no. 1 (2006): 82–96.

320 *she replied that:* Alice H. Lichtenstein, interview with author, September 7, 2007.

321 *their advice became even more draconian:* Robert H. Eckel et al., "2013 AHA/ACC Guideline on Lifestyle Management to Reduce Cardiovascular Risk: A Report of the American College of Cardiology/American Heart Association Task Force on Practice Guidelines," *Circulation* (2013), epub ahead of print, doi: 10.1161/ 01.cir.0000437740 .48606.d1.

321 *DASH and OmniHeart:* Eva Obarzanek et al., "Effects on Blood Lipids of a Blood Pressure–Lowering Diet: The Dietary Approaches to Stop Hypertension (DASH) Trial," *American Journal of Clinical Nutrition* 74 (2001): 80–89; Lawrence Appel et al., "Effects of Protein, Monounsaturated Fat, and Carbohydrate Intake on Blood Pressure and Serum Lipids: Results of the OmniHeart Randomized Trial," *Journal of the American Medical Association* 294, no. 19 (2005): 2455–2464.

323 *"became disenchanted":* Krauss, interview, August 20, 2012.

324 *as had others before him:* Smith and Pinckney, *Diet, Blood Cholesterol and Coronary Heart Disease*. Before Taubes's book, this self-published compendium was the most important reference for doubters of the diet-heart hypothesis. See also Michael F. Oliver, "It Is More Important to Increase the Intake of Unsaturated Fats than to Decrease the Intake of Saturated Fats: Evidence from Clinical Trials Relating to Ischemic Heart Disease," *American Journal of Clinical Nutrition* 66, no. 4, suppl. (1997): 980S–986S.

324 *"a long row to hoe":* Krauss, email message to author, January 4, 2009.

324 *Krauss told me:* Krauss, email message to author, June 14, 2009.

324 *"agonizing series" . . . five "major permutations":* Ibid.

324 *For the first paper:* Patty W. Siri-Tarino et al., "Saturated Fat, Carbohydrate, and Cardiovascular Disease," *American Journal of Clinical Nutrition* 91.3 (2010): 502.

325 *In his editorial:* Jeremiah Stamler, "Diet-Heart: A Problematic Revisit," *American Journal of Clinical Nutrition* 91, no. 3 (2010): 497–499.

325 *Dariush Mozaffarian, announced:* Dariush Mozaffarian, "The Great Fat Debate: Taking the Focus off of Saturated Fat," *Journal of the American Dietetic Association* 111, no. 5 (2011): 665.

326 *Americans have reduced their consumption:* Centers for Disease Control and Prevention, "Trends in Intake of Energy and Macronutrients, 1971–2000," 80–82.

327 *total cholesterol levels ... have fallen ... "high" cholesterol:* National Cholesterol Education Program, "Program Description," accessed October 29 2013, http://www.nhlbi.nih.gov/about/ncep/ncep_pd.htm.

327 *due to declines in LDL-cholesterol:* Nancy D. Ernst et al., "Consistency between US Dietary Fat Intake and Serum Total Cholesterol Concentrations: The National Health and Nutrition Examination Surveys," *American Journal of Clinical Nutrition* 66, no. 4, suppl. (1997): 965S–972S.

327 *he predicted that if "mankind ...":* Edgar V. Allen, "Clinical Progress: Atherosclerosis. A Symposium," *Circulation* 5, no. 1 (1952): 99.

327 *not clear that the actual* occurrence *of heart disease has declined:* Wayne D. Rosamond et al., "Trends in the Incidence of Myocardial Infarction and in Mortality Due to Coronary Heart Disease, 1987 to 1994," *New England Journal of Medicine* 339, no. 13 (1998): 861–867; Hugh Tunstall-Pedoe et al., "Contribution of Trends in Survival and Coronary-Event Rates to Changes in Coronary Heart Disease Mortality: 10-Year Results from 37 WHO MONICA Project Populations. Monitoring Trends and Determinants in Cardiovascular Disease," *Lancet* 353, no. 9164 (1999): 1547–1557.

327 *"very few" of whom "currently follow":* Dietary Guidelines Advisory Committee, *Report of the Dietary Guidelines Advisory Committee,* 72.

327 *most recent set of AHA dietary guidelines:* Alice H. Lichtenstein et al., "Diet and Lifestyle Recommendations Revision 2006: A Scientific Statement from the American Heart Association Nutrition Committee," *Circulation* 114, no. 1 (2006): 82–96.

328 *prohibitions against saturated fats remain strong:* Dietary Guidelines Advisory Committee, *Report of the Dietary Guidelines Advisory Committee,* 4 and 13, among others.

328 *"healthy diets are high in carbohydrates":* Ibid., 311.

329 *6 percent per year:* Caroline Scott-Thomas, "Low-Fat Trend Continues to Grow Fat Replacer Sales," *FoodNavigatorusa.com,* March 7, 2012, last accessed February 14, 2014, http://www.foodnavigator-usa.com/Markets/Low-fat-trend-continues-to-grow-fat-replacer-sales-says-GIA.

Conclusion

331 *"You may be making yourself miserable":* Edward R. Pinckney and Cathey Pinckney, *The Cholesterol Controversy* (Los Angeles, Shelbourne Press, 1973), 3.

333 *expert panels ... recently recommended:* Robert H. Eckel et al., "2013 AHA/ACC Guideline on Lifestyle Management to Reduce Cardiovascular Risk: A Report of the American College of Cardiology/American Heart Association Task Force on Practice Guidelines," *Circulation* (2013), doi: 10.1161/ 01.cir.0000437740.48606.d1.

335 *"genetics would point at nothing":* David B. Goldstein, "Common Genetic Variation and Human Traits," *New England Journal of Medicine* 360 no. 17 (2009): 1696–1698; David B. Goldstein, email message to author, November 26, 2013.

Glossary

AAP—American Academy of Pediatrics, the leading professional society of pediatricians.

AHA—American Heart Association, the nation's oldest voluntary organization dedicated to fighting heart disease and stroke; also the largest not-for-profit group in the country.

Case control study—a type of epidemiological study where subjects diagnosed with a disease or condition are compared to healthy controls and risk factors (e.g., diet, exercise, serum cholesterol) are assessed, usually retroactively. This type of study can be relatively inexpensive, since subjects are often assessed only once and are not followed over time.

Clinical trial—a type of study in which participants are assigned to receive one or more interventions so that researchers can evaluate the effects of the interventions on health-related outcomes. A "randomized" trial is one that assigns participants to different study arms by chance. A "controlled" trial has a control group that does not receive the intervention(s). A "randomized controlled clinical trial" is considered the gold standard of clinical trials and of scientific evidence generally.

Dietary Goals for the United States—the five goals issued by the US Senate Select Committee on Nutrition and Human Needs in 1977 (the "McGovern report").

Dietary Guidelines for Americans—periodic reports, starting in 1980, issued jointly by the US Department of Agriculture and US Department of Health and Human Services, that advise Americans about nutrition for good health. The USDA food pyramid was based on these guidelines.

Double bond—a chemical term referring to the way that two atoms are linked together. A double bond is like a double handshake between atoms. Fatty acid molecules with one or more double bonds are called "unsaturated" and are the dominant type found in olive oil and vegetable oils, while fatty acids without double bonds are called "saturated" and prevail in the fats found in animal foods. Double bonds come in two formations, "trans" and "cis."

Epidemiological study—a type of study that identifies the incidence of disease or some other condition across a population. Nutritional epidemiology involves assessing the diet of a population, sometimes periodically, and correlating that information with eventual health outcomes. These studies can demonstrate associations but not causation. Also known as an "observational" study.

Fatty acids—chains of carbon atoms surrounded by hydrogen atoms. Individual fatty acids can be saturated or unsaturated. Three fatty acids bound together like a pitchfork are called triglycerides.

FDA—Food and Drug Administration, which is part of the US Department of Health and Human Services. The FDA is entrusted with protecting the nation's food supply.

HDL-cholesterol—the type of cholesterol in high density lipoproteins that is known as "good" because people with higher levels tend to have a lower risk for heart disease. HDL-cholesterol is a fraction of total cholesterol.

LDL-cholesterol—the type of cholesterol in low density lipoproteins that is known as "bad" because people with very high levels tend to have a higher risk of heart disease.

Low-fat diet—a regime usually defined as one with between 25 percent and 35 percent of total calories as fat. The low-fat diet is different from the "prudent" diet, which restricts only saturated fats as well as the dietary cholesterol found in eggs, animal foods, and shellfish, but does not restrict fat overall.

Monounsaturated fats—fats in which the fatty acids contain only one double bond. The most common monounsaturated fat is called "oleic," the type most abundant in olive oil.

NCEP—National Cholesterol Education Program, a program managed by the National Heart, Lung, and Blood Institute within the National Institutes of Health. NCEP was created in 1985 with the objective of instructing Americans about how to avoid atherosclerotic cardiovascular disease. Until 2013, NCEP periodically published the nation's most important guidelines for doctors on how to lower cholesterol with diet and/or drugs.

NHI—National Heart Institute, an agency in the National Institutes of Health devoted to fighting cardiovascular disease. Founded by President Harry S. Truman in 1948, it was renamed the National Heart, Lung, and Blood Institute (NHLBI) in 1969.

NHLBI—National Heart, Lung, and Blood Institute, the agency at the National Institutes of Health devoted to the prevention and treatment of heart, lung and blood diseases, including cardiovascular disease. Formerly the National Heart Institute (NHI).

NIH—National Institutes of Health, the US government's primary agency responsible for biomedical and health-related research, located in Bethesda, Maryland.

Nurses Health Study—the largest and longest epidemiological study in the United States. Begun in 1976, the study ("Nurses I") was expanded in 1989 ("Nurses II") and has altogether follow more than 200,000 women. "Food frequency questionnaires" on diet and lifestyle are sent out every two years, with responses being voluntary. The study is funded by the NIH and directed by Walter C. Willett at the Harvard School of Public Health.

Polyunsaturated fats—fats in which the fatty acids contain multiple double bonds. Polyunsaturated fats include vegetable oils, such as soybean, corn, safflower, sunflower, cottonseed and rapeseed, the main oil in Canola.

Prudent diet—the first officially recommended diet for the prevention of heart disease, widely employed in the United States from the late 1940s through the 1970s, at which point, the low-fat diet took precedence. The prudent diet restricted saturated fats and the dietary cholesterol found in eggs, animal foods and shellfish but unlike the "low-fat diet," did not restrict fat overall. Prudent diets typically had 40 percent of total calories as fat.

Saturated fats—the fats that have no double bonds in the fatty acids they contain. These fats are found predominantly in animal foods, such as eggs, dairy, and meat, as well as in palm and coconut oils.

Trans fats—the fats that contain fatty acids with a double bond in the "trans" configuration. A "trans" bond creates a molecule in a zigzag shape, allowing adjacent fatty acids to lie neatly against each other, resulting in a fat that can be a solid at room temperature. The other type of double bond, called "cis," creates U-shaped molecules that cannot stack together and therefore create oils.

Triglycerides—a form of fatty acids circulating in the blood. Triglycerides are comprised of three fatty acids joined together at their ends by a glycerol molecule, in the shape of a pitchfork. Since the 1940s, high triglycerides have been considered a biomarker for heart disease.

Unsaturated fats—the fats with fatty acids that contain either one double bond (monounsaturated) or more (polyunsaturated).

USDA—United States Department of Agriculture. Since 1980, the USDA has been the co-author of the *Dietary Guidelines for Americans*. From 1992–2011, the USDA published its food pyramid based on these guidelines. The pyramid was then replaced by a graphic called "My Plate."

WHI—Women's Health Initiative. The largest-ever clinical trial of the low-fat diet, conducted on nearly fifty thousand women over seven years, with results published in 2006. The NIH-funded study, estimated to cost upwards of $700 million, was conducted by health centers across the country and had three arms with different interventions: hormone replacement therapy, calcium/vitamin D supplementation, and the low-fat diet.

WHO—World Health Organization, an agency of the United Nations devoted to international public health.

Bibliography

Aaes-Jørgensen, E., J. P. Funch, P. F. Engel, and H. Dam. "The Role of Fat in the Diet of Rats." *British Journal of Nutrition* 10, no. 04 (1956): 317–324.

"About the Foundation." http://www.atkinsfoundation.org/about.asp, last accessed October 11, 2013.

Accurso, Anthony, Richard K. Bernstein, Annika Dahlqvist, et al. "Dietary Carbohydrate Restriction in Type 2 Diabetes Mellitus and Metabolic Syndrome: Time for a Critical Appraisal." *Nutrition & Metabolism* 5 (April 8, 2008): 9.

Adams, Charles Darwin, trans. *The Genuine Works of Hippocrates.* New York: Dover, 1868.

Adams, Ronald J., and Kenneth M. Jennings. "Media Advocacy: A Case Study of Philip Sokolof's Cholesterol Awareness Campaigns." *Journal of Consumer Affairs* 27, no. 1 (Summer 1993): 145–165.

Ahrens, Edward H. Jr. "The Management of Hyperlipidemia: Whether, Rather than How." *Annals of Internal Medicine* 85, no. 1 (July 1976): 87–93.

———. "The Evidence Relating Six Dietary Factors to the Nation's Health. Introduction." *American Journal of Clinical Nutrition* 32, no. 12 (December 1979): 2627–2631.

———. "After 40 Years of Cholesterol-Watching." *Journal of Lipid Research* 25, no. 13 (December 15, 1984): 1442–1449.

———. "The Diet-Heart Question in 1985: Has It Really Been Settled?" *Lancet* 1, no. 8437 (May 11, 1985): 1085–1087.

———. "Carbohydrates, Plasma Triglycerides, and Coronary Heart Disease." *Nutrition Reviews* 44, no. 2 (February 1986): 60–64.

Ahrens, Edward H. Jr., David H. Blankenhorn, and Theodore T. Tsaltas. "Effect on Human Serum Lipids of Substituting Plant for Animal Fat in Diet." *Proceedings for the Society of Experimental Biology and Medicine* 86, no. 4 (August–September 1954): 872–878.

Ahrens, Edward H. Jr., Jules Hirsch, William Insull Jr., Theodore T. Tsaltas, Rolf Blomstrand, and Malcolm L. Peterson. "Dietary Control of Serum Lipids in Relation to Atherosclerosis." *Journal of the American Medical Association* 164, no. 17 (August 24, 1957): 1905–1911.

Ahrens, Edward H. Jr., Jules Hirsch, Kurt Oette, John W. Farquhar, and Yechezkiel Stein. "Carbohydrate-Induced and Fat-Induced Lipemia." *Transactions of the Association of American Physicians* 74 (1961): 134–146.

Ahrens, Edward H. Jr., William Insull Jr., Rolf Blomstrand, Jules Hirsch, Theodore T. Tsaltas, and Malcolm L. Peterson. "The Influence of Dietary Fats on Serum-Lipid Levels in Man." *Lancet* 272, no. 6976 (May 11, 1957): 943–953.

Akiya, Toshimi, Chuji Araki, and Kiyoko Igarashi. "Novel Methods of Evaluation Deterioration and Nutritive Value of Oxidized Oil." *Lipids* 8, no. 6 (June 1973): 348–352.

Alberti-Fidanza, Adalberta. "Mediterranean Meal Patterns." *Bibliotheca Nutritio et Dieta* 45 (1990): 59–71.

Albrink, Margaret J. "Triglycerides, Lipoproteins, and Coronary Artery Disease." *Archives of Internal Medicine* 109, no. 3 (March 1962): 345–359.

———. "The Significance of Serum Triglycerides." *Journal of the American Dietetic Association* 42 (January 1963): 29–31.

Aldana, Steven G., Roger Greenlaw, Audrey Salberg, Ray M. Merrill, Ron Hager, Rick B. Jorgensen. "The Effects of an Intensive Lifestyle Modification Program on Carotid Artery Intima-Media Thickness: A Randomized Trial." *American Journal of Health Promotion* 21, no. 6 (July–August 2007): 510–516.

Allbaugh, Leland Girard. *Crete: A Case Study of an Underdeveloped Area.* Princeton, NJ: Princeton University Press, 1953.

Allen, Edgar V., Louis N. Katz, Ancel Keys, and John W. Gofman, "Atherosclerosis: A Symposium," *Circulation* 5, no. 1 (January 1952): 98–134.

Al-Marzouki, Sanaa, Stephen Evans, Tom Marshall, and Ian Roberts. "Are These Data Real? Statistical Methods for the Detection of Data Fabrication in Clinical Trials." *British Medical Journal* 331, no. 7511 (July 30, 2005): 267–270.

Alonso, Alvaro, and Miguel Ángel Martínez-González. "Olive Oil Consumption and Reduced Incidence of Hypertension: The SUN Study." *Lipids* 39, no. 12 (December 2004): 1233–1238.

Alonso, Alvaro, Valentina Ruiz-Gutierrez, and Miguel Ángel Martínez-González. "Monounsaturated Fatty Acids, Olive Oil and Blood Pressure: Epidemiological, Clinical and Experimental Evidence." *Public Health Nutrition* 9, no. 2 (April 2005): 251–257.

American Academy of Pediatrics, Committee on Nutrition. "Prudent Life-style for Children: Dietary Fat and Cholesterol." *Pediatrics* 78, no. 3 (September 1, 1986): 521–525.

———. "Cholesterol in Childhood." *Pediatrics* 101, no. 1, part 1 (January 1998): 141–147.

American Diabetes Association. "Position Statement. Nutrition Recommendations and Interventions for Diabetes." *Diabetes Care* 31, suppl. 1 (January 2008): S61–S78.

American Heart Association. *An Eating Plan for Healthy Americans: Our American Heart Association Diet.* Dallas: American Heart Association, 1995.

———. Committee on Nutrition. "Diet and Heart Disease." New York: American Heart Association, 1968.

———. "Diet and Coronary Heart Disease." New York: American Heart Association, 1973.

———. "Diet and Coronary Heart Disease." New York: American Heart Association, 1978.

Anderson, Joseph T., Francisco Grande, and Ancel Keys. "Hydrogenated Fats in the Diet and Lipids in the Serum of Man." *Journal of Nutrition* 75 (1961): 388–394.

Anderson, Joseph T., Ancel Keys, and Francisco Grande. "The Effects of Different Food Fats on Serum Cholesterol Concentration in Man." *Journal of Nutrition* 62, no. 3 (July 10, 1957); 421–424.

Anderson, Keaven M., William P. Castelli, and Daniel Levy. "Cholesterol and Mortality: 30 Years of Follow-up from the Framingham Study." *Journal of the American Medical Association* 257, no. 16 (April 24, 1987): 2176–2180.

Anderson, Sue Ann. "Guidelines for Use of Dietary Intake Data." *Journal of the American Dietetic Association* 88, no. 10 (October 1988): 1258–1260.

Andrews, John S., Wendell H. Griffith, James F. Mead, and Robert A. Stein. "Toxicity of Air-Oxidized Soybean Oil." *Journal of Nutrition* 70, no. 2 (February 1, 1960): 199–210.

Anitschkow, Nikolai N. and S. Chalatow, "Ueber Experimentelle Cholester-insteatose und ihre Bedeutehung für die Entstehung Einiger Pathologischer Prozesse." *Zentralblatt für Allgemeine Pathologie und Pathologische Anatomie* 24 (1913): 1–9.

Anon. "The Fat of the Land." *Time* 67 no. 3 (January 13, 1961): 48–52.

————. "Beauty: Vogue's Take It Off, Keep It Off Super Diet . . . Devised with the Guidance of Dr. Robert Atkins." *Vogue* 155, no. 10 (1970): 84–85.

————. "A Few Kind Words for Cholesterol." *Time*, June 9, 1980.

————. "Focus." *Journal of the American Oil Chemists' Society* 61, no. 9 (1984): 1434.

————. "Sorry, It's True: Cholesterol Really Is a Killer." *Time*, January 23, 1984.

————. "New Findings on Palm Oil." *Nutrition Reviews* 45, no. 9 (1987): 205–207.

————. "Tropical Fats Labeling: Malaysians Counterattack ASA Drive." *Journal of the American Oil Chemists' Society* 64, no. 12 (December 1987): 1596–1598.

————. "FASEB Nutrition Study Using 'Flawed Data,' Researcher Charges." *Food Chemical News* (January 25, 1988): 52–54.

————. "Congress Hears Cholesterol Debate." Associated Press, December 9, 1989.

————. "The Battle of Pork Rind Hill," *Newsweek*, March 5, 2000.

————. "Death of a Diet Doctor." Snopes.com, last modified February 11, 2004, http://www.snopes.com/medical/doctor/atkins.asp.

Antar, Mohamed A., Margaret A. Ohlson, and Robert E. Hodges. "Perspectives in Nutrition: Changes in Retail Market Food Supplies in the United States in the Last Seventy Years in Relation to the Incidence of Coronary Heart Disease, with Special Reference to Dietary Carbohydrates and Essential Fatty Acids." *American Journal of Clinical Nutrition* 14 (March 1964): 169–178.

Appel, Lawrence J., Frank M. Sacks, Vincent J. Carey, et al. "Effects of Protein, Monounsaturated Fat, and Carbohydrate Intake on Blood Pressure and Serum Lipids: Results of the OmniHeart Randomized Trial." *Journal of the American Medical Association* 294, no. 19 (November 16, 2005): 2455–2464.

Applewhite, Thomas H. " 'Statistical Correlations' Relating Trans-Fats to Cancer: A Commentary." *Federation Proceedings* 38, no. 11 (1979): 2435.

————. "Nutritional Effects of Isomeric Fats: Facts and Fallacies." In *Dietary Fats and Health*. Edited by Edward George Perkins and W. J. Visek. Chicago: American Oil Chemists' Society (1983).

————. "Trans Isomers, Serum Lipids and Cardiovascular Disease: Another Point of View." *Nutrition Reviews* 51, no. 11 (November 1993): 344–345.

Aravanis, Christos. "The Classic Risk Factors for Coronary Heart Disease: Experience in Europe." *Preventive Medicine* 12, no. 1 (January 1983): 16–19.

Aro, Antti, Matti Jauhiainen, Raija Partanen, Irma Salminen, and Marja Mutanen. "Stearic Acid, Trans Fatty Acids, and Dairy Fat: Effects on Serum and Lipoprotein Lipids, Apolipoproteins, Lipoprotein(a), and Lipid Transfer Proteins in Healthy Subjects." *American Journal of Clinical Nutrition* 65, no. 5 (May 1997): 1419–1426.

Aro, Antti, I. Salminen, J. K. Huttunen, et al. "Adipose Tissue Isomeric *Trans* Fatty Acids and Risk of Myocardial Infarction in Nine Countries: the EURAMIC Study." *Lancet* 345, no. 8945 (February 4, 1995): 273–278.

Ascherio, Alberto, Martijn B. Katan, Peter L. Zock, Meir J. Stampfer, and Walter C. Willett. "Trans Fatty Acids and Coronary Heart Disease." *New England Journal of Medicine* 340, no. 25 (June 24, 1999): 1994–1998.

Association of Schools of Public Health. "Health Revolutionary: The Life and Work of Ancel Keys." Public Health Leadership Film. Last accessed February 14, 2014. http://www.asph.org/document.cfm?page=793.

Astrup, Arne, Jørn Dyerberg, Peter Elwood, et al. "The Role of Reducing Intakes of Saturated Fat in the Prevention of Cardiovascular Disease: Where Does the Evidence Stand in 2010?" *American Journal of Clinical Nutrition* 93, no. 4 (April 2011): 684–688.

Astrup, Arne, Peter Marckmann, and John Blundell. "Oiling of Health Messages in Marketing of Food." *The Lancet* 356, no. 9244 (November 25, 2000): 1786.

Atkins, Robert C. *Dr. Atkins' Diet Revolution: The High-Calorie Way to Stay Thin Forever.* Philadelphia: David McKay Co., 1972.

———. Interview with Larry King. *Larry King Live.* CNN, January 6, 2003.

Austin, Peter C., Muhammad M. Mamdani, David N. Juurlink, and Janet E. Hux. "Testing Multiple Statistical Hypotheses Resulted in Spurious Associations: A Study of Astrological Signs and Health." *Journal of Clinical Epidemiology* 59, no. 9 (September 2006): 964–969.

Bach, Anna, Lluís Serra-Majem, Josep L. Carrasco, et al. "The Use of Indexes Evaluating the Adherence to the Mediterranean Diet in Epidemiological Studies: A Review." *Public Health Nutrition* 9, no. 1A (February 2006): 132–146.

Bacon, Francis. *Novum Organum Scientiarum*, England, 1620, Book 1: XXXIV.

Bailar, John C. "Dietary Fat and Cancer Trends—A Further Critique." *Federation Proceedings* 38, no. 11 (October 1979): 2435–2436.

Ball, Richard A., and J. Robert Lilly. "The Menace of Margarine: The Rise and Fall of a Social Problem." *Social Problems* 29, no. 5 (June 1982): 488–498.

Banting, William. *Letter on Corpulence. Addressed to the Public.* London, 1863. Reprinted: New York: Cosimo Classics, 2005.

Barbour, Andrew D. "The Deposition and Utilization of Hydrogenation Isooleic Acid in the Animal Body." *The Journal of Biological Chemistry* 101, no. 1 (June 1933): 63–72.

Barker, J. Ellis. *Cancer.* London: John Murray, 1924.

Bauer, Bob. Letter Responding to the Health Claim Petition (Docket No. 2003Q-0559). Office of Nutritional Products, Labeling and Dietary Supplements, US Food and Drug Administration, November 1, 2004.

Baum, Seth J., Penny M. Kris-Etherton, Walter C. Willett, et al. "Fatty Acids in Cardiovascular Health and Disease: A Comprehensive Update." *Journal of Clinical Lipidology* 6, no. 3 (May 2012): 216–234.

Beaglehole, Robert, Mary A. Foulkes, Ian A. M. Prior, and Elaine F. Eyles. "Cholesterol and Mortality in New Zealand Maoris." *British Medical Journal* 280, no. 6210 (February 2, 1980): 285–287.

Beauchamp, Gary K., Russell S. J. Keast, Diane Morel, et al. "Phytochemistry: Ibuprofen-like Activity in Extra-Virgin Olive Oil." *Nature* 437, no. 7055 (September 1, 2005): 45–46.

Beckles, G. L., C. F. Chou, Centers for Disease Control and Prevention, "Diabetes—United States, 2006 and 2010," *Morbidity and Mortality Weekly Report* 62, suppl. 3 (2012): 99–104.

Bekelman, Justin E., Yan Li, and Cary P. Gross. "Scope and Impact of Financial Conflicts of Interest in Biomedical Research; A Systematic Review." *Journal of the American Medical Association* 289, no. 4 (January 22–29, 2003): 454–465.

Bendsen, N. T., R. Christensen, E. M. Bartels, and A. Astrup. "Consumption of Industrial and Ruminant Trans Fatty Acids and Risk of Coronary Heart Disease: A Systematic Review and Meta-Analysis of Cohort Studies." *European Journal of Clinical Nutrition* 65, no. 7 (July 2011): 773–783.

Beresford, Shirley A. A., Karen C. Johnson, et al. "Low-Fat Dietary Pattern and Risk of Colorectal Cancer: The Women's Health Initiative Randomized Controlled Dietary Modification Trial." *Journal of the American Medical Association* 295, no. 6 (February 8, 2006): 643–654.

Bier, Dennis M., J. T. Brosnan, J. P. Flatt, et al. "Report of the IDECG Working Group on Lower and Upper Limits of Carbohydrate and Fat Intake." *European Journal of Clinical Nutrition* 53, no. 1 suppl. (April 1999): S177–S178.

Bier, Dennis M., Ronald M. Lauer, and Olli Simell. "Summary." *The American Journal of Clinical Nutrition* 72, no. 5 suppl. (November 2000): 1410S–1413S.

Bierenbaum, Marvin L., Donald P. Green, Alvin Florin, Alan Fleischman, and Anne B. Caldwell. "Modified-Fat Dietary Management of the Young Male with Coronary Disease," *Journal of the American Medical Association* 202, no. 13 (1967): 59–63.

Biesalski, Hans Konrad. "Meat and Cancer: Meat as a Component of a Healthy Diet." *European Journal of Clinical Nutrition* 56, suppl. 1 (March 2002): S2–S11.

Bingham, Sheila A. "Limitations of the Various Methods for Collecting Dietary Intake Data." *Annals of Nutrition and Metabolism* 35, no. 3 (1991): 117–127.

Biss, Kurt, Kang-Jey Ho, Belma Mikkelson, Lena Lewis, and C. Bruce Taylor. "Some Unique Biologic Characteristics of the Masai of East Africa." *New England Journal of Medicine* 284, no. 13 (April 1971): 694–699.

Bistrian, Bruce R., George L. Blackburn, Jean-Pierre Flatt, Jack Sizer, Nevin S. Scrimshaw, and Mindy Sherman. "Nitrogen Metabolism and Insulin Requirements in Obese Diabetic Adults on a Protein-Sparing Modified Fast." *Diabetes* 25, no. 6 (June 1976): 494–504.

Bittman, Mark. "No Meat, No Dairy, No Problem." *New York Times Sunday Magazine*, January 1, 2012.

Blackburn, G. L. "Mechanisms of Nitrogen Sparing with Severe Calorie Restricted Diets." *International Journal of Obesity* 5, no. 3 (1981): 215–216.

Blackburn, Henry. "The Low Risk Coronary Male." *American Journal of Cardiology* 58, no. 1 (July 1986): 161.

———. "Ancel Keys Lecture: The Three Beauties: Bench, Clinical, and Population Research." *Circulation* 86, no. 4 (October 1992): 1323–1331.

Blackburn, Henry, and Darwin Labarthe. "Stories for the Evolution of Guidelines for Casual Interference in Epidemiologic Associations: 1953–1965." *American Journal of Epidemiology* 176, no. 12 (December 5, 2012): 1071–1077.

Blakeslee, Alton, and Jeremiah Stamler. *Your Heart Has Nine Lives: Nine Steps to Heart Health.* New York: Pocket Books, 1966.

Blasbalg, Tanya L., Joseph R. Hibbeln, Christopher E. Ramsden, Sharon F. Majchrzak, and Robert R. Rawlings. "Changes in Consumption of Omega-3 and Omega-6 Fatty Acids in the United States During the 20th Century." *American Journal of Clinical Nutrition* 93, no. 5 (May 2011): 950–962.

Blondheim, S. H., T. Horne, R. Davidovich, J. Kapitulnik, S. Segal, and N. A. Kaufmann. "Unsaturated Fatty Acids in Adipose Tissue of Israeli Jews." *Israel Journal of Medical Sciences* 12, no. 7 (July 1976): 658–661.

Blume, Elaine. "The Truth About Trans: Hydrogenated Oils Aren't Guilty as Charged." *Center for Science in the Public Interest: Nutrition Action Healthletter* 15, no. 2 (March 1, 1988): 8–10.

Bogani, Paola, Claudio Galli, Marco Villa, and Francesco Visioli. "Postprandial Anti-inflammatory and Antioxidant Effects of Extra Virgin Olive Oil." *Atherosclerosis* 190, no. 1 (January 2007): 181–186.

Boniface, D. B., and M. E. Tefft, "Dietary Fats and 16-year Coronary Heart Disease Mortality in a Cohort of Men and Women in Great Britain." *European Journal of Clinical Nutrition* 56, no. 8 (August 2002): 786–792.

Bostock, John, and H. T. Riley. *The Natural History of Pliny.* London: Taylor and Francis, 1855.

Böttiger, Lars-Erik, and Lars A. Carlson. "Serum Glucoproteins in Men with Myocardial Infarction." *Journal of Atherosclerosis Research* 1, no. 3 (May 6, 1961): 184–188.

Breslow, Jan L. "Why You Should Support the American Heart Association!" *Circulation* 94, no. 11 (December 1, 1996): 3016–3022.

Broad, William James. "NIH Deals Gingerly with Diet-Disease Link." *Science* 204, no. 4398 (June 15, 1979): 1175–1178.

———. "Academy Says Curb on Cholesterol Not Needed." *Science* 208, no. 4450 (June 20, 1980): 1354–1355.

Brobeck, John R. "Mechanisms in the Development of Obesity in Animals with Hypothalamic Lesions." *Physiological Reviews* 26, no. 4 (October 1, 1946): 541–559.

Brody, Jane E. *Jane Brody's Good Food Book: Living the High Carbohydrate Way.* New York: W. W. Norton, 1985.

Brown, Michael S., and Joseph L. Goldstein. "How LDL Receptors Influence Cholesterol and Atherosclerosis." *Scientific American* 251, no. 5 (November 1984): 58–66.

Byers, Tim. "Hardened Fats, Hardened Arteries?" *New England Journal of Medicine* 337, no. 21 (November 20, 1997): 1544–1545.

Caballero, Benjamin, Theresa Clay, Sally M. Davis, et al. "Pathways: A School-Based, Randomized Controlled Trial for the Prevention of Obesity in American Indian Schoolchildren." *American Journal of Clinical Nutrition* 78, no. 5 (November 2003): 1030–1038.

Campbell, T. Colin, and Chen Junshi. "Diet and Chronic Degenerative Diseases: Perspectives from China." *American Journal of Clinical Nutrition* 59, no. 5 suppl. (May 1994): 1153S–1161S.

Campbell, T. Colin, Banoo Parpia, and Junshi Chen. "Diet, Lifestyle, and the Etiology of Coronary Artery Disease: The Cornell China Study." *American Journal of Cardiology* 82, no. 10B (November 26, 1998): 18T–21T.

Canadian Pediatric Society and Health Canada, Joint Working Group. *Nutrition Recommendations Update: Dietary Fat and Children.* Ottowa, Ontario: Health Canada, 1993.

Cannon, Geoffrey. *Food and Health: The Experts Agree.* London: Consumers' Association, 1992.

Capewell, Simon, and Martin O'Flaherty. "What Explains Declining Coronary Mortality? Lessons and Warnings." *Heart* 94, no. 9 (September 2008): 1105–1108.

Carlson, Lars A., Lars E. Böttiger, and P. E. Åhdfeldt. "Risk Factors for Myocardial Infarction in the Stockholm Prospective Study." *Acta Medica Scandinavica* 206, no. 5 (1979): 351–360.

Cassady, Bridget A., Nicole L. Charboneau, Emily E. Brys, Kristin A. Crouse, Donald C. Beitz, and Ted Wilson. "Effects of Low Carbohydrate Diets High in Red Meats or Poultry, Fish and Shellfish on Plasma Lipids and Weight Loss." *Nutrition & Metabolism* 4, no. 23 (October 31, 2007). doi:10.1186/1743-7075-4-23.

Castelli, William P. "Concerning the Possibility of a Nut . . ." *Archives of Internal Medicine* 152, no. 7 (July 1992): 1371–1372.

Castelli, William P., Joseph T. Doyle, Tavia Gordon, et al. "HDL Cholesterol and Other Lipids in Coronary Heart Disease: The Cooperative Lipoprotein Phenotyping Study." *Circulation* 55, no. 5 (May 1977): 767–772.

Center for Food Safety and Applied Nutrition, US Food and Drug Administration. "FDA Issues Draft Guidance for Industry on How to Reduce Acrylamide in Certain Foods." *CFSAN Constituent Update,* November 14, 2013, http://www.fda.gov/Food/NewsEvents/ConstituentUpdates/ucm374601.htm.

Center for Science in the Public Interest. *Saturated Fat Attack.* Washington, DC: Center for Science in the Public Interest, 1988.

———. "Building a Healthier America, 35th Anniversary Report." Washington, DC: Center for Science in the Public Interest, 2006.

Centers for Disease Control and Prevention. "Trends in Intake of Energy and Macronutrients in the United States, 1971–2000." *Morbidity and Mortality Weekly Report* 53, no. 4 (February 6, 2004): 80–82.

———. National Health Examination Survey, 1960–1962. Available at http://www.cdc.gov/nchs/nhanes.htm.

Central Committee for Medical and Community Program, American Heart Association. "Dietary Fat and Its Relation to Heart Attacks and Strokes: Report by the Central Committee for Medical and Community Program of the American Heart Association." *Journal of the American Medical Association* 175 (February 4, 1961): 389–391.

Chamberlin, Thomas C. "The Method of Multiple Working Hypotheses." (Repr. *Journal of Geology,* 1897.) *Science* 148, no. 3671 (May 7, 1965): 754–759.

Charles, Dan. "The Making of Meat Eating America." Morning Edition, National Public Radio, June 26, 2012.

Chlebowski, Rowan T., George L. Blackburn, Cynthia A. Thomson, et al. "Dietary Fat Reduction and Breast Cancer Outcome: Interim Efficacy Results from the Women's Intervention Nutrition Study." *Journal of the National Cancer Institute* 98, no. 24 (December 20, 2006): 1767–1776.

Christakis, George, Seymour H. Rinzler, Morton Archer, and Arthur Kraus. "Effect of the Anti-Coronary Club Program on Coronary Heart Disease: Risk Factor Status." *Journal of the American Medical Association* 198, no. 6 (November 7, 1966): 597–604.

Christakis, George, Seymour H. Rinzler, Morton Archer, and Ethel Maslansky. "Summary of the Research Activities of the Anti-Coronary Club." *Public Health Reports* 81, no. 1 (January 1966): 64–70.

Clarke, William R., Helmut G. Schrott, Paul E. Leaverton, William E. Connor, and Ronald M. Lauer. "Tracking of Blood Lipids and Blood Pressures in School Age Children: The Muscatine Study." *Circulation* 58, no. 4 (October 1978): 626–634.

Claxson, Andrew W. D., Geoffrey E. Hawkes, David P. Richardson, et al. "Generation of Lipid Peroxidation Products in Culinary Oils and Fats During Episodes of Thermal Stressing: A High Field 1H NMR Study." *FEBS Letters* 355, no. 1 (November 21, 1994): 81–90.

Clayton, Paul, and Judith Rowbotham. "How the Mid-Victorian Worked, Ate and Died." *International Journal of Environmental Research and Public Health* 6, no. 3 (March 2009): 1235–1253.

Cleave, Thomas L., and George D. Campbell. *Diabetes, Coronary Thrombosis, and the Saccharine Disease.* Bristol: John Wright & Sons, 1966.

Cobe, P., J. M. Lang, T. H. Strenk, and D. Tanyeri. "Best Do-Over That We'll All Be Doing Soon." *Restaurant Business,* April 6, 2007.

Coggon, D., B. Pannett, C. Osmond, and E. D. Acheson. "A Survey of Cancer and Occupation in Young and Middle Aged Men. I. Cancers of the Respiratory Tract." *British Journal of Industrial Medicine* 43, no. 5 (May 1986): 332–338.

Combined Staff Clinic. "Obesity." *American Journal of Medicine* 19, no. 1 (July 1955): 115–125.

Committee of Principal Investigators. "A Co-operative Trial in the Primary Prevention of Ischaemic Heart Disease Using Clofibrate: A Report from the Committee of Principal Investigators." *British Heart Journal* 40 (October 1978): 1069–1118.

Conklin, Daniel J., Oleg A. Barski, Jean-Francois Lesgards, et al. "Acrolein Consumption Induces Systemic Dyslipidemia and Lipoprotein Modification." *Toxicology and Applied Pharmacology* 243, no. 1 (February 15, 2010): 1–12.

Conklin, Daniel J., Russell A. Prough, Peter Juvan, et al. "Acrolein-Induced Dyslipidemia and Acute-Phase Response Are Independent of HMG-CoA Reductase." *Molecular Nutrition and Food Research* 55, no. 9 (September 2011): 1411–1422.

Cooper, Thomas. *Some Information Respecting America.* London: J. Johnson, 1794.

———. *The Chainbearer.* Oxford: Oxford University, 1845.

Cordain, Loren, Janette Brand Miller, S. Boyd Eaton, Neil Mann, Susanne H. Holt, and John D. Speth. "Plant-animal Subsistence Ratios and Macronutrient Energy Estimations in Worldwide Hunter-gatherer Diets." *American Journal of Clinical Nutrition* 71, no. 3 (March 2000): 682–692.

Cowley, Geoffrey. "Healer of Hearts: Dean Ornish's Low-Tech Methods Could Transform American Medicine. But the Doctor Is Still Striving to Transform Himself." *Newsweek,* March 16, 1998.

Crampton, E. W., R. H. Common, E. T. Pritchard, and Florence A. Farmer. "Studies to Determine the Nature of the Damage to the Nutritive Value of Some Vegetable Oils from Heat Treatment: IV. Ethyl Esters of Heat Polymerized Linseed, Soybean and Sunflower Seed Oils." *Journal of Nutrition* 60, no. 1 (September 10, 1956): 13–24.

Crawford, Michael A. "Fatty-Acid Ratios in Free-Living and Domestic Animals." *Lancet* 291, no. 7556 (June 22, 1968): 1329–1333.

Csallany, A. Saari, I. Han, D.W. Shoeman, and C. Chen. "4-Hydroxynonenal (HNE), a Toxic Aldehyde in French Fries from Fast Food Restaurants." Poster presentation at the HNE Symposium of the 16th Bi-Annual Conference of the Free Radical Society and HNE Symposium, London, September 1–9, 2012.

Cummings, Richard Osborn. *The American and His Food: A History of Food Habits in the United States.* Chicago: The University of Chicago Press, 1940.

Damas, David. *Arctic Migrants/Arctic Villagers: The Transformation of Inuit Settlement in the Central Arctic.* Quebec: McGill-Queen's Press, 2002.

Damasceno, N. R., A. Pérez-Heras, M. Serra, et al. "Crossover Study of Diets Enriched with Virgin Olive Oil, Walnuts or Almonds. Effects on Lipids and Other Cardiovascular Risk Markers." *Nutrition Metabolism Cardiovascular Disease* 21, no. 1 suppl. (2011): 14S–20S.

Daniel, Carrie R., Amanda J. Cross, Corinna Koebnick, and Rashmi Sinha. "Trends in Meat Consumption in the USA." *Public Health Nutrition* 14, no. 4 (2011): 575–583.

Davidson, Alan. "Lard" in *The Penguin Companion to Food.* New York: Penguin Books, 2002, 530–531.

Day, Ivan. *Cooking in Europe 1650–1850.* Westport, CT: Greenwood Press, 2009.

Day, José, Malcolm Carruthers, Alan Bailey, and David Robinson. "Anthropometric, Physiological and Biochemical Differences Between Urban and Rural Masai." *Atherosclerosis* 23, no. 2 (1976): 357–361.

Dayton, Seymour, and Morton Lee Pearce. "Diet and Atherosclerosis." *Lancet* 295, no. 7644 (February 28, 1970): 473–474.

Dayton, Seymour, Morton Lee Pearce, Sam Hashimoto, Wilfrid J. Dixon, and Uwamie Tomiyasu. "A Controlled Clinical Trial of a Diet High in Unsaturated Fat in Preventing Complications of Atherosclerosis." *Circulation* 40, no. 1, suppl. 2 (1969): II-1–II-63.

Decker, Walter J., and Walter Mertz. "Effects of Dietary Elaidic Acid on Membrane Function in Rat Mitochondria and Erythrocytes." *Journal of Nutrition* 91, no. 3 (March 1967): 324–330.

DeHaven, Joseph, Robert Sherwin, Rosa Hendler, and Philip Felig. "Nitrogen and Sodium Balance and Sympathetic-Nervous-System Activity in Obese Subjects Treated With a Low-Calorie Protein or Mixed Diet." *New England Journal of Medicine* 302, no. 9 (February 28, 1980): 477–482.

Després, Jean-Pierre. "Bringing JUPITER Down to Earth." *Lancet* 373, no. 9670 (April 4, 2009): 1147–1148.

Deuel, Harry J. Jr. "The Butter-Margarine Controversy." *Science* 103, no. 2668 (February 15, 1946): 183–187.

Deuel, Harry J. Jr., Samuel M. Greenberg, Evelyn E. Savage, and Lucien A. Bavetta. "Studies on the Comparative Nutritive Value of Fats: XIII. Growth and Reproduction Over 25 Generations on Sherman Diet B Where Butterfat was Replaced by Margarine Fat, Including a Study of Calcium Metabolism." *Journal of Nutrition* 42, no. 2 (1950): 239–255.

Deuel, Harry J. Jr., Eli Movitt, and Lois F. Hallman. "Studies of the Comparative Nutritive Value of Fats: IV. The Negative Effect of Different Fats on Fertility and Lactation in the Rat." *Journal of Nutrition* 27, no. 6 (June 1944): 509–513.

Deuel, Harry J. Jr., Eli Movitt, Lois F. Hallman, Fred Mattson, and Evelyn Brown. "Studies of the Comparative Nutritive Value of Fats: I. Growth Rate and Efficiency of Conversion of Various Diets to Tissue." *Journal of Nutrition* 27, no. 1 (January 1944): 107–121.

Dietary Guidelines Advisory Committee. Prepared for the Agricultural Research Service, US Department of Agriculture and US Department of Health and Human Services. *Report of the Dietary Guidelines Advisory Committee on the Dietary Guidelines for Americans, 2010. To the Secretary of Agriculture and the Secretary of Health and Human Services.* Washington, DC: US Government Printing Office, June 15, 2010.

DISC Collaborative Research Group. "Dietary Intervention Study in Children (DISC) with Elevated Low Density Lipoprotein Cholesterol: Design and Baseline Characteristics." *Annals of Epidemiology* 3, no. 4 (July 1993): 393–402.

Doll, R., R. Peto, K. Wheatley, R. Gray, and I. Sutherland. "Mortality in Relation to Smoking: 40 Years' Observations on Male British Doctors." *British Medical Journal* 309, no. 6959 (October 8, 1994): 901–911.

Donaldson, Blake F. *Strong Medicine.* New York: Cassell, 1963.

Dreon, Darlene M., Harriett A. Fernstrom, Paul T. Williams, and Ronald M. Krauss. "A Very-Low-Fat Diet Is Not Associated with Improved Lipoprotein Profiles in Men with a Predominance of Large, Low-Density Lipoproteins." *American Journal of Clinical Nutrition* 69, no. 3 (March 1999): 411–418.

Drewnowski, Adam. "The Cost of U.S. Foods as Related to Their Nutritive Value." *American Journal of Clinical Nutrition* 92, no. 5 (Nov, 2010): 1181–1188.

Dupré, Ruth. " 'If It's Yellow, It Must be Butter': Margarine Regulation in North America Since 1886." *Journal of Economic History* 59, no. 2 (June 1999): 353–371.

Duthie, Susan J. "Soybean Growers Move to Label Palm Oil as Unhealthy, Bringing Rivalry to a Boil." *Wall Street Journal,* August 31, 1987.

Eckel, Robert H., J. M. Jakicic, V. S. Hubbard, et al. "2013 AHA/ACC Guideline on Lifestyle Management to Reduce Cardiovascular Risk: A Report of the American College of Cardiology/American Heart Association Task Force on Practice Guidelines." *Circulation,* (2013), doi:10.1161/01.cir.0000437740.48606.d1.

Editors. "Coronary Heart Disease and Carbohydrate Metabolism." *Journal of the American Medical Association* 201, no. 13 (September 25, 1967): 164.

———. "Diet and Atherosclerosis." *Lancet* 2, no. 7627 (November 1, 1969): 939–940.

———. "Can I Avoid a Heart Attack?" *Lancet* 303, no. 7858 (April 6, 1974): 605–607.

———. "Trans Fatty Acids Dispute Rages in Letters to FASEB." *Food Chemical News* (May 30, 1988): 6–10.

———. "Expression of Concern." *British Medical Journal* 331, no. 7511 (July 30, 2005): 266.

Enig, Mary G. *Trans Fatty Acids in the Food Supply: A Comprehensive Report Covering 60 Years of Research,* 2nd Edition. Silver Spring, MD: Enig Associates, 1995.

Enig, Mary G., S. Atal, M. Keeney, and J. Sampugna. "Isomeric Trans Fatty Acids in the U.S. Diet." *Journal of the American College of Nutrition* 9, no. 5 (October 1990): 471–486.

Enig, Mary G., R. Munn, and M. Keeney, "Dietary Fat and Cancer Trends—A Critique." *Federation Proceedings* 37, no. 9 (July 1978): 2215–2220.

Ernst, Nancy D., C. T. Sempos, R. R. Briefel, and M. B. Clark. "Consistency Between US Dietary Fat Intake and Serum Total Cholesterol Concentrations: The National Health and Nutrition Examination Surveys." *American Journal of Clinical Nutrition* 66, no. 4 suppl. (October 1997): 965S–972S.

Esposito, Katherine, Raffaele Marfella, Miryam Ciotola, et al. "Effect of a Mediterranean-Style Diet on Endothelial Dysfunction and Markers of Vascular Inflammation in the Metabolic Syndrome: A Randomized Trial." *Journal of the American Medical Association* 292, no. 12 (September 22, 2004): 1440–1446.

Esterbauer, Hermann. "Cytotoxicity and Genotoxicity of Lipid-Oxidation Products." *American Journal of Clinical Nutrition* 57, no. 5 suppl. (May 1993): 779S–786S.

Esterbauer, Hermann, K. H. Cheeseman, M. U. Dianzani, G. Poli, and T. F. Slater. "Separation and Characterization of the Aldehydic Products of Lipid Peroxidation Stimulated by ADP-Fe2+ in Rat Liver Microsomes." *Biochemical Journal* 208, no. 1 (October 15, 1982): 129–140.

Esterbauer, Hermann, Günther Jürgens, Oswald Quehenberger, and Ernst Koller. "Autoxidation of Human Low Density Lipoprotein: Loss of Polyunsaturated Fatty Acids and Vitamin E and Generation of Aldehydes." *Journal of Lipid Research* 28, no. 5 (May 1987): 495–509.

Esterbauer, Hermann, Rudolf Jörg Schaur, and Helmward Zollner. "Chemistry and Biochemistry of 4-Hydroxynonenal, Malonaldehyde and Related Aldehydes." *Free Radical Biology & Medicine* 11, no. 1 (1991): 81–128.

Estruch, Ramón, Emilio Ros, Jordi Salas-Salvadó, et al. "Primary Prevention of Cardiovascular Disease with a Mediterranean Diet." *New England Journal of Medicine* 368, no. 14 (April 4, 2013): 1279–1290.

European Food Safety Authority. "Analysis of Occurrence of 3 monochloropropane 1,2 diol (3 MCPD) in Food in Europe in the Year 2009–2011 and Preliminary Exposure Assessment." *EFSA Journal* 11, no. 9 (2013): 3381. doi:10.2903/j.efsa.2013.3381.

Expert Panel on Trans Fatty Acids and Coronary Heart Disease. "Trans Fatty Acids and Coronary Heart Disease Risk." *American Journal of Clinical Nutrition* 62, no. 3 suppl. (1995): 655S–708S.

Falta, Wilhelm. *Endocrine Diseases, Including Their Diagnosis and Treatment.* Philadelphia: P. Blakiston's Sons, 1923.

Federal Trade Commission, Complaint, "In the Matter of Standard Brands, Inc., et al.: Consent Order, Etc., In Regard to the Alleged Violation of the Federal Trade Commission Act." Docket C-2377, April 9, 1973.

Fehily, A. M., J. W. G. Yarnell, P. M. Sweetnam, and P. C. Elwood. "Diet and Incident of Ischaemic Heart Disease: The Caerphilly Study." *British Journal of Nutrition* 69, no. 2 (March 1993): 303–314.

Feinleib, Manning. "On a Possible Inverse Relationship Between Serum Cholesterol and Cancer Mortality." *American Journal of Epidemiology* 114, no. 1 (July 1981): 5–10.

———. "Summary of a Workshop on Cholesterol and Noncardiovascular Disease Mortality." *Preventive Medicine* 11, no. 3 (May 1982): 360–367.

Feron, V. J., H. P. Til, Flora de Vrijer, et al. "Aldehydes: Occurrence, Carcinogenic Potential, Mechanism of Action and Risk Assessment." *Mutation Research* 259, no. 3–4 (March–April 1991): 363–385.

Ferro-Luzzi, Anna, and Francesco Branca. "Mediterranean Diet, Italian-Style: Prototype of a Healthy Diet." *American Journal of Clinical Nutrition* 61, no. 6 suppl. (June 1995): 1338S–1345S.

Ferro-Luzzi, Anna, Philip James, and Anthony Kafatos. "The High-Fat Greek Diet: a Recipe for All?" *European Journal of Clinical Nutrition* 56, no. 9 (September 2002): 796–809.

———. "Response to Letter: Response to the Letter Submitted by D. Trichopoulos entitled, 'In Defense of the Mediterranean Diet.' " *European Journal of Clinical Nutrition* 56, no. 9 (September 2002): 930–931.

Ferro-Luzzi, Anna, and Stefania Sette. "The Mediterranean Diet: An Attempt to Define Its Present and Past Composition." *European Journal of Clinical Nutrition* 43, no. 2 suppl. (1989): 13–29.

Ferro-Luzzi, Anna, Pasquale Strazzullo, Cristina Scaccini, et al. "Changing the Mediterranean Diet: Effects on Blood Lipids." *American Journal of Clinical Nutrition* 40, no. 5 (November 1984): 1027–1037.

Fiedorowicz, Jess G., and William G. Haynes. "Cholesterol, Mood, and Vascular Health: Untangling the Relationship. Does Low Cholesterol Predispose to Depression and Suicide, or Vice Versa?" *Current Psychiatry* 9, no. 7 (July 2010): 17–22.

Finegan, Aileen, Noel Hickey, Brian Maurer, and Risteárd Mulcahy. "Diet and Coronary Heart Disease: Dietary Analysis on 100 Male Patients." *American Journal of Clinical Nutrition* 21, no. 2 (February 1968): 143–148.

———. "Diet and Coronary Heart Disease: Dietary Analysis on 50 Female Patients." *American Journal of Clinical Nutrition* 22, no. 1 (January 1969): 8–9.

Firestone, David. "Worldwide Regulation of Frying Fats and Oils." *Inform* 4 (1993): 1366–1371.

Fischer, Louis, and Julian L. Rogatz. "Insulin in Malnutrition." *Archives of Pediatrics & Adolescent Medicine* 31, no. 3 (March 1926): 363–372.

Fitó, M., M. Cladellas, R. de la Torre, et al. "Anti-Inflammatory Effect of Virgin Olive Oil in Stable Coronary Disease Patients: A Randomized, Crossover, Controlled Trial." *European Journal of Clinical Nutrition* 62, no. 4 (April 2004): 570–574.

Flavell, C. M. "Women and Coronary Heart Disease." *Progress in Cardiovascular Nursing* 9, no. 4 (Fall 1994): 18–27.

Flint, Austin. *A Practical Treatise on the Diagnosis, Pathology, and Treatment of Diseases of the Heart.* Philadelphia: Blanchard and Lea, 1859.

Flock, M. R., J. A. Fleming, and Penny M. Kris-Etherton. "Macronutrient Replacement Options for Saturated Fat: Effects on Cardiovascular Health." *Current Opinion in Lipidology* 25, no. 1 (February 2014): 67–74.

Fogliano, Vincenzo, and Raffaele Sacchi. "Oleocanthal in Olive Oil: Between Myth and Reality." *Molecular Nutrition & Food Research* 50, no. 1 (January 2006): 5–6.

Food and Agriculture Organization of the United Nations. "Fats and Fatty Acids in Human Nutrition: Report of an Expert Consultation. 10–14 November 2008." *FAO Food and Nutrition Paper* 91. Rome: Food and Agriculture Organization of the United Nations, 2010.

Food and Drug Administration, US Department of Health and Human Services. "Food Labeling: Trans Fatty Acids in Nutrition Labeling, Nutrient Content Claims, and Health Claims; Proposed Rule." Washington, DC: US Government Printing Office, 1999.

———. "Food Labeling: *Trans* Fatty Acids in Nutrition Labeling, Nutrient Content Claims, and Health Claims, Final and Proposed Rule." *Federal Register* 68, no. 133. Washington, DC: US Government Printing Office, July 11, 2003.

Food and Nutrition Board, Division of Biological Sciences, Assembly of Life Sciences, The National Research Council, National Academy of Sciences. *Toward Healthful Diets.* Washington, DC: National Academy Press, 1980.

Foppa, Ivo, and Christoph E. Minder. "Oral, Pharyngeal and Laryngeal Cancer as a Cause of Death Among Swiss Cooks." *Scandinavian Journal of Work, Environment & Health* 18, no. 5 (October 1992): 287–292.

Forbes, Hamish. "Ethnoarchaeology and the Place of the Olive in the Economy of the Southern Argolid, Greece." In *La Production du Vin et l'Huile en Méditerranée.* Edited by M.-C. Amouretti and J.-P. Brun, 213–226. Paris: Ecole Française d'Athenes, 1993.

Forsythe, Cassandra E., Stephen D. Phinney, Richard D. Feinman, et al. "Limited Effect of Dietary Saturated Fat on Plasma Saturated Fat in the Context of a Low Carbohydrate Diet." *Lipids* 45, no. 10 (October 2010): 947–962.

Foster, Gary D., Holly R. Wyatt, James O. Hill, et al. "Weight and Metabolic Outcomes After 2 Years on a Low-Carbohydrate Versus Low-Fat Diet: A Randomized Trial." *Annals of Internal Medicine* 153, no. 3 (August 3, 2010): 147–157.

Frank, Charles W., Eve Weinblatt, and Sam Shapiro. "Angina Pectoris in Men." *Circulation* 42, no. 3 (March 1973): 509–517.

Frantz, Ivan D., Emily A. Dawson, Patricia L. Ashman, et al. "Test of Effect of Lipid Lowering by Diet on Cardiovascular Risk. The Minnesota Coronary Survey." *Arteriosclerosis, Thrombosis, and Vascular Biology* 9, no. 1 (January–February 1989): 129–135.

Fraser, Gary E. "Determinants of Ischemic Heart Disease in Seventh-Day Adventists: A Review." *American Journal of Clinical Nutrition* 48, no. 3 suppl. (September 1988): 833–836.

Fraser, Gary E., Joan Sabaté, and W. Lawrence Beeson. "The Application of Results of Some Studies of California Seventh-Day Adventists to the General Population." *Archives of Internal Medicine* 153, no. 4 (February 22, 1993): 533–534.

Fredrickson, Donald S. "Mutants, Hyperlipoproteinaemia, and Coronary Artery Disease." *British Medical Journal* 2, no. 5755 (April 24, 1971): 187–192.

Freedman, David S., Charles L. Shear, Sathanur R. Srinivasan, Larry S. Webber, and Gerald S. Berenson. "Tracking of Serum Lipids and Lipoproteins in Children Over an 8-year Period: The Bogalusa Heart Study." *Preventive Medicine* 14, no. 2 (March 1985): 203–216.

Fullanana, Andres, Angel A. Carbonell-Barrachina, and Sukh Sidhu. "Comparison of Volatile Aldehydes Present in the Cooking Fumes of Extra Virgin Olive, Olive, and Canola Oils." *Journal of Agriculture and Food Chemistry* 52, no. 16 (August 11, 2004): 5207–5214.

Galan, Pilar, Emmanuelle Kesse-Guyot, Sébastien Czernichow, Serge Briancon, Jacques Blacher, and Serge Hercberg. "Effects of B Vitamins and Omega 3 Fatty Acids on Cardiovascular Disease: A Randomised Placebo Controlled Trial." *British Medical Journal* 341 (November 29, 2010): 1–9.

Gammal, Elias B., Kenneth K. Carroll, and Earl R. Plunkett. "Effects of Dietary Fat on the Uptake and Clearance of 7,12 Dimethylbenz(α)anthracene by Rat Mammary Tissue." *Cancer Research* 28, no. 2 (February 1968): 384–385.

Garcia-Palmieri, Mario R., Paul D. Sorlie, Raul Costas, Jr., and Richard J. Havlik. "An Apparent Inverse Relationship Between Serum Cholesterol and Cancer Mortality in Puerto Rico." *American Journal of Epidemiology* 114, no. 1 (July 1981): 29–40.

Gardner, Christopher D., Alexandre Kiazand, Sofiya Alhassan, et al. "Comparison of the Atkins, Zone, Ornish, and LEARN Diets for Change in Weight and Related Risk Factors Among Overweight Premenopausal Women: The A TO Z Weight Loss Study: A Randomized Trial." *Journal of the American Medical Association* 297, no. 9 (March 7, 2007): 969–977.

Garg, Rekha, Jennifer H. Madans, and Joel C. Kleinman. "Regional Variation in Ischemic Heart Disease Incidence." *Journal of Clinical Epidemiology* 45, no. 2 (February 1992): 149–156.

German, J. Bruce, Robert A. Gibson, Ronald M. Krauss, et al. "A Reappraisal of the Impact of Dairy Foods and Milk Fat on Cardiovascular Disease Risk." *European Journal of Nutrition* 48, no. 4 (2009): 191–203.

Gertler, Menard M., Paul D. White, Raoul Simon, and Lida G. Gottsch. "Long-Term Follow-up of Young Coronary Patients." *American Journal of Medical Sciences* 247, no. 2 (February 1964): 145–155.

Gibbons, Gary H., John Gordon Harold, Mariell Jessup, Rose Marie Robertson, and William Oetgen. "The Next Steps in Developing Clinical Practice Guidelines for Prevention." *Circulation* 128, no. 15 (October 8, 2013): 1716–1717.

Gilchrist, A. Rae. "The Edinburgh Tradition in Clinical Cardiology." *Scottish Medical Journal* 17, no. 8 (August 1972): 282–287.

Ginsberg, Henry N., Penny Kris-Etherton, Barbara Dennis, et al. "Effects of Reducing Dietary Saturated Fatty Acids on Plasma Lipids and Lipoproteins in Healthy Subjects: The DELTA Study, Protocol 1." *Arteriosclerosis, Thrombosis, and Vascular Biology* 18, no. 3 (March 1998): 441–449.

GISSI-Prevenzione Investigators (Gruppo Italiano per lo Studio della Sopravvivenza nell'Infarto Miocardico). "Dietary Supplementation with n-3 Polyunsaturated Fatty Acids and Vitamin E after Myocardial Infarction: Results of the GISSI-Prevenzione Trial." *Lancet* 354, no. 9177 (August 7, 1999): 447–455.

Glazer, M. D., and J. W. Hurst. "Coronary Atherosclerotic Heart Disease: Some Important Differences Between Men and Women." *American Journal of Noninvasive Cardiology* 61, no. 1 (1987).

Gofman, John W., Frank Lindgren, Harold Elliott, et al. "The Role of Lipids and Lipoproteins in Atherosclerosis." *Science* 111, no. 2877 (February 17, 1950): 166–186.

Gofman, John W., Alex Y. Nichols, and E. Virginia Dobbin. *Dietary Prevention and Treatment of Heart Disease.* New York: Putnam, 1958.

Gogoi, Palavi. "Atkins Gets Itself in a Stew." *Bloomberg Businessweek,* August 1, 2005.

Goldbourt, U., S. Yaari, and J. H. Medalie. "Factors Predictive of Long-Term Coronary Heart Disease Mortality Among 10,059 Male Israeli Civil Servants and Municipal Employees. A 23-Year Mortality Follow-up in the Israeli Ischemic Heart Disease Study." *Cardiology* 82, nos. 2–3 (1993): 100–121.

Gordon, Edgar S., Marshall Goldberg, and Grace J. Chosy. "A New Concept in the Treatment of Obesity." *Journal of the American Medical Association* 186, no. 1 (October 5, 1963): 156–166.

Gordon, Robert S., and Amelia Cherkes. "Unesterified Fatty Acid in Human Blood Plasma." *Journal of Clinical Investigation* 35, no. 2 (February 1956): 206–212.

Gordon, Tavia, William P. Castelli, Marthana C. Hjortland, William B. Kannel, and Thomas R. Dawber. "High Density Lipoprotein as a Protective Factor Against Coronary Heart

Disease: The Framingham Study." *American Journal of Medicine* 62, no. 5 (May 1977): 707–714.

Gould, K. Lance, Dean Ornish, Larry Scherwitz, et al. "Changes in Myocardial Perfusion Abnormalities by Positron Emission Tomography after Long-Term, Intense Risk Factor Modification." *Journal of the American Medical Association* 274, no. 11 (September 20, 1995): 894–901.

Gould, R. Gordon. "Lipid Metabolism and Atherosclerosis." *American Journal of Medicine* 11, no. 2 (August 1951): 209–227.

Gould, R. Gordon, C. Bruce Taylor, Joanne S. Hagerman, Irving Warner, and Donald J. Campbell. "Cholesterol Metabolism: I. Effect of Dietary Cholesterol on the Synthesis of Cholesterol in Dog Tissue in Vitro." *Journal of Biological Chemistry* 201, no. 2 (April 1, 1953): 519–528.

Greenberg, Samuel M., and A. C. Frazer. "Some Factors Affecting the Growth and Development of Rats Fed Rancid Fat." *Journal of Nutrition* 50, no. 4 (August 1953): 421–440.

Greenblatt, James M. "Low Cholesterol and Its Psychological Effects: Low Cholesterol Is Linked to Depression, Suicide, and Violence." *Psychology Today*, June 10, 2011. Accessed January 2, 2014. http://www.psychologytoday.com/blog/the-breakthrough-depression -solution/201106/low-cholesterol-and-its-psychological-effects.

Griel, Amy E., and Penny Kris-Etherton. "Brief Critical Review: Beyond Saturated Fat: The Importance of the Dietary Fatty Acid Profile on Cardiovascular Disease." *Nutrition Reviews* 64, no. 5 (May 2006): 257–262.

Grigg, David. "Olive Oil, the Mediterranean and the World." *GeoJournal* 53, no. 2 (February 2001): 163–172.

Groen, J., B. K. Tjiong, C. E. Kamminga, and A. F. Willebrands. "Influence of Nutrition, Individual, and Some Other Factors, Including Various Forms of Stress, on Serum Cholesterol; Experiment of Nine Months' Duration in 60 Normal Human Volunteers." *Voeding* 13 (October 1952): 556–587.

Grootveld, Martin, Christopher J. L. Silwood, Paul Addis, Andrew Claxson, Bartolomé Bonet Serra, and Marta Viana. "Health Effects of Oxidized Heated Oils." *Foodservice Research International* 13, no. 1 (October 2001): 41–55.

Grootveld, Martin, Christopher J. L. Silwood, and Andrew W. D. Claxson. "Letter to the Editor. Warning: Thermally-Stressed Polyunsaturates Are Damaging to Health." *Food Chemistry* 67 (1999): 211–213.

Grundy, Scott, David Bilheimer, Henry Blackburn, et al. "Rationale of the Diet-Heart Statement of the American Heart Association." *Circulation* 65, no. 4 (April 1982): 839A–854A.

Grune, Tilman, Neven Zarkovic, and Kostelidou Kalliopi. "Lipid Peroxidation Research in Europe and the COST B35 Action 'Lipid Peroxidation Associated Disorders." *Free Radical Research* 44, no. 10 (October 2010): 1095–1097.

Guberan, E. "Surprising Decline of Cardiovascular Mortality in Switzerland: 1951–1976." *Journal of Epidemiology and Community Health* 33, no. 2 (June 1979): 114–120.

Halperin, M., Jerome Cornfield, and S. C. Mitchell. "Letters to the Editor: Effect of Diet on Coronary-Heart-Disease Mortality." *Lancet* 302, no. 7826 (August 25, 1973): 438–439.

Hamilakis, Yannis. "Food Technologies/Technologies of the Today: The Social Context of Wine and Oil Production and Consumption in Bronze Age Crete." *World Archeology* 31, no. 1 (June 1999): 38–54.

Han, In Hwa, and A. Saari Csallany. "Formation of Toxic α-β-Unsaturated 4-Hydroxy-Aldehydes in Thermally Oxidized Fatty Acid Methyl Esters." *Journal of the American Oil Chemists' Society* 86, no. 3 (March 2009): 253–260.

———. "Temperature Dependence of HNE Formation in Vegetable Oils and Butter Oil." *Journal of the American Oil Chemists' Society* 85, no. 8 (August 2008): 777–782.

Han, Paul W., and Lawrence A. Frohman. "Hyperinsulinemia in Tube-fed Hypophysectomized Rats Bearing Hypothalamic Lesions." *American Journal of Physiology* 219, no. 6 (1970): 1632–1636.

Hankins, Gerald W. *Sunrise Over Pangnirtung: The Story of Otto Schaefer, M.D.* Calgary, Canada: The Arctic Institute of North America of the University of Calgary, 2000.

Hansen, Anders. "Swedish Health Advisory Body Says Too Much Carbohydrate, Not Fat, Leads to Obesity." *British Medical Journal* 347 (November 15, 2013). doi: 10.1136/bmj.f6873.

Hanssen, Per. "Treatment of Obesity by a Diet Relatively Poor in Carbohydrates." *Acta Medica Scandinavica* 88, no. 1 (January 1936): 97–106.

Hardinge, Mervyn G., and Fredrick J. Stare. "Nutritional Studies of Vegetarians. 2. Dietary and Serum Levels of Cholesterol." *American Journal of Clinical Nutrition* 2, no. 2 (March 1954): 83–88.

Hardy, Stephen C., and Ronald E. Kleinman. "Fat and Cholesterol in the Diet of Infants and Young Children: Implications for Growth, Development, and Long-Term Health." *Journal of Pediatrics* 125, no. 5, part 2 (November 1994): S69–S77.

Harman, Denham. "Letter to the Editor. Atherosclerosis: Possible Ill-Effects of the Use of Highly Unsaturated Fats to Lower Serum Cholesterol Levels." *Lancet* 275, no. 7005 (November 30, 1957): 1116–1117.

Harris, Maureen I. "Prevalence of Noninsulin-Dependent Diabetes and Impaired Glucose Tolerance." In *Diabetes in America: Diabetes Data Compiled in 1984*, 1–31. US Department of Health and Human Services, Public Health Service, August 1985.

Harris, William S., Dariush Mozaffarian, Eric Rimm, et al. "Omega-6 Fatty Acids and Risk for Cardiovascular Disease. A Science Advisory from the American Heart Association Nutrition Subcommittee of the Council of Nutrition, Physical Activity, and Metabolism; Council on Cardiovascular Nursing; and Council on Epidemiology and Prevention." *Circulation* 119, no. 6 (February 17, 2009): 902–907.

Hayes, Kenneth C., for the Expert Panel. "Fatty Acid Expert Roundtable: Key Statements about Fatty Acids." *Journal of the American College of Nutrition* 29, no. 3 suppl. (2010): 285S–288S.

Hays, James H., Angela DiSabatino, Robert T. Gorman, Simi Vincent, and Michael E. Stillabower. "Effect of a High Saturated Fat and No-Starch Diet on Serum Lipid Subfractions in Patients with Documented Atherosclerotic Cardiovascular Disease." *Mayo Clinic Proceedings* 78, no. 11 (November 2003): 1331–1336.

Hayward, Rodney A., and Harlan M. Krumholz. "Three Reasons to Abandon Low-Density Lipoprotein Targets: An Open Letter to the Adult Treatment Panel IV of the National Institute of Health." *Circulation: Cardiovascular Quality and Outcomes* 5, no. 1 (January 2012): 2–5.

Haywood, Rachel M., Andrew W. D. Claxson, Geoffrey W. Hawkes, et al. "Detection of Aldehydes and Their Conjugated Hydroperoxydiene Precursors in Thermally-Stressed Culinary Oils and Fats: Investigations Using High Resolution Proton NMR Spectroscopy." *Free Radical Research* 22, no. 5 (May 1995): 441–482.

Hecht, Harvey S., and H. Robert Superko. "Electron Beam Tomography and National Cholesterol Education Program Guidelines in Asymptomatic Women." *Journal of the American College of Cardiology* 37, no. 6 (May 2001): 1506–1511.

Hegsted, Mark. "Washington—Dietary Guidelines." Preventing Heart Attack and Stroke: A History of Cardiovascular Disease Epidemiology, ed. Henry Blackburn, last accessed January 29, 2014, http://www.epi.umn.edu/cvdepi/pdfs/Hegstedguidelines.pdf.

Helsing, Elisabet, and Antonia Trichopoulou, eds. "The Mediterranean Diet and Food Culture—a Symposium." *European Journal of Clinical Nutrition* 43, suppl. 2 (1989): 1–92.

Hetherington, A. W., and S. W. Ranson. "The Spontaneous Activity and Food Intake of Rats with Hypothalamic Lesions." *American Journal of Physiology* 136, no. 4 (1942): 609–617.

Hibbeln, Joseph R., and Norman Salem, Jr. "Dietary Polyunsaturated Fatty Acids and Depression: When Cholesterol Does Not Satisfy." *American Journal of Clinical Nutrition* 62, no. 1 (July 1995): 1–9.

Hibbeln, Joseph R., John C. Umhau, David T. George, and Norman Salem, Jr. "Do Plasma Polyunsaturates Predict Hostility and Violence?" In *Nutrition and Fitness: Metabolic and Behavior Aspects in Health and Disease, World Review of Nutrition and Diatetics*. Edited by A. P. Simopoulos and K. N. Pavlou. Basel, Switzerland: Karger, 1996, 175–186.

Hilditch, Thomas Percy, and N. L. Vidyarthi. "The Products of Partial Hydrogenation of Higher Monoethylenic Esters." *Proceedings of the Royal Society of London. Series A, Mathematical, Physical and Engineering Sciences* 122, no. 790 (February 1, 1929): 552–570.

Hirsch, Jules, and Edward H. Ahrens, Jr. "The Separation of Complex Lipide Mixtures by the Use of Silic Acid Chromatography." *Journal of Biological Chemistry* 233, no. 2 (August 1958): 311–320.

Hite, Adele H., Richard David Feinman, Gabriel E. Guzman, Morton Satin, Pamela A. Schoenfeld, and Richard J. Wood. "In the Face of Contradictory Evidence: Report of the Dietary Guidelines for Americans Committee." *Nutrition* 26, no. 10 (October 2010): 915–924.

Hoffman, William. "Meet Monsieur Cholesterol." Update. University of Minnesota, 1979. Accessed January 2, 2013. http://mbbnet.umn.edu/hoff/hoff_ak.html.

Holmes, Michelle D., David J. Hunter, Graham A. Colditz, et al. "Association of Dietary Intake of Fat and Fatty Acids with Risk of Breast Cancer." *Journal of the American Medical Association* 281, no. 10 (March 10, 1999): 914–920.

Hooper, Lee, Paul A. Kroon, Eric B. Rimm, et al. "Flavonoids, Flavonoid-Rich Foods, and Cardiovascular Risk: a Meta-Analysis of Randomized Controlled Trials." *American Journal of Clinical Nutrition* 88, no. 1 (July 2008). 38–50.

Hopkins, Paul N. "Effects of Dietary Cholesterol on Serum Cholesterol: A Meta-Analysis and Review." *American Journal of Clinical Nutrition* 55, no. 6 (June 1992): 1060–1070.

Hornstra, Gerard, and Anna Vendelmans-Starrenburg. "Induction of Experimental Arterial Occlusive Thrombi in Rats." *Atherosclerosis* 17, no. 3 (May–June 1973): 369–382.

Horowitz, Roger. *Putting Meat on the American Table: Taste, Technology, Transformation.* Baltimore, MD: Johns Hopkins University Press, 2006.

Horton, Richard. "Expression of Concern: Indo-Mediterranean Diet Heart Study." *The Lancet* 366, no. 9483 (July 30, 2005): 354–356.

Howard, Barbara V., JoAnn E. Manson, Marcia L. Stefanick, et al. "Low-Fat Dietary Pattern and Weight Change Over 7 Years: The Women's Health Initiative Dietary Modification Trial." *Journal of the American Medical Association* 295, no. 1 (January 4, 2006): 39–49.

Howard, Barbara V., Linda Van Horn, Judith Hsia, et al. "Low-Fat Dietary Pattern and Risk of Cardiovascular Disease: The Women's Health Initiative Randomized Controlled Dietary Modification Trial." *Journal of the American Medical Association* 295, no. 6 (February 8, 2006): 655–666.

Hrdlička, Aleš. Physiological and Medical Observations Among the Indians of Southwestern United States and Northern Mexico, No. 34. Washington, DC: US Government Printing Office, 1908.

Hu, Frank B. "The Mediterranean Diet and Mortality—Olive Oil and Beyond." *New England Journal of Medicine* 348, no. 26 (June 26, 2003): 2595–2596.

Hu, Frank B., JoAnn E. Manson, and Walter C. Willett. "Types of Dietary Fat and Risk of Coronary Heart Disease: A Critical Review." *Journal of American College of Nutrition* 20, no. 1 (February 2001): 5–19.

Hulley, Stephen B., Judith M. B. Walsh, and Thomas B. Newman. "Health Policy on Blood Cholesterol. Time to Change Directions." *Circulation* 86, no. 3 (September 1992): 1026–1029.

Hunter, Beatrice Trum. *Consumer Beware.* New York: Simon & Schuster, 1971.

Hunter, David J., Eric B. Rimm, Frank M. Sacks, Meir J. Stampfer, Graham A. Colditz, Lisa B. Litin, and Walter C. Willett. "Comparison of Measures of Fatty Acid Intake by Subcutaneous Fat Aspirate, Food Frequency Questionnaire, and Diet Records in a Free-Living Population of US Men." *American Journal of Epidemiology* 135, no. 4 (February 15, 1992): 418–427.

Hunter, J. Edward. "Dietary *trans* Fatty Acids: Review of Recent Human Studies and Food Industry Responses." *Lipids* 41, no. 11 (November 2006): 967–992.

Hunter, J. Edward, and Thomas H. Applewhite. "Isomeric Fatty Acids in the US Diet: Levels and Health Perspectives." *American Journal of Clinical Nutrition* 44, no. 6 (December 1986): 707–717.

Hustvedt, B. E., and A. Løvø. "Correlation between Hyperinsulinemia and Hyperphagia in Rats with Ventromedial Hypothalamic Lesions." *Acta Physiologica Scandinavica* 84, no. 1 (January 1972): 29–33.

Institute of Medicine of the National Academies, Panel on Macronutrients, Panel on the Definition of Dietary Fiber, Subcommittee on Upper Reference Levels of Nutrients, Subcommittee on Interpretation and Uses of Dietary Reference Intakes, and the Standing Committee on the Scientific Evaluation of Dietary Reference Intakes. "Dietary Fats: Total Fat and Fatty Acids." In *Dietary Reference Intakes for Energy, Carbohydrate, Fiber, Fat, Fatty Acids, Cholesterol, Protein, and Amino Acids, part 1.* Washington, DC: National Academies Press, 2002.

———. "Letter Report on Dietary Reference Intakes for Trans Fatty Acids." In *Dietary Reference Intakes for Energy, Carbohydrate, Fiber, Fat, Fatty Acids, Cholesterol, Protein, and Amino Acids, part 1.* Washington, DC: National Academies Press, 2002.

Instituto Nazionale di Statistica. "Statistical Analysis on Young Conscripts" (Analisi Statistica sui Giovani Iscritti nelle Liste di Leva). ISTAT Notiziario Serie 4 Foglio 41 (1993): 1–10.

International Agency for Research on Cancer, World Health Organization. "Household Use of Solid Fuels and High-Temperature Frying." *IARC Monographs on the Evaluation of Carcinogenic Risks to Humans*, vol. 95. Lyon, France: IARC, 2006.

Jacobs, David, Henry Blackburn, Millicent Higgins, et al. "Report of the Conference on Low Blood Cholesterol: Mortality Associations." *Circulation* 86, no. 3 (January 1992): 1046–1060.

Jacobson, Michael F., and Sarah Fritschner. *The Fast-Food Guide: What's Good, What's Bad, and How to Tell the Difference*. New York: Workman, 1986.

Jochim, Michael A. *Strategies for Survival: Cultural Behavior in an Ecological Context*. New York: Academic Press, 1981.

Johnson, Richard J. *The Fat Switch*. Mercola.com, 2012.

Johnston, Patricia V., Ogden C. Johnson, and Fred A. Kummerow. "Occurrence of Trans Fatty Acids in Human Tissue." *Science* 126, no. 3276 (October 11, 1957): 698–699.

———. "Deposition in Tissues and Fecal Excretion of Trans Fatty Acids in the Rat." *Journal of Nutrition* 65, no. 1 (May 10, 1958): 13–23.

Jolliffe, Norman, Seymour H. Rinzler, and Morton Archer. "The Anti-Coronary Club: Including a Discussion of the Effects of a Prudent Diet on the Serum Cholesterol Level of Middleaged Men." *The American Journal of Clinical Nutrition* 7, no. 4 (July 1959): 451–462.

Jones, David S. "Visions of a Cure: Visualization, Clinical Trials, and Controversies in Cardiac Therapeutics, 1968–1998." *Isis* 91, no. 3 (September 2000): 504–541.

Joslin, Elliot Proctor. *A Diabetic Manual for the Mutual Use of Doctor and Patient*. Philadelphia: Lea & Febiger, 1919.

Judd, Joseph T., Beverly A. Clevidence, Richard A. Muesing, Janet Wittes, Matthew E. Sunkin, and John J. Podczasy. "Dietary Trans Fatty Acids: Effects on Plasma Lipids and Lipoproteins of Healthy Men and Women." *American Journal of Clinical Nutrition* 59, no. 4 (April 1994): 861–868.

Kaaks, Rudolf, Nadia Slimani, and Elio Riboli. "Pilot Phase Studies on the Accuracy of Dietary Intake Measurements in the EPIC Project: Overall Evaluation of Results." *International Journal of Epidemiology* 26, no. 1 suppl. (1997): S26–36.

Kagan, Abraham, Jordan Popper, Dwayne M. Reed, Charles J. MacLean, and John S. Grove. "Trends in Stroke Incidence and Mortality in Hawaiian Japanese Men." *Stroke* 25, no. 6 (June 1994): 1170–1175.

Kaminer, Benjamin, and W. P. W. Lutz. "Blood Pressure in Bushmen of the Kalahari Desert." *Circulation* 22, no. 2 (August 1960): 289–295.

Kannel, William B. "Metabolic Risk Factors for Coronary Heart Disease in Women: Perspective from the Framingham Study." *American Heart Journal* 114, no. 2 (August 1987): 413–419.

Kannel, William B., William P. Castelli, Tavia Gordon, and Patricia M. McNamara. "Serum Cholesterol, Lipoproteins, and the Risk of Coronary Heart Disease, The Framingham Study." *Annals of Internal Medicine* 74, no. 1 (January 1, 1971): 1–12.

Kannel, William B., Thomas R. Dawber, Abraham Kagan, Nicholas Revotskie, and Joseph Stokes. "Factors of Risk in the Development of Coronary Heart Disease—Six-Year Follow-up Experience. The Framingham Study." *Annals of Internal Medicine* 55, no. 1 (July 1961): 33–50.

Kannel, William B., and Tavia Gordon. "The Framingham Study: An Epidemiological Investigation of Cardiovascular Disease." Section 24, unpublished paper. Washington, DC: National Heart, Lung, and Blood Institute, 1987.

Kaplan, Robert M. *Disease, Diagnosis and Dollars.* New York: Copernicus Books, 2009.

Kaplan, Robert M., and Michelle T. Toshima. "Does a Reduced Fat Diet Cause Retardation in Child Growth?" *Preventive Medicine* 21, no. 1 (January 1992): 33–52.

Kark, J. D., A. H. Smith, and C. G. Hames. "The Relationship of Serum Cholesterol to the Incidence of Cancer in Evans County, Georgia." *Journal of Chronic Diseases* 33, no. 5 (1980): 311–322.

Katan, Martijn B. "High-oil Compared with Low-Fat, High-Carbohydrate Diets in the Prevention of Ischemic Heart Disease." *American Journal of Clinical Nutrition* 66, no. 4 suppl. (1997): 974S–979S.

Katan, Martijn B., Scott M. Grundy, and Walter C. Willett. "Should a Low-Fat, High-Carbohydrate Diet Be Recommended for Everyone? Beyond Low-Fat Diets." *New England Journal of Medicine* 337, no. 8 (August 21, 1997): 563–566.

Katan, Martijn B., Peter L. Zock, and Ronald P. Mensink. "Dietary Oils, Serum Lipoproteins, and Coronary Heart Disease." *American Journal of Clinical Nutrition* 61, no. 6 (1995): 1368S–1373S.

Kato, Hiroo, Jeanne Tillotson, Milton Z. Nichaman, George G. Rhoads, and Howard B. Hamilton. "Epidemiologic Studies of Coronary Heart Disease and Stroke in Japanese Men Living in Japan, Hawaii and California." *American Journal of Epidemiology* 97, no. 6 (June 1973): 372–385.

Katritsis, Demosthenes G., and John P. A. Ioannidis. "Percutaneous Coronary Intervention Versus Conservative Therapy in Nonacute Coronary Artery Disease: A Meta-Analysis." *Circulation* 111, no. 22 (June 7, 2005): 2906–2912.

Katsouyanni, Klea, Eric B. Rimm, Charalambos Gnardellis, Dimitrio Trichopoulos, Evangelos Polychronopoulos, and Antonia Trichopoulou. "Reproducibility and Relative Validity of an Extensive Semi-Quantitative Food Frequency Questionnaire Using Dietary Records and Biochemical Markers among Greek Schoolteachers." *International Journal of Epidemiology* 26, no. 1, suppl. 1 (1997): S118–S127.

Kaunitz, Hans. "Importance of Lipids in Arteriosclerosis: An Outdated Theory," in Select Committee on Nutrition and Human Needs of the United States Senate, *Dietary Goals for the United States—Supplemental Views.* 42–54. Washington, DC: US Government Printing Office, 1977.

Kaunitz, Hans, and Ruth E. Johnson. "Exacerbation of the Heart and Liver Lesions in Rats by Feeding Various Mildly Oxidized Fats." *Lipids* 8, no. 6 (June 1973): 329–336.

Kelleher, Philip C., Stephen D. Phinney, Ethan A. H. Sims, et al. "Effects of Carbohydrate-Containing and Carbohydrate-Restricted Hypocaloric and Eucaloric Diets on Serum Concentrations of Retinol-Binding Protein, Thyroxine-Binding Prealbumin and Transferrin." *Metabolism* 32, no. 1 (January 1983): 95–101.

Key, Timothy J., Paul N. Appleby, Elizabeth A. Spencer, Ruth C. Travis, Andrew W. Roddam, and Naomi E. Allen. "Mortality in British Vegetarians: Results from the European Prospective Investigation into Cancer and Nutrition (EPIC-Oxford)." *American Journal of Clinical Nutrition* 89, no. 5 suppl. (May 2009): 1613S–1619S.

Keys, Ancel. "Human Atherosclerosis and the Diet." *Circulation* 5, no. 1 (1952): 115–118.

———. "Atherosclerosis: A Problem in Newer Public Health." *Journal of the Mount Sinai Hospital, New York* 20, no. 2 (July–August 1953): 118–139.

———. "The Diet and Development of Coronary Heart Disease." *Journal of Chronic Disease* 4, no. 4 (October 1956): 364–380.

———. "Diet and the Epidemiology of Coronary Heart Disease." *Journal of the American Medical Association* 164, no. 17 (August 24, 1957): 1912–1919.

———. "Epidemiologic Aspects of Coronary Artery Disease." *Journal of Chronic Diseases* 6, no. 5 (November 1957): 552–559.

———. "Arteriosclerotic Heart Disease in Roseto, Pennsylvania." *Journal of the American Medical Association* 195, no. 2 (January 10, 1966): 137–139.

———. "Sucrose in the Diet and Coronary Heart Disease." *Atherosclerosis* 14, no. 2 (September–October 1971): 193–202.

———. "Letter: Sucrose in the Diet and Coronary Heart Disease." *Atherosclerosis* 18, no. 2 (September–October 1973): 352.

———. "Letter to the Editors." *Atherosclerosis* 18, no. 2 (September–October 1973): 352.

———. "Coronary Heart Disease—The Global Picture." *Atherosclerosis* 22, no. 2 (September–October 1975): 149–192.

———. *Seven Countries: A Multivariate Analysis of Death and Coronary Heart Disease.* Cambridge, MA: Harvard University Press, 1980.

———. "From Naples to Seven Countries—A Sentimental Journey." In *Progress in Biochemical Parmacology* 19. Edited by R. J. Hegyeli, 1–30. Basel, Switzerland: Karger, 1983.

———. "Mediterranean Diet and Public Health." *American Journal of Clinical Nutrition* 61, no. 6 suppl. (June 1995): 1321S–1323S.

Keys, Ancel, ed. "Coronary Heart Disease in Seven Countries." *Circulation* 41 and 42, no. 1 suppl. 1, American Heart Association Monograph No. 29 (April 1970): 1–211.

Keys, Ancel, and Joseph T. Anderson. "The Relationship of the Diet to the Development of Atherosclerosis in Man." In *Symposium on Atherosclerosis*. Publication 338. Washington, DC: National Academy of Sciences–National Research Council, 1954, 181–196.

Keys, Ancel, Joseph T. Anderson, Flaminio Fidanza, Margaret Haney Keys, and Bengt Swahn. "Effects of Diet on Blood Lipids In Man, Particularly Cholesterol and Lipoproteins." *Clinical Chemistry* 1, no. 1 (February 1955): 34–52.

Keys, Ancel, Joseph T. Anderson, and Francisco Grande. "Fats and Disease." *Lancet* 272, no. 6796 (May 11, 1957): 992–993.

———. "Prediction of Serum Cholesterol Responses of Man to Changes in Fats in the Diet." *Lancet* 273, no. 7003 (November 16, 1957): 959–966.

———. "Serum Cholesterol in Man: Diet Fat and Intrinsic Responsiveness." *Circulation* 19, no. 2 (1959): 201–214.

Keys, Ancel, Christos Aravanis, and Helen Sdrin. "The Diets of Middle-aged Men in Two Rural Areas of Greece." *Voeding* 27, no. 11 (1966): 575–586.

Keys, Ancel, Flaminio Fidanza, Vicenzo Scardi, Gino Bergami, Margaret Haney Keys, and Ferruccio Di Lorenzo. "Studies on Serum Cholesterol and Other Characteristics of Clinically Healthy Men in Naples." *Archives of Internal Medicine* 93, no. 3 (March 1954): 328–336.

Keys, Ancel, and Francisco Grande. "Role of Dietary Fat in Human Nutrition: III. Diet and the Epidemiology of Coronary Heart Disease." *American Journal of Public Health and the Nation's Health* 47, no. 12 (December 1957): 1520–1530.

Keys, Ancel, Francisco Grande, and Joseph T. Anderson. "Bias and Misrepresentation Revisited: 'Perspective' on Saturated Fat." *The American Journal of Clinical Nutrition* 27, no. 2 (February 1974): 188–212.

Keys, Ancel, and Margaret Keys. *Eat Well and Stay Well.* New York: Doubleday, 1959.

———. *How to Eat Well and Stay Well the Mediterranean Way.* Garden City, NY: Doubleday, 1975.

Keys, Ancel, and Noboru Kimora. "Diets of Middle-Aged Farmers in Japan." *American Journal of Clinical Nutrition* 23, no. 2 (February 1970): 212–223.

Keys, Ancel, Alessandro Menotti, Christos Aravanis, et al. "The Seven Countries Study: 2,289 Deaths in 15 Years." *Preventive Medicine* 13, no. 2 (March 1984): 141–154.

Keys, Ancel, Alessandro Menotti, Mariti J. Karvonen, et al. "The Diet and 15-year Death Rate in the Seven Countries Study." *American Journal of Epidemiology* 124, no. 6 (December 1986): 903–915.

Keys, Ancel, Francisco Vivanco, J. L. Rodriguez Miñon, Margaret Haney Keys, and H. Castro Mendoza. "Studies on the Diet, Body Fatness and Serum Cholesterol in Madrid, Spain." *Metabolism Clinical and Experimental* 3, no. 3 (May 1954): 195–212.

Khosla, Pramod. "Palm Oil: A Nutritional Overview." *Journal of Agriculture and Food Industry* 17 (2000): 21–23.

Khosla, Pramod, and Kalyana Sundram, eds. "A Supplement on Palm Oil." *Journal of the American College of Nutrition* 29, no. 3 suppl. (June 2010): 237S–239S.

Kim, Song-Suk, Daniel D. Gallaher, and A. Saari Csallany. "Lipophilic Aldehydes and Related Carbonyl Compounds in Rat and Human Urine." *Lipids* 34, no. 5 (May 1999): 489–495.

Kimura, Noboru. "Changing Patterns of Coronary Heart Disease, Stroke, and Nutrient Intake in Japan." *Preventive Medicine* 12, no. 1 (January 1983): 222–227.

Kinsell, Lawrence W., J. Partridge, Lenore Boling, S. Margen, and G. Michaels. "Dietary Modification of Serum Cholesterol and Phospholipid Levels." *Journal of Clinical Endocrinology and Metabolism* 12, no. 7 (July 1952): 909–913.

Kinsella, John E., Geza Bruckner, J. Mai, and J. Shimp. "Metabolism of Trans Fatty Acids with Emphasis on the Effects of Trans, Trans-Octadecadienoate on Lipid Composition, Essential Fatty Acid, and Prostaglandins: An Overview." *American Journal of Clinical Nutrition* 34, no. 10 (October 1981): 2307–2318.

Knittle, J. L., and Edward H. Ahrens, Jr. "Carbohydrate Metabolism in Two Forms of Hyperglyceridemia." *Journal of Clinical Investigation* 43 (March 1964): 485–495.

Knopp, Robert H., Pathmaja Paramsothy, Barbara M. Retzlaff, et al. "Gender Differences in Lipoprotein Metabolism and Dietary Response: Basis in Hormonal Differences and Implications for Cardiovascular Disease." *Current Atherosclerosis Reports* 7, no. 6 (November 2005): 472–479.

———. "Sex Differences in Lipoprotein Metabolism and Dietary Response: Basis in Hormonal Differences and Implications for Cardiovascular Disease." *Current Cardiology Reports* 8, no. 6 (November 2006): 452–459.

Knopp, Robert H., Barbara Retzlaff, Carolyn Walden, Brian Fish, Brenda Buck, and Barbara McCann. "One-Year Effects of Increasingly Fat-Restricted, Carbohydrate-Enriched Diets on Lipoprotein Levels in Free-living Subjects." *Proceedings for the Society of Experimental Biology and Medicine* 225, no. 3 (December 2000): 191–199.

Koeth, Robert A., Zeneng Wang, Bruce S. Levison, et al. "Intestinal Microbiota Metabolism of L-Carnitine, a Nutrient in Red Meat, Promotes Atherosclerosis." *Nature Medicine* 19, no. 5 (May 2013): 576–585.

Kolata, Gina. "Heart Panel's Conclusions Questioned." *Science* 227, no. 4682 (January 4, 1985): 40–41.

———. "Culprit in Heart Disease Goes Beyond Meat's Fat." *New York Times*, April 8, 2013: A14.

———. "Eggs, Too, May Provoke Bacteria to Raise Heart Risk." *New York Times*, April 25, 2013: A14.

Koletzko, Berthold, Katharina Dokoupil, Susanne Reitmayr, Barbara Weimert-Harendza, and Erich Keller. "Dietary Fat Intakes of Infants and Primary School Children in Germany." *American Journal of Clinical Nutrition* 72, no. 5 suppl. (November 2000): 1329S–1398S.

Korányi, A. "Prophylaxis and Treatment of the Coronary Syndrome." *Therapia Hungarica* 12 (1963): 17.

Kozarevic, Djordje, D. L. McGee, N. Vojvodic, et al. "Serum Cholesterol and Mortality: The Yugoslavia Cardiovascular Disease Study." *American Journal of Epidemiology* 114, no. 1 (1981): 21–28.

Krauss, Ronald M. "Dietary and Genetic Probes of Atherogenic Dyslipidemia." *Arteriosclerosis, Thrombosis, and Vascular Biology* 25, no. 11 (November 2005): 2265–2272.

Krauss, Ronald M., Patricia J. Blanche, Robin S. Rawlings, Harriett S. Fernstrom, and Paul T. Williams. "Separate Effects of Reduced Carbohydrate Intake and Weight Loss on Atherogenic Dyslipidemia." *American Journal of Clinical Nutrition* 83, no. 5 (May 2006): 1025–1031.

Krauss, Ronald M., and Darlene M. Dreon. "Low-density-lipoprotein Subclasses and Response to a Low-fat Diet in Healthy Men." *American Journal of Clinical Nutrition* 62, no. 2 suppl. (August 1995): 478S–487S.

Krauss, Ronald M., Robert H. Eckel, Barbara Howard, et al. "AHA Dietary Guidelines Revision 2000: A Statement for Healthcare Professionals from the Nutrition Committee of the American Heart Association." *Circulation* 102, no. 18 (October 31, 2000): 2284–2299.

Krieger, James W., Harry S. Sitren, Michael J. Daniels, and Bobbi Langkamp-Henken. "Effects of Variation in Protein and Carbohydrate Intake on Body Mass and Composition During Energy Restriction: A Meta-Regression." *American Journal of Clinical Nutrition* 83, no. 2 (February 2006): 260–274.

Kris-Etherton, Penny M., Robert H. Eckel, Barbara V. Howard, Sachiko St. Jeor, and Terry L. Bazzarre. "Lyon Diet Heart Study Benefits of a Mediterranean-Style, National Cholesterol Education Program/American Heart Association Step I Dietary Pattern on Cardiovascular Disease." *Circulation* 103, no. 13 (April 3, 2001): 1823–1825.

Kris-Etherton, Penny M., and Robert J. Nicolosi. "Trans Fatty Acids and Coronary Heart Disease Risk." *American Journal of Clinical Nutrition* 62, no. 3 suppl. (1995): 655S–708S.

Kris-Etherton, Penny M., Denise Shaffer Taylor, Shaomei Ya-Poth, et al. "Polyunsaturated Fatty Acids in the Food Chain in the United States." *American Journal of Clinical Nutrition* 71, no. 1 suppl. (January 2000): 179S–188S.

Kristal, Alan R., Ulrike Peters, and John D. Potter. "Is It Time to Abandon the Food Frequency Questionnaire?" *Cancer Epidemiology, Biomarkers and Prevention* 14, no. 12 (December 2005): 2826–2828.

Kromhout, Daan, and Bennie Bloemberg. "Diet and Coronary Heart Disease in the Seven Countries Study." In *Prevention of Coronary Heart Disease: Diet, Lifestyle and Risk Factors in the Seven Countries Study*. Edited by Daan Kromhout, Alessandro Menotti, and Henry Blackburn. Dordrecht, The Netherlands: Kluwer Academic Publishers, 2002, 43–70.

Kromhout, Daan, Erik J. Giltay, and Johanna M. Geleijnse. "n-3 Fatty Acids and Cardiovascular Events after Myocardial Infarction." *New England Journal of Medicine* 363, no. 21 (November 18, 2010): 2015–2026.

Kromhout, Daan, Ancel Keys, Christ Aravanis, et al. "Food Consumption Patterns in the 1960s in Seven Countries." *American Journal of Clinical Nutrition* 49, no. 5 (May 1989): 889–894.

Kromhout, Daan, Alessandro Menotti, and Henry W. Blackburn, eds. *The Seven Countries Study: A Scientific Adventure in Cardiovascular Disease Epidemiology*. Bilthoven, The Netherlands, privately published, 1993.

Kronmal, Richard A. "Commentary on the Published Results of the Lipid Research Clinics Coronary Primary Prevention Trial." *Journal of the American Medical Association* 253, no. 14 (April 12, 1985): 2091–2093.

Krumholz, Harlan M. "Editorial: Target Cardiovascular Risk Rather than Cholesterol Concentration." *British Medical Journal* 347 (2013). doi:10.1136/bmj.f7110.

Kummerow, Fred A., T. Mizuguchi, T. Arima, B. H. S. Cho, W. J. Huang, and R. Tracey. "The Influence of Three Sources of Dietary Fats and Cholesterol on Lipid Composition of Swine Serum Lipids and Aorta Tissue." *Artery* 4 (1978): 360–384.

Kummerow, Fred A., Sherry Q. Zhou, and Mohamedain M. Mahfouz. "Effects of Trans Fatty Acids on Calcium Influx into Human Arterial Endothelial Cells." *American Journal of Clinical Nutrition* 70, no. 5 (November 1999): 832–838.

Kuo, Peter T., Louise Feng, Norman N. Cohen, William T. Fitts, and Leonard D. Miller. "Dietary Carbohydrates in Hyperlipemia (Hyperglyceridemia); Hepatic and Adipose Tissue Lipogenic Activities." *American Journal of Clinical Nutrition* 20, no. 2 (February 1967): 116–125.

Kurlansky, Mark. "Essential Oil." *Bon Appétit*. September 30, 2008. http://www.bonappetit.com/trends/article/essential-oil.

Kushi, Lawrence H., and Edward Giovannucci. "Dietary Fat and Cancer." *American Journal of Medicine* 113, no. 9, suppl. B (December 30, 2002): 63S–70S.

Kushi, Lawrence H., Elizabeth B. Lenart, and Walter C. Willett. "Health Implications of Mediterranean Diets in Light of Contemporary Knowledge. 1. Plant Foods and Dairy Products." *American Journal of Clinical Nutrition* 61, no. 6 suppl. (June 1995): 1407S–1415S.

———. "Health Implications of Mediterranean Diets in Light of Contemporary Knowledge. 2. Meat, Wine, Fats and Oils." *American Journal of Clinical Nutrition* 61, no. 6 suppl. (June 1995): 1416S–1427S.

L'Abbé, M. R., Steen Stender, C. M. Skeaff, B. Ghafoorunissa, and M. Tavella. "Approaches to Removing *Trans* Fats from the Food Supply in Industrialized and Developing Countries." *European Journal of Clinical Nutrition* 63, suppl. (2009): S50–S67.

Lamarche, Benoit, A. Tchernof, Sital Moorjani, et al. "Small, Dense Low-Density Lipoprotein Particles as a Predictor of the Risk of Ischemic Heart Disease in Men: Prospective Results From the Quebec Cardiovascular Study." *Circulation* 95, no. 1 (January 7, 1997): 69–75.

Lands, William E. M., M. Blank, L. J. Nutter, and O. Privett. "A Comparison of Acyltransferase Activities in Vitro with the Distribution of Fatty Acids in Lecithins and Triglycerides in Vivo." *Lipids* 1, no. 3 (May 1966): 224–229.

Lapinleimu, Helena, Jorma Vilkari, Eero Jokinen, et al. "Prospective Randomised Trial in 1062 Infants of Diet Low in Saturated Fat and Cholesterol." *Lancet* 345, no. 8948 (February 25, 1995): 471–476.

LaRosa, John C., Scott M. Grundy, David D. Waters, et al. "Intensive Lipid Lowering with Atorvastatin in Patients with Stable Coronary Disease." *New England Journal of Medicine* 352, no. 14 (April 7, 2005): 1425–1435.

Laskarzewski, Peter, John A. Morrison, I. deGroot, et al. "Lipid and Lipoprotein Tracking in 108 Children Over a Four-Year Period." *Pediatrics* 64, no. 5 (November 1979): 584–591.

Lawson, Larry D., and Fred A. Kummerow. "B-Oxidation of the Coenzyme A Esters of Vaccenic, Elaidic, and Petroselaidic Acids by Rat Heart Mitochondria." *Lipids* 14, no. 5 (May 1979): 501–503.

Lee, Patrick Y., Karen P. Alexander, Bradley G. Hammill, Sara K. Pasquali, and Eric D. Peterson. "Representation of Elderly Persons and Women in Published Randomized Trials of Acute Coronary Syndromes." *Journal of the American Medical Association* 286, no. 6 (August 8, 2001): 708–713.

Lehzen, George, and Karl Knauss. "Über Xanthoma Multiplex Planum, Tuberosum, Mollusciformis." *Archiv A, Pathological Anatomy and Histology* 116 (1889): 85–104.

Leren, Paul. "The Effect of Plasma Cholesterol Lowering Diet in Male Survivors of Myocardial Infarction: A Controlled Clinical Trial." *Acta Medica Scandinavica Supplementum* 466 (1966): 1–92.

Lesser, Lenard I., Cara B. Ebbeling, Merrill Goozner, David Wypij, and David S. Ludwig. "Relationship between Funding Source and Conclusion among Nutrition-Related Scientific Articles." *PLoS Medicine* 4, no. 1 (January 2007): 41–46.

Levenstein, Harvey. *Paradox of Plenty: A Social History of Eating in Modern America*. Berkeley, CA: University of California Press, 2003.

Levine, Deborah. "Corpulence and Correspondence: President William H. Taft and the Medical Management of Obesity." *Annals of Internal Medicine* 159, no. 8 (2013): 565–570.

Levine, Janet M. "Hearts and Minds: The Politics of Diet and Heart Disease." In *Consuming Fears: The Politics of Product Risks*. Edited by Henry M. Sapolsky. New York: Basic Books, 1986, 40–79.

Li, Zhengling, James D. Otvos, Stefania Lamon-Fava, et al. "Men and Women Differ in Lipoprotein Response to Dietary Saturated Fat and Cholesterol Restriction." *Journal of Nutrition* 133, no. 11 (November 2003): 3428–3433.

List, Gary R., and M. A. Jackson. "Giants of the Past: The Battle Over Hydrogenation (1903–1920)." *Inform* 18, no. 6 (June 2007): 403–405.

Lichtenstein, Alice H., Lawrence J. Appel, Michael Brands, et al. "Diet and Lifestyle Recommendations, Revision 2006: A Scientific Statement from the American Heart Association Nutrition Committee." *Circulation* 114, no. 1 (July 4, 2006): 82–96.

Lichtenstein, Alice H., Lynne M. Ausman, Wanda Carrasco, Jennifer L. Jenner, Jose M. Ordovas, and Ernst J. Schaefer. "Hydrogenation Impairs the Hypolipidemic Effect of Corn Oil in Humans. Hydrogenation, Trans Fatty Acids, and Plasma Lipids." *Arteriosclerosis, Thrombosis, and Vascular Biology* 13, no. 2 (February 1993): 154–161.

Lichtenstein, Alice H., and Linda Van Horn. "Very Low Fat Diets." *Circulation* 98, no. 9 (1998): 935–939.

Lieb, Clarence W. "The Effects on Human Beings of a Twelve Months' Exclusive Meat Diet: Based on Intensive Clinical and Laboratory Studies on Two Arctic Explorers Living Under Average Conditions in a New York Climate." *Journal of the American Medical Association* 93, no. 1 (July 6, 1929): 20–22.

Lieb, Clarence W., and Edward Tolstoi. "Effect of an Exclusive Meat Diet on Chemical Constituents of the Blood." *Proceedings of the Society for Experimental Biology and Medicine* 26, no. 4 (January 1929): 324–325.

Liebman, Bonnie. "Just the Mediterranean Diet Facts." *Nutrition Action Health Letter* 21, no. 10 (1994).

Life Sciences Research Center, Federation of American Societies for Experimental Biology. Prepared for the Bureau of Foods, Food and Drug Administration. *Evaluation of the Health Aspects of Hydrogenated Soybean Oil as a Food Ingredient.* Bethesda, MD: Federation of American Societies for Experimental Biology, 1976.

Lifshitz, Fima, and Nancy Moses. "Growth Failure. A Complication of Dietary Treatment of Hypercholesterolemia." *American Journal of Diseases of Children* 143, no. 5 (May 1989): 537–542.

Lionis, Christos D., Antonis D. Koutis, Nikos Antonakis, Åke Isacsson, Lars H. Lindholm, and Michael Fioretos. "Mortality Rates in a Cardiovascular 'Low -Risk' Population in Rural Crete." *Family Practice* 10, no. 3 (September 1993): 300–304.

Lloyd-Jones, Donald, R. J. Adams, T. M. Brown, et al. "Heart Disease and Stroke Statistics—2010 Update: A Report from the American Heart Association." *Circulation* 121, no. 7 (February 23, 2010): 46–215.

Lloyd-Jones, Donald, Robert Adams, Mercedes Carnethon, et al. "Heart Disease and Stroke Statistics—2009 Update: A Report from the American Heart Association Statistics Committee and Stroke Statistics Subcommittee." *Circulation* 119, no. 3 (2009): 480–486.

De Lorgeril, Michel, Serge Renaud, P. Salen, et al. "Mediterranean Alpha-Linolenic Acid-Rich Diet in Secondary Prevention of Coronary Heart Disease." *Lancet* 343, no. 8911 (June 11, 1994): 1454–1459.

De Lorgeril, Michael, P. Salen, E. Caillat-Vallet, M. T. Hanauer, J. C. Barthelemy, and N. Mamelle. "Control of Bias in Dietary Trial to Prevent Coronary Recurrences: The Lyon Diet Heart Study." *European Journal of Clinical Nutrition* 51, no. 2 (February 1997): 116–122.

Lowenstein, Frank W. "Blood-pressure in Relation to Age and Sex in the Tropics and Subtropics: A Review of the Literature and an Investigation in Two Tribes of Brazil Indians." *Lancet* 277, no. 7173 (February 18, 1961): 389–392.

———. "Epidemiologic Investigations in Relation to Diet in Groups Who Show Little Atherosclerosis and Are Almost Free of Coronary Ischemic Heart Disease." *American Journal of Clinical Nutrition* 15, no. 3 (1964): 175–186.

LRC Study Group. "The Lipid Research Clinics Coronary Primary Prevention Trial Results. I: Reduction in Incidence of Coronary Heart Disease." *Journal of the American Medical Association* 251, no. 3 (January 20, 1984): 351–364.

———. "The Lipid Research Clinics Coronary Primary Prevention Trial Results. II: The Relationship of Reduction in Incidence of Coronary Heart Disease to Cholesterol Lowering." *Journal of the American Medical Association* 251, no. 3 (January 20, 1984): 365–374.

Lund, E., and J. K. Borgan. "Cancer Mortality Among Cooks." *Tidsskrift for Den Norske Legeforening* 107 (1987): 2635–2637.

Lundberg, George D. "MRFIT and the Goals of the Journal." *Journal of the American Medical Association* 248, no. 12 (September 24, 1982): 1501.

Mabrouk, Ahmed Fahmy, and J. B. Brown. "The Trans Fatty Acids of Margarines and Shortenings." *Journal of the American Oil Chemists' Society* 33, no. 3 (March 1956): 98–102.

Mahabir, S., D. J. Baer, C. Giffen, et al. "Calorie Intake Misreporting by Diet Record and Food Frequency Questionnaire Compared to Doubly Labeled Water Among Postmenopausal Women." *European Journal of Clinical Nutrition* 60, no. 4 (April 2005): 561–565.

Mahfouz, Mohamedain M., T. L. Smith, and Fred A. Kummerow. "Effect of Dietary Fats on Desaturase Activities and the Biosynthesis of Fatty Acids in Rat-Liver Microsomes." *Lipids* 19, no. 3 (March 1984): 214–222.

Malhotra, S. L. "Geographical Aspects of Acute Myocardial Infarction in India with Special Reference to Patterns of Diet and Eating." *British Heart Journal* 29, no. 3 (May 1967): 337–344.

———. "Epidemiology of Ischaemic Heart Disease in Southern India with Special Reference to Causation." *British Heart Journal* 29, no. 6 (November 1967): 895–905.

———. "Dietary Factors and Ischemic Heart Disease." *American Journal of Clinical Nutrition* 24, no. 10 (1971): 1195–1198.

Malmros, Haqvin. "The Relation of Nutrition to Health: A Statistical Study of the Effect of the War-Time on Arteriosclerosis Cardiosclerosis, Tuberculosis and Diabetes." *Acta Medica Scandinavica Supplementum* 246 (1950): 137–153.

Mann, George V. "Epidemiology of Coronary Heart Disease." *American Journal of Medicine* 23, no. 3 (1957): 463–480.

———. "Diet and Coronary Heart Disease." *Archives of Internal Medicine* 104 (1959): 921–929.

———. "Diet-Heart: End of an Era." *New England Journal of Medicine* 297, no. 12 (September 22, 1977): 644–650.

———. "Coronary Heart Disease—the Doctor's Dilemma." *American Heart Journal* 96, no. 5 (November 1978): 569–571.

———. "A Short History of the Diet/Heart Hypothesis." In *Coronary Heart Disease: The Dietary Sense and Nonsense. An Evaluation by Scientists.* Edited by George V. Mann for the Veritas Society. London: Janus, 1993, 1–17.

Mann, George V., Georgiana Pearson, Tavia Gordon, Thomas R. Dawber, Lorna Lyell, and Dewey Shurtleff. "Diet and Cardiovascular Disease in the Framingham Study I. Measurement of Dietary Intake." *American Journal of Clinical Nutrition* 11, no. 3 (September 1962): 200–225.

Mann, George V., R. D. Shaffer, R. S. Anderson, et al. "Cardiovascular Disease in the Masai." *Journal of Atherosclerosis Research* 4, no. 4 (1964): 289–312.

Mann, George V., Anne Spoerry, Margarete Gary, and Debra Jarashow. "Atherosclerosis in the Masai." *American Journal of Epidemiology* 95, no. 1 (1972): 26–37.

Mann, George V., and Fredrick J. Stare. "Nutrition and Atherosclerosis." In *Symposium on Atherosclerosis*. Publication 338. Washington, DC: National Academy of Sciences–National Research Council, 1954, 169–180.

Marcy, Randolph B. *The Prairie Traveler: A Handbook for Overland Expeditions*. London: Trubner, 1863.

Marmot, M. G., Sherman L. Syme, Abraham Kagan, Hiroo Kato, J. B. Cohen, and J. Belsky. "Epidemiologic Studies of Coronary Heart Disease and Stroke in Japanese Men Living in Japan, Hawaii and California: Prevalence of Coronary and Hypertensive Heart Disease and Associated Risk Factors." *American Journal of Epidemiology* 102, no. 6 (December 1975): 514–525.

Marshall, Joseph M. III. *The Day the World Ended at Little Bighorn: A Lakota History*. New York: Penguin Books, 2006.

Massiello, F. J. "Changing Trends in Consumer Margarines." *Journal of the American Oil Chemists' Society* 55, no. 2 (February 1978): 262–265.

Masterjohn, Chris. "The China Study by Colin T. Campbell." *Wise Traditions in Food, Farming, and the Healing Arts* 6, no. 1 (Spring 2005): 41–45.

————. "Does Carnitine from Red Meat Contribute to Heart Disease Through Intestinal Bacterial Metabolism to TMAO?" *Mother Nature Obeyed* (blog). April 10, 2013.

Mattson, Fred H. and Scott M. Grundy. "Comparison of Effects of Dietary Saturated, Unsaturated, and Polyunsaturated Fatty Acids on Plasma Lipids and Lipoproteins in Man." *Journal of Lipid Research* 26, no. 2 (February 1985): 194–202.

Mauer, Alvin M. "Should There Be Intervention to Alter Serum Lipids in Children?" *Annual Review of Nutrition* 11 (July 1991): 375–391.

Mazhar, D., and J. Waxman. "Dietary Fat and Breast Cancer." *Quarterly Journal of Medicine* 99, no. 7 (2006): 469–473.

McCarrison, Robert. *Nutrition and National Health: The Cantor Lectures*. London: Faber and Faber Limited, 1936.

McClellan, Walter S., Virgil R. Rupp, and Vincent Toscani. "Prolonged Meat Diets with a Study of the Metabolism of Nitrogen, Calcium, and Phosporus." *Journal of Biological Chemistry* 87, no. 3 (July 1930): 669–680.

McCollum, Elmer Verner. *The Newer Knowledge of Nutrition*. New York: MacMillan, 1921.

McConnell, Kenneth P. and Robert Gordon Sinclair. "Passage of Elaidic Acid Through the Placenta and Also into the Milk of the Rat." *Journal of Biological Chemistry* 118, no. 1 (1937): 123–129.

McGill, Henry C., C. Alex McMahan, Edward E. Herderick, Gray T. Malcom, Richard E. Tracy, and Jack P. Strong. "Origin of Atherosclerosis in Childhood and Adolescence." *American Journal of Clinical Nutrition* 72, no. 5 suppl. (November 2000): 1307S–1315S.

McMichael, John. "Prevention of Coronary Heart-Disease." *Lancet* 308, no. 7985 (September 11, 1976): 569.

McOsker, Don E., Fred H. Mattson, H. Bruce Sweringen, and Albert M. Kligman. "The Influence of Partially Hydrogenated Dietary Fats on Serum Cholesterol Levels." *Journal of the American Medical Association* 180, no. 5 (May 5, 1962): 380–385.

Meadows, Bob, M. Morehouse, and M. Simmons. "The Problem with Low-Fat Diets." *People*, February 27, 2006, 89–90.

Meckling, Kelly A., Caitriona O'Sullivan, and Dayna Saari. "Comparison of a Low-Fat Diet to a Low-Carbohydrate Diet on Weight Loss, Body Composition, and Risk Factors for Diabetes and Cardiovascular Disease in Free-Living, Overweight Men and Women." *Journal of Clinical Endocrinology & Metabolism* 89, no. 6 (June 2004): 2717–2723.

Medalie, Jack H., Harold A. Kahn, Henry N. Neufeld, Egon Riss, and Uri Goldbourt. "Five-Year Myocardial Infarction Incidence—II. Association of Single Variables to Age and Birthplace." *Journal of Chronic Diseases* 26, no. 6 (1973): 329–349.

Medical News. "Questions Surround Treatment of Children with High Cholesterol." *Journal of American Medical Association* 214, no. 10 (1970): 1783–1785.

Menotti, Alessandro, Daan Kromhout, Henry Blackburn, Flaminio Fidanza, Ratko Buzina, and Aulikki Nissinen. "Food Intake Patterns and 25-Year Mortality from Coronary Heart Disease: Cross-Cultural Correlations in the Seven Countries Study." *European Journal of Epidemiology* 15, no. 6 (1999): 507–515.

Mensink, Ronald P., and Martijn B. Katan. "Effect of Dietary Trans Fatty Acids on High-Density and Low-Density Lipoprotein Cholesterol Levels in Healthy Subjects." *New England Journal of Medicine* 323, no. 7 (August 16, 1990): 439–445.

Meyer, W. H. "Dietary Fat and Cancer Trends—Further Comments." *Federation Proceedings* 38, no. 11 (November 1979): 2436–2437.

Michaels, Leon. "Ætiology of Coronary Artery Disease: An Historical Approach." *British Heart Journal* 28, no. 2 (March 1966): 258–264.

———. *The Eighteenth-Century Origins of Angina Pectoris: Predisposing Causes, Recognition and Aftermath,* Medical History, suppl. 21. London: The Wellcome Trust Centre for the History of Medicine at UCL, 2001.

Michels, Karin, and Frank Sacks. "Trans Fatty Acids in European Margarines." *New England Journal of Medicine* 332, no. 8 (February 23, 1995): 541–542.

Miettinen, Matti, Martti Karvonen, Osmo Turpeinen, Reino Elosuo, and Erkki Paavilainen. "Effect of Cholesterol-Lowering Diet on Mortality from Coronary Heart-Disease and Other Causes: A Twelve-Year Clinical Trial in Men and Women." *Lancet* 300, no. 7782 (October 1972): 835–838.

———. "Effect of Diet on Coronary-Heart-Disease Mortality." *Lancet* 302, no. 7840 (1973): 1266–1267.

Miller, Seth R., Paul I. Tartter, Angelos E. Papatestas, Gary Slater, and Arthur H. Aufses. "Serum Cholesterol and Human Colon Cancer." *Journal of the National Cancer Institute* 67, no. 2 (August 1981): 297–300.

Mills, Barbara K. "The Nutritionist Who Prepared the Pro-Cholesterol Report Defends It Against Critics." *People*, June 16, 1980.

Mills, Paul K., W. Lawrence Beeson, Roland L. Phillips, and Gary E. Fraser. "Cancer Incidence Among California Seventh-Day Adventists, 1976–1982." *American Journal of Clinical Nutrition* 59, no. 5 suppl. (May 1994): 1136S–1142S.

Montanari, Massimo. *The Culture of Food.* Translated by Carl Ipsen. Cambridge, MA: Wiley-Blackwell, 1996.

Moore, Thomas J. "The Cholesterol Myth." *The Atlantic* 264, no. 3 (September 1989): 37.

———. *Heart Failure: A Critical Inquiry into American Medicine and the Revolution in Heart Care.* New York: Simon and Schuster, 1989.

Moore, William W. *Fighting for Life: A History of the American Heart Association 1911–1975.* Dallas: American Heart Association, 1983.

Moreno, Luis A., Antonio Sarría, Aurora Lázaro, and Manuel Bueno. "Dietary Fat Intake and Body Mass Index in Spanish Children." *American Journal of Clinical Nutrition* 72, no. 5 suppl. (November 2000): 1399S–1403S.

Morgan, Jane B., A. C. Kimber, A. M. Redfern, and B. J. Stordy. "Healthy Eating for Infants—Mothers' Attitudes." *Acta Paediatrica* 84, no. 5 (May 1995): 512–515.

Morrell, Sally Fallon and Mary Enig. "Guts and Grease: The Diet of Native Americans," *Wise Traditions in Food, Farming and the Healing Arts* 2, no. 1 (Spring 2001): 40–47.

Mozaffarian, Dariush. "The Great Fat Debate: Taking the Focus Off of Saturated Fat." *Journal of the American Dietetic Association* 111, no. 5 (May 2011): 665–666.

Mozaffarian, Dariush, Martijn B. Katan, Alberto Ascherio, Meir J. Stampfer, and Walter C. Willett. "Trans Fatty Acids and Cardiovascular Disease." *New England Journal of Medicine* 354, no. 15 (April 13, 2006): 1601–1613.

Mulcahy, Risteard, Noel Hickey, Ian Graham, and Gilbert McKenzie. "Factors Influencing Long-Term Prognosis in Male Patients Surviving a First Coronary Attack." *British Heart Journal* 37, no. 2 (February 1975): 158–165.

Muldoon, Matthew F., Stephen B. Manuck, and Karen A. Matthews. "Lowering Cholesterol Concentrations and Mortality: A Quantitative Review of Primary Prevention Trials." *British Medical Journal* 301, no. 6747 (August 11, 1990): 309–314.

Multiple Risk Factor Intervention Trial Research Group. "Multiple Risk Factor Intervention Trial: Risk Factor Changes and Mortality Results." *Journal of American Medicine* 248, no. 12 (September 24, 1982): 1465–1477.

Murata, Mitsunori. "Secular Trends in Growth and Changes in Eating Patterns of Japanese Children." *American Journal of Clinical Nutrition* 72, no. 5 suppl. (November 2000): 1379S–1383S.

Murphy, Suzanne P., and Rachel K. Johnson. "The Scientific Basis of Recent US Guidance on Sugars Intake," *American Journal of Clinical Nutrition* 78, no. 4 (2003): 827S–833S.

Napoli, Claudio, Christopher K. Glass, Joseph L. Witztum, Reena Deutsch, Francesco P. D'Armiento, and Wulf Palinski. "Influence of Maternal Hypercholesterolaemia During Pregnancy on Progression of Early Atherosclerotic Lesions in Childhood: Fat of Early Lesions in Children (FELIC) Study." *Lancet* 354, no. 9186 (October 9, 1999): 1234–1241.

Naska, Androniki, Eleni Oikonomou, Antonia Trichopoulou, Theodora Psaltopoulou, and Dimitrios Trichopoulos. "Siesta in Healthy Adults and Coronary Mortality in the General Population." *Archives of Internal Medicine* 167, no. 3 (February 12, 2007): 296–301.

———. Author reply to "Siesta, All-Cause Mortality, and Cardiovascular Mortality: Is There a "Siesta" at Adjudicating Cardiovascular Mortality?" by Sripal Bangalore, Sabrina Sawhney, and Franz H. Messerli. *Archives of Internal Medicine* 167, no. 19 (October 22, 2007): 2143–2144.

National Cholesterol Education Program. *Third Report of the National Cholesterol Education Program (NCEP). Expert Panel on Detection, Evaluation, and Treatment of High Blood Cholesterol in Adults: (Adult Treatment Panel III) Final Report.* NIH Publication No. 02-5215. Washington, DC: NIH, 2002.

National Diet-Heart Study Research Group. "The National Diet Heart Study Final Report." *American Heart Association Monograph* 18 in *Circulation* 37 and 38, suppl. 1 (March 1968): I-ix-I-428.

National Institutes of Health. "Lowering Blood Cholesterol to Prevent Heart Disease." *NIH Consensus Statement* 5, no. 7 (December 10–12, 1984): 1–11.

National Research Council, Division of Medical Sciences. *Symposium on Atherosclerosis.* Publication 338. Washington, DC: National Academy of Sciences–National Research Council, March, 1954.

National Toxicology Program, US Public Health Service, US Department of Health and Human Services. "Report on Carcinogens: 12th Edition." Washington, DC: US Government Printing Office, 2011.

Negre-Salvayre, Anne, Nathalie Auge, Victoria Ayala, et al. "Pathological Aspects of Lipid Peroxidation." *Free Radical Research* 44, no. 10 (October 2010): 1125–1171.

Ness, Andy R., J. Hughes, P. C. Elwood, E. Whitley, G. D. Smith, and M. L. Burr. "The Long-Term Effect of Dietary Advice in Men with Coronary Disease: Follow-Up of the Diet and Reinfarction Trial (DART)." *European Journal of Clinical Nutrition* 56, no. 6 (June 2002): 512–518.

Nestel, Paul J., and Andrea Poyser. "Changes in Cholesterol Synthesis and Excretion When Cholesterol Intake Is Increased." *Metabolism* 25, no. 12 (December 1976): 1591–1599.

Nestle, Marion. "Mediterranean Diets: Historical and Research Overview." *American Journal of Clinical Nutrition* 61, no. 6 suppl. (June 1995): 1313S–1320S.

———. "The Mediterranean (Diet and Disease Prevention)." In *Cambridge World History of Food 2.* Edited by Kenneth Kiple and Kriemhild Coneè Ornelas. Cambridge, England: Cambridge University Press, 2000, 1193–1203.

———. *Food Politics.* Berkeley, CA: University of California Press, 2002.

Nestle, Marion, ed. "Mediterranean Diets." *American Journal of Clinical Nutrition* 61, no. 6 suppl. (1995): ix–1427S.

Nicklas, Theresa A., Larry S. Webber, MaryLynn Koschak, and Gerald S. Berenson. "Nutrient Adequacy of Low Fat Intakes for Children: The Bogalusa Heart Study." *Pediatrics* 89, no. 2 (February 1, 1992): 221–228.

Niinikoski, Harri, Hanna Lagström, Eero Jokinen, et al. "Impact of Repeated Dietary Counseling Between Infancy and 14 Years of Age on Dietary Intakes and Serum Lipids and Lipoproteins: The STRIP Study." *Circulation* 116, no. 9 (August 13, 2007): 1032–1040.

Niinikoski, Harri, Jorma Viikari, Tapani Rönnemaa, et al. "Regulation of Growth of 7- to 36-Month-Old Children by Energy and Fat Intake in the Prospective, Randomized STRIP Baby Trial." *Pediatrics* 100, no. 5 (November 1997): 810–816.

Noakes, Tim D. "The Women's Health Initiative Randomized Controlled Dietary Modification Trial: An Inconvenient Finding and the Diet-Heart Hypothesis." *South African Medical Journal* 103, no. 11 (September 30, 2013): 824–825.

Nordmann, Alain J., Katja Suter-Zimmermann, Heiner C. Bucher, et al. "Meta-Analysis Comparing Mediterranean to Low-Fat Diets for Modification of Cardiovascular Risk Factors." *American Journal of Medicine* 124, no. 9 (September 2011): 841–851.

Nydegger, Uris E., and René E. Butler. "Serum Lipoprotein Levels in Patients with Cancer." *Cancer Research* 32, no. 8 (August 1972): 1756–1760.

Obarzanek, Eva, Sally A. Hunsberger, Linda Van Horn, et al. "Safety of a Fat-Reduced Diet: The Dietary Intervention Study in Children (DISC)." *Pediatrics* 100, no. 1 (July 1997): 51–59.

Obarzanek, Eva, Frank M. Sacks, William M. Vollmer, et al. "Effects on Blood Lipids of a Blood Pressure-Lowering Diet: The Dietary Approaches to Stop Hypertension (DASH) Trial." *American Journal of Clinical Nutrition* 74, no. 1 (2001): 80–89.

O'Brien, Patrick. "Dietary Shifts and Implications for US Agriculture." *American Journal of Clinical Nutrition* 61, no. 6 suppl. (1995): 1390S–1396S.

Office of the Surgeon General, US Public Health Service, US Department of Health and Human Services. "Healthy People: The Surgeon General's Report on Health Promotion and Disease Prevention." Docket number 79-55071, Washington DC: US Government Printing Office, 1979.

Ohfuji, Takehi Ko, and Takashi Kaneda. "Characterization of Toxic Components in Thermally Oxidized Oil." *Lipids* 8 (1973): 353–359.

Oliver, Michael Francis. "Ischaemic Heart Disease: A Secondary Prevention Trial Using Clofibrate." *Pharmacological Control of Lipid Metabolism* 26 (1972): 255–259.

———. "Dietary Cholesterol, Plasma Cholesterol and Coronary Heart Disease." *British Heart Journal* 38, no. 3 (March 1976): 214–218.

———. "It Is More Important to Increase the Intake of Unsaturated Fats than to Decrease the Intake of Saturated Fats: Evidence from Clinical Trials Relating to Ischemic Heart Disease." *American Journal of Clinical Nutrition* 66, no. 4 suppl. (October 1997): 980S–986S.

Opie, Lionel H. "Letter to the Editor: Mediterranean Diet for the Primary Prevention of Heart Disease." *New England Journal of Medicine* 369, no. 7 (August 15, 2013): 672–673.

Orchard, Trevor J., Richard P. Donahue, Lewis H. Kuller, Patrick N. Hodge, and Allan L. Drash. "Cholesterol Screening in Childhood: Does It Predict Adult Hypercholesterolemia? The Beaver County Experience." *Journal of Pediatrics* 103, no. 5 (November 1983): 687–691.

Ornish, Dean. "Avoiding Revascularization with Lifestyle Changes: The Multicenter Lifestyle Demonstration Project." *American Journal of Cardiology* 82, no. 10B (November 26, 1998): 72–76.

Ornish, Dean, Shirley E. Brown, J. H. Billings, et al. "Can Lifestyle Changes Reverse Coronary Heart Disease? The Lifestyle Heart Trial." *Lancet* 336, no. 8708 (July 21, 1990): 129–133.

Ornish, Dean, Larry W. Scherwitz, James H. Billings, et al. "Intensive Lifestyle Changes for Reversal of Coronary Heart Disease." *Journal of the American Medical Association* 280, no. 23 (December 16, 1998): 2001–2007.

Orr, John B., and John L. Gilks. *Studies of Nutrition: The Physique and Health of Two African Tribes.* Medical Research Council. Special Report Series. No. 155. London: Stationery Office, 1931.

Osler, William. *The Principles and Practice of Medicine.* 1892. Reprint, RareBooksClub.com, 2012.

Ozonoff, David. "The Political Economy of Cancer Research." *Science and Nature* 2 (1979): 14–16.

Page, Irvine H., Edgar V. Allen, Francis L. Chamberlain, Ancel Keys, Jeremiah Stamler, and Fredrick J. Stare. "Dietary Fat and Its Relation to Heart Attacks and Strokes." *Circulation* 23, no. 1 (1961): 133–136.

Page, Irvine H., Fredrick J. Stare, A. C. Corcoran, Herbert Pollack, and Charles F. Wilkinson. "Atherosclerosis and the Fat Content of the Diet." *Circulation* 16, no. 2 (August 1957): 163–178.

Pagoto, Sherry L., and Bradley M. Appelhans. "A Call for an End to the Diet Debates." *Journal of the American Medical Association* 310, no. 7 (2013): 687–688.

Palmieri, Luigi, Kathleen Bennett, Simona Giampaoli, and Simon Capewell. "Explaining the Decrease in Coronary Heart Disease Mortality in Italy between 1980 and 2000." *American Journal of Public Health* 100, no. 4 (April 2010): 684–692.

Pan, An, Qi Sun, Adam M. Bernstein, et al. "Red Meat Consumption and Mortality: Results from 2 Prospective Cohort Studies." *Archives of Internal Medicine* 172, no. 7 (April 9, 2012): 555–563.

Park, Youngmee K., and Elizabeth A. Yetley. "Trench Changes in Use and Current Intakes of Tropical Oils in the United States." *American Journal of Clinical Nutrition* 51, no. 5 (1990): 738–748.

Patek, Arthur J., Forrest E. Kendall, Nancy M. deFritsch, and Robert L. Hirsch. "Cirrhosis-Enhancing Effect of Corn Oil." *Archives of Pathology* 82, no. 6 (December 1966): 596–601.

Patel, Sanjay R. "Is Siesta More Beneficial than Nocturnal Sleep?" *Archives of Internal Medicine* 167, no. 19 (October 22, 2007): 2143–2144.

Pearce, Morton Lee, and Seymour Dayton. "Incidence of Cancer in Men on a Diet High in Polyunsaturated Fat." *Lancet* 297, no. 7697 (March 6, 1971): 464–467.

Pennington, Alfred W. "Obesity in Industry: The Problem and Its Solution." *Industrial Medicine & Surgery* 18, no. 6 (June 1949): 259.

———. "Obesity." *Medical Times* 80, no. 7 (July 1952): 389–398.

———. "An Alternate Approach to the Problem of Obesity." *American Journal of Clinical Nutrition* 1, no. 2 (1953): 100–106.

———. "A Reorientation on Obesity." *New England Journal of Medicine* 248, no. 23 (June 4, 1953): 959–964.

———. "Treatment of Obesity with Calorically Unrestricted Diets." *Journal of Clinical Nutrition* 1, no. 5 (July–August 1953): 343–348.

———. "Obesity: Overnutrition or Disease of Metabolism?" *American Journal of Digestive Diseases* 20, no. 9 (September 1953): 268–274.

———. "Treatment of Obesity: Developments of the Past 150 Years." *American Journal of Digestive Diseases* 21, no. 3 (March 1954): 65–69.

Pernetti, Mimma, Kees van Malssen, Daniel Kalnin, and Eckhard Flöter. "Structuring Edible Oil with Lecithin and Sorbitan Tri-Stearate." *Food Hydrocolloids* 21, nos. 5–6 (July–August 2007): 855–861.

Phillips, Roland L., Frank R. Lemon, W. Lawrence Beeson, and Jan W. Kuzma. "Coronary Heart Disease Mortality Among Seventh-Day Adventists with Differing Dietary Habits: A Preliminary Report." *American Journal of Clinical Nutrition* 31, no. 10 suppl. (October 1978): S191–S198.

Phinney, Stephen D., Bruce R. Bistrian, R. R. Wolfe, and G. L. Blackburn. "The Human Metabolic Response to Chronic Ketosis Without Caloric Restriction: Physical and Biochemical Adaption." *Metabolism* 32, no. 8 (August 1983): 757–768.

Phinney, Stephen D., Edward S. Horton, Ethan A. H. Sims, John S. Hanson, Elliot Danforth Jr., and Betty M. Lagrange. "Capacity for Moderate Exercise in Obese Subjects after Adaptation to a Hypocaloric, Ketogenic Diet." *Journal of Clinical Investigation* 66, no. 5 (November 1980): 1152–1161.

Phinney, Stephen D., and Jeff S. Volek. *New Atkins for a New You: The Ultimate Diet for Shedding Weight and Feeling Great*. New York: Touchstone, 2010.

Phinney, Stephen D., James A. Wortman, and Douglas Bibus. "Oolichan Grease: A Unique Marine Lipid and Dietary Staple of the North Pacific Coast." *Lipids* 44, no. 1 (January 2009): 47–51.

Pickat, A. K. "The Nutritive Value of Margarine and Soy Bean-Oil." *Voprosy Pitaniia* 2, no. 5 (1933): 34–60.

Pinckney, Edward R., and Cathey Pinckney. *The Cholesterol Controversy*. Los Angeles: Sherbourne Press, 1973.

Plourde, Mélanie, and Stephen C. Cunnane. "Extremely Limited Synthesis of Long Chain Polyunsaturates in Adults: Implications for Their Dietary Essentiality and Use as Supplements." *Applied Physiology, Nutrition and Metabolism* 32, no. 4 (August 2007): 619–634.

Plumb, Robert K. "Diet Linked to Cut in Heart Attacks." *New York Times*, May 17, 1962, 39.

Poli, Giuseppi, and Rudolph Jörg Schaur. "4-Hydroxynonenal: A Lipid Degradation Product Provided with Cell Regulatory Functions." *Molecular Aspects of Medicine* 24, nos. 4–5 suppl. (August–October 2003): 147–313.

Poli, Giuseppi, Rudolph Jörg Schaur, W. G. Sterns, and G. Leonnarduzzi. "4-Hydroxynonenal: A Membrane Lipid Oxidation Product of Medicinal Interest." *Medicinal Research Reviews* 28, no. 4 (July 2008): 569–631.

Popper, Karl. *Objective Knowledge: An Evolutionary Approach*. Revised edition. Oxford: Clarendon Press, 1979.

Porter, Eugene O. "Oleomargarine: Pattern for State Trade Barriers." *Southwestern Social Science Quarterly* 29 (1948): 38–48.

Poustie, Vanessa J., and Patricia Rutherford. "Dietary Treatment for Familial Hypercholesterolaemia." *Cochrane Database of Systematic Reviews*, no. 2 (2001): CD001918.

Powley, Terry L. "The Ventromedial Hypothalamic Syndrome, Satiety and a Cephalic Phase Hypothesis." *Psychological Review* 84, no. 1 (1977): 89–126.

Prentice, Andrew M., and Alison A. Paul. "Fat and Energy Needs of Children in Developing Countries." *American Journal of Clinical Nutrition* 72, no. 5 suppl. (November 2000): 1253s-1265s.

Prentice, George. "Cancer Among Negroes." *British Medical Journal* 2, no. 3285 (December 15, 1923): 1181.

Prentice, Ross L., Bette Caan, Rowan T. Chlebowski, et al. "Low-Fat Dietary Pattern and Risk of Invasive Breast Cancer: The Women's Health Initiative Randomized Controlled Dietary Modification Trial." *Journal of the American Medical Association* 295, no. 6 (February 8, 2006): 629–642.

Prentice, Ross L., Cynthia A. Thomson, Bette Caan, et al. "Low-Fat Dietary Pattern and Cancer Incidence in the Women's Health Initiative Dietary Modification Randomized

Controlled Trial." *Journal of the National Cancer Institute* 99, no. 20 (October 17, 2007): 1534–1543.

Price, Weston A. *Nutrition and Physical Degeneration*. 1939. Reprinted. La Mesa, CA: The Price-Pottenger Nutrition Foundation, 2004.

Prior, Ian A., Flora Davidson, Clare E. Salmond, and Z. Czochanska. "Cholesterol, Coconuts, and Diet on Polynesian Atolls: A Natural Experiment: The Pukapuka and Tokelau Island Studies." *American Journal of Clinical Nutrition* 34, no. 8 (August 1981): 1552–1561.

The Procter & Gamble Company. "The Story of Crisco." In *The Story of Crisco: 250 Tested Recipes*, by Marion Harris Neil. Cincinnati, OH: Procter & Gamble, 1914, 5–17.

Psaltopoulou, Theodora, Androniki Naska, Philoppos Orfanos, Dimitrios Trichopoulos, Theodoros Mountokalakis, and Antonia Trichopoulou. "Olive Oil, the Mediterranean Diet, and Arterial Blood Pressure: The Greek European Prospective Investigation into Cancer and Nutrition (EPIC) Study." *American Journal of Clinical Nutrition* 80, no. 4 (October 1, 2004): 1012–1018.

Qintão, Eder, Scott Grundy, and Edward H. Ahrens, Jr. "Effects of Dietary Cholesterol on the Regulation of Total Body Cholesterol in Man." *Journal of Lipid Research* 12, no. 2 (March 1971): 233–247.

Ramsden, Christopher E., Joseph R. Hibbeln, Sharon F. Majchrzak, and John M. Davis. "N-6 Fatty Acid-Specific and Mixed Polyunsaturate Dietary Interventions Have Different Effects on CHD Risk: A Meta-Analysis of Randomised Controlled Trials." *British Journal of Nutrition* 104, no. 11 (December 2010): 1586–1600.

Ramsden, Christopher E., Daisy Zamora, Boonseng Leelarthaepin, et al. "Use of Dietary Linoleic Acid for Secondary Prevention of Coronary Heart Disease and Death: Evaluation of Recovered Data from the Sydney Diet Heart Study and Updated Meta-Analysis." *British Medical Journal* 346 (February 4, 2013): doi:10.1136/bmj.e8707.

Rand, Margaret L., Adje A. Hennissen, and Gerard Hornstra. "Effects of Dietary Palm Oil on Arterial Thrombosis, Platelet Responses and Platelet Membrane Fluidity in Rats." *Lipids* 23, no. 11 (November 1988): 1019–1023.

Ravnskov, Uffe. *The Cholesterol Myths: Exposing the Fallacy that Saturated Fat and Cholesterol Cause Heart Disease*. Washington, DC: New Trends, 2000.

Ray, Kausik K., Sreenivasa Rao Kondapally Seshasai, Sebhat Erqou, et al. "Statins and All-Cause Mortality in High-Risk Primary Prevention: A Meta-Analysis of 11 Randomized Controlled Trials Involving 65,229 Participants." *Archives of Internal Medicine* 170, no. 12 (June 28, 2010): 1024–1031.

Reeves, Robert M. Letter to the Editor. "Effect of Dietary Trans Fatty Acids on Cholesterol Levels." *New England Journal of Medicine* 324, no. 5 (January 31, 1991): 338–340.

———. Presentation at a conference hosted by the Institute of Shortening and Edible Oils, Las Vegas, August 2007.

Reid, D. D., and G. A. Rose. "Preliminary Communications: Assessing the Comparability of Mortality Statistics." *British Medical Journal* 2, no. 5422 (December 5, 1964): 1437–1439.

Reiser, Raymond. "Saturated Fat in the Diet and Serum Cholesterol Concentration: A Critical Examination of the Literature." *American Journal of Clinical Nutrition* 26, no. 5 (May 1973): 524–555.

———. "Saturated Fat: A Rebuttal." *American Journal of Clinical Nutrition* 27, no. 3 (March 1974): 228–229.

Research Committee. "Low-Fat Diet in Myocardial Infarction: A Controlled Trial." *Lancet* 2, no. 7411 (September 11, 1965): 501–504.

Riepma, S. F. *The Story of Margarine*. Washington, DC: Public Affairs Press, 1970.

Rillamas-Sun, Eileen, Andrea Z. LaCroix, Molly E. Warring, et al. "Obesity and Late-Age Survival Without Major Disease or Disability in Older Women." *Journal of the American Medical Association, Internal Medicine* 174, no. 1 (January 2014): 98–106.

Rittenberg, D., and Rudolf Schoenheimer. "Deuterium as an Indicator in the Study of Intermediary Metabolism: XI. Further Studies on the Biological Uptake of Deuterium into Organic Substances, with Special Reference to Fat and Cholesterol Formation." *Journal of Biological Chemistry* 121, no. 1 (October 1, 1937): 235–253.

Rivellese, Angela A., Rosalba Giacco, Giovanni Annuzzi, et al. "Effects of Monounsaturated vs. Saturated Fat on Postprandial Lipemia and Adipose Tissue Lipases in Type 2 Diabetes." *Clinical Nutrition* 27, no. 1 (February 2008): 133–141.

Robe, Karl. "Focus Gets Clearer on Confused Food Oil Picture." *Food Processing*, December 1961, 62–68.

Roberts, T. L., D. A. Wood, R. A. Riemersma, P. J. Gallagher, and Fiona C. Lampe. "Trans Isomers of Oleic and Linoleic Acids in Adipose Tissue and Sudden Cardiac Death." *Lancet* 345, no. 8945 (February 4, 1995): 278–282.

Rogers, Adrianne E., and Matthew P. Longnecker. "Biology of Disease: Dietary and Nutritional Influences on Cancer—A Review of Epidemiological and Experimental Data." *Laboratory Investigation* 59, no. 6 (1988): 729–759.

Rony, H. R. *Obesity and Leanness*. Philadelphia: Lea and Febiger, 1940.

Root, Waverley, and Richard De Rochemont. *Eating in America: A History*. New York: Morrow, 1976.

Rosamond, Wayne D., Lloyd E. Chambless, Aaron R. Folsom, et al. "Trends in the Incidence of Myocardial Infarction and in Mortality Due to Coronary Heart Disease, 1987 to 1994." *New England Journal of Medicine* 339, no. 13 (September 24, 1998): 861–867.

Rose, Geoffrey, Henry Blackburn, Ancel Keys, et al. "Colon Cancer and Blood-Cholesterol." *Lancet* 303, no. 7850 (February 9, 1974): 181–183.

Rose, Geoffrey, W. B. Thompson, and R. T. Williams. "Corn Oil in Treatment of Ischaemic Heart Disease." *British Medical Journal* 1, no. 5449 (June 12, 1965): 1531–1533.

Ross, Russell. "The Pathogenesis of Atherosclerosis—An Update." *New England Journal of Medicine* 314, no. 8 (February 20, 1986): 488–500.

Rothstein, William G. *Public Health and the Risk Factor: A History of an Uneven Medical Revolution*. Rochester Studies in Medical History 3. Rochester, NY: University of Rochester Press, 2003.

Rouja, Philippe Max, Éric Dewailly, and Carole Blanchet. "Fat, Fishing Patterns, and Health Among the Bardi People of North Western Australia." *Lipids* 38, no. 4 (April 2003): 399–405.

Roussouw, Jacques E., Loretta Finnegan, William R. Harlan, Vivian W. Pinn, Carolyn Clifford, and Joan A. McGowan. "The Evolution of the Women's Health Initiative: Perspectives from the NIH." *Journal of the American Medical Women's Association* 50, no. 2 (March/April 1995): 50–55.

Rubba, Paolo, F. Mancini, M. Gentile, and M. Mancini. "The Mediterranean Diet in Italy: An Update." *World Review of Nutrition and Dietetics* 97 (2007): 85–113.

Ruiz-Canela, Miguel, and Miguel A. Martínez-González. "Olive Oil in the Primary Prevention of Cardiovascular Disease." *Maturitas* 68, no. 3 (March 2011): 245–250.

Sacks, Frank M., George A. Bray, Vincent J. Carey, et al. "Comparison of Weight-Loss Diets with Different Compositions of Fat, Protein, and Carbohydrates." *New England Journal of Medicine* 360, no. 9 (February 26, 2009): 859–873.

Sacks, Frank M., and Lisa Litlin. "Trans-Fatty-Acid Content of Common Foods." *New England Journal of Medicine* 329, no. 26 (December 23, 1993): 1969–1970.

Samaha, Frederick F., Nayyar Iqbal, Prakash Seshadri, et al. "A Low-Carbohydrate as Compared with a Low-Fat Diet in Severe Obesity." *New England Journal of Medicine* 348, no. 21 (May 22, 2003): 2074–2081.

Samuel, Paul, Donald J. McNamara, and Joseph Shapiro. "The Role of Diet in the Etiology and Treatment of Atherosclerosis." *Annual Review of Medicine* 34, no. 1 (1983): 179–194.

Sarri, Katerina, and Anthony Kafatos. Letter to the Editor. "The Seven Countries Study in Crete: Olive Oil, Mediterranean Diet or Fasting?" *Public Health Nutrition* 8, no. 6 (2005): 666.

Sarri, Katerina, Manolis K. Linardakis, Frosso N. Bervanaki, Nikolaos E. Tzanakis, and Anthony G. Kafatos. "Greek Orthodox Fasting Rituals: A Hidden Characteristic of the Mediterranean Diet of Crete." *British Journal of Nutrition* 92, no. 2 (2004): 277–284.

Schaefer, Ernst J., Joi L. Augustin, Mary M. Schaefer, et al. "Lack of Efficacy of a Food-frequency Questionnaire in Assessing Dietary Macronutrient Intakes in Subjects Consuming Diets of Known Composition." *American Journal of Clinical Nutrition* 71, no. 3 (March 2000): 746–751.

Schaefer, Otto. "Medical Observations and Problems in the Canadian Arctic: Part II." *Canadian Medical Association Journal* 81, no. 5 (September 1, 1959): 386–393.

———. "Glycosuria and Diabetes Mellitus in Canadian Eskimos: A Preliminary Report and Hypothesis." *Canadian Medical Association Journal* 99, no. 5 (August 3, 1968): 201–206.

———. "When the Eskimo Comes to Town." *Nutrition Today* 6, no. 6 (November–December 1971): 8–16.

Schatzkin, Arthur, Peter Greenwald, David P. Byar, and Carolyn K. Clifford. "The Dietary Fat–Breast Cancer Hypothesis Is Alive." *Journal of the American Medical Association* 261, no. 22 (June 9, 1989): 3284–3287.

Schatzkin, Arthur, Victor Kipnis, Raymond J. Carroll, et al. "A Comparison of a Food Frequency Questionnaire with a 24-hour Recall for Use in an Epidemiological Cohort Study: Results from the Biomarker-based Observing Protein and Energy Nutrition (OPEN) Study." *International Journal of Epidemiology* 32, no. 6 (December 2003): 1054–1062.

Schettler, Gotthard. "Atherosclerosis During Periods of Food Deprivation Following World Wars I and II." *Preventive Medicine* 12, no. 1 (1983): 75–83.

Schleifer, David. "Reforming Food: How Trans Fats Entered and Exited the American Food System." PhD dissertation. New York University, 2010.

———. "The Perfect Solution: How Trans Fats Became the Healthy Replacement for Saturated Fats." *Technology and Culture* 53, no. 1 (January 2012): 94–119.

Seinfeld, Jerry. *I'm Telling You for the Last Time*. Broadhurst Theatre, New York, NY, August 6–9, 1998.

Seiz, Keith. *Dietary Goals for the United States,* Ninety-Fifth Congress (Washington, DC: US Government Printing Office, 1977).

———. "Formulations: Sourcing Ideal Trans-Free Oils." *Functional Foods & Neutraceuticals* (July 2005): 36–37.

Seltzer, Carl C. "The Framingham Heart Study Shows No Increases in Coronary Heart Disease Rates from Cholesterol Values of 205–264 mg/dL." *Giornale Italiano di Cardiologia* (Padua) 21, no. 6 (1991): 683.

Senti, Frederic R., ed. Prepared for the Center for Food Safety and Applied Nutrition, Food and Drug Administration. *Health Aspects of Dietary Trans-Fatty Acids.* Bethesda, MD: Life Sciences Research Office, Federation of American Societies for Experimental Biology, August 1985.

Seppanen, C. M., and A. Saari Csallany. "Simultaneous Determination of Lipophilic Aldehydes by High-Performance Liquid Chromatography in Vegetable Oil." *Journal of the American Oil Chemists' Society* 78, no. 12 (December 1, 2001): 1253–1260.

———. "Formation of 4-Hydroxynonenal, a Toxic Aldehyde, in Soybean Oil at Frying Temperature." *Journal of the American Oil Chemists' Society* 79, no. 10 (October 1, 2002): 1033–1038.

Serra-Majem, Lluís, J. Ngo de la Cruz, L. Ribas, and L. Salleras. "Mediterranean Diet and Health: Is All the Secret in Olive Oil?" *Pathophysiology of Haemostasis and Thrombosis* 33, nos. 5–6 (September–December 2003/2004): 461–465.

Serra-Majem, Lluís, Lourdes Ribas, Ricard Tresserras, Joy Ngo, and Llufs Salleras. "How Could Changes in Diet Explain Changes in Coronary Heart Disease Mortality in Spain? The Spanish Paradox." *American Journal of Clinical Nutrition* 61, no. 6 suppl. (June 1995): 1351S–1359S.

Serra-Majem, Lluís, Blanca Roman, and Ramón Estruch. "Scientific Evidence of Interventions Using the Mediterranean Diet: A Systematic Review." *Nutritional Reviews* 64, no. 2 (February 2006): S27–S47.

Serra-Majem, Lluís, Antonia Trichopoulou, Joy Ngo de la Cruz, et al. "Does the Definition of the Mediterranean Diet Need to be Updated?" *Public Health Nutrition* 7, no. 7 (October 2004): 927–929.

Shai, Iris, Dan Schwarzfuchs, Yaakov Henkin, et al. "Weight Loss with a Low-Carbohydrate, Mediterranean, or Low-Fat Diet." *New England Journal of Medicine* 359, no. 3 (July 17, 2008): 229–241.

Shaper, A. Gerald. "Cardiovascular Studies in the Samburu Tribe of Northern Kenya." *American Heart Journal* 63, no. 4 (April 1962): 437–442.

———. Interview with Henry Blackburn. In "Preventing Heart Attack and Stroke: A History of Cardiovascular Disease Epidemiology," last accessed February 14, 2014. http://www .epi.umn.edu/cvdepi/interview.asp?id=64.

Sharman, Matthew J., Ana L. Gómez, William J. Kraemer, and Jeff S. Volek. "Very Low-Carbohdryate and Low-Fat Diets Affect Fasting Lipids and Postprandial Lipemia Differently in Overweight Men." *Journal of Nutrition* 134, no. 4 (April 1, 2004): 880–885.

Shaten, Barbara J., Lewis H. Kuller, Marcus O. Kjelsberg, et al. "Lung Cancer Mortality After 16 Years in MRFIT Participants in Intervention and Usual-Care Groups." *Annals of Epidemiology* 7, no. 2 (February 1997): 125–136.

Shekelle, Richard B., Anne MacMillan Shryock, Oglesby Paul, et al. "Diet, Serum Cholesterol, and Death from Coronary Heart Disease: The Western Electric Study." *New England Journal of Medicine* 304, no. 2 (January 8, 1981): 65–70.

Shekelle, Richard, and Salim Yusuf. "Report of the Conference on Low Blood Cholesterol: Mortality Associations." *Circulation* 86, no. 3 (1992): 1046–1060.

Shi, Z., X. Hu, B. Yuan, G. Hu, X. Pan, Y. Dai, J. E. Byles, and G. Holmboe-Ottesen. "Vegetable-Rich Food Pattern Is Related to Obesity in China." *International Journal of Obesity* 32, no. 6 (2008): 975–984.

Shields, David S. "Prospecting for Oil." *Gastronomica* 10, no. 4 (2010): 25–34.

Shin, Ju Young, Jerry Suls, and René Martin. "Are Cholesterol and Depression Inversely Related? A Meta-Analysis of the Association Between Two Cardiac Risk Factors." *Annals of Behavioral Medicine* 36, no. 1 (August 2008): 33–43.

Siampos, George S. *Recent Population Change Calling for Policy Action: With Special Reference to Fertility and Migration.* Athens: National Statistical Service of Greece, 1980.

Sieri, Sabina, Vittorio Krogh, Pietro Ferrari, et al. "Dietary Fat and Breast Cancer Risk in the European Prospective Investigation into Cancer and Nutrition." *American Journal of Clinical Nutrition* 88, no. 5 (November 2008): 1304–1312.

Silwood, Christopher J. L., and Martin C. Grootveld. "Application of High-Resolution, Two-Dimensional H and C Nuclear Magnetic Resonance Techniques to the Characterization of Lipid Oxidation Products in Autoxidized Linoleoyl Linolenoylglycerols." *Lipids* 34, no. 7 (July 1999): 741–756.

Simell, Olli, Harri Niinikoski, Tapani Rönnemaa, et al. "Special Turku Coronary Risk Factor Intervention Project for Babies (STRIP)." *American Journal of Clinical Nutrition* 72, no. 5 suppl. (November 2000): 1316S–1331S.

Simons, Leon A., Yechiel Friedlander, John McCallum, and Judith Simons. "Risk Factors for Coronary Heart Disease in the Prospective Dubbo Study of Australian Elderly." *Atherosclerosis* 117, no. 1 (1995): 107–118.

Sinclair, Hugh M. "The Diet of Canadian Indians and Eskimos." *Proceedings of the Nutrition Society* 12, no. 1 (1953): 74.

Singh, Ram B., Shanti S. Rastogi, Rakesh Verma, Laxmi Bolaki, and Reema Singh. "An Indian Experiment with Nutritional Modulation in Acute Myocardial Infarction." *American Journal of Cardiology* 69, no. 9 (April 1, 1992): 879–885.

Singh, Ram B., Shanti S. Rastogi, Rakesh Verma, L. Bolaki, Reema Singh, S. Ghosh, and Mohammad A. Niaz. "Randomised Controlled Trial of Cardioprotective Diet in Patients with Recent Acute Myocardinal Infarction: Results of One Year Follow Up." *British Medical Journal* 304, no. 6833 (April 18, 1992): 1015–1019.

Siri-Tarino, Patty W., Qi Sun, Frank B. Hu, and Ronald M. Krauss. "Saturated Fat, Carbohydrate, and Cardiovascular Disease." *American Journal of Clinical Nutrition* 91, no. 3 (March 2010): 502–509.

Slining, Meghan M., Kevin C. Mathias, and Barry M. Popkin. "Trends in Food and Beverage Sources among US Children and Adolescents: 1989–2010." *Journal of the Academy of Nutrition and Dietetics* 113, no. 12 (December 2013): 1683–1694.

Smith, Jane, and Fiona Godlee. "Investigating Allegations of Scientific Misconduct." *British Medical Journal* 331, no. 7511 (July 30, 2005): 245–246.

Smith, Leland L. "The Autoxidation of Cholesterol." In *Autoxidation in Food and Biological Systems.* Edited by Michael G. Simic and Marcus Karel. New York: Springer Science+Business Media, 1980, 119–132.

Smith, Russell Lesley, and Edward Robert Pinckney. *Diet, Blood Cholesterol, and Coronary Heart Disease: A Critical Review of the Literature.* Santa Monica, CA: privately published, July 1988.

Soman, C. R. "Correspondence: Indo-Mediterranean Diet and Progression of Coronary Artery Disease." *Lancet* 366, no. 9483 (July 30, 2005): 365–366.

Spencer, Colin. *Vegetarianism: A History.* London: Grub Street, 2000.

Speth, John D. *Bison Kills and Bone Counts: Decision Making by Ancient Hunters.* Chicago: University of Chicago Press, 1983.

Squires, Sally. "Hearts and Minds." *Washington Post,* July 24, 2001.

Stamler, Jeremiah. "Diet-Heart: A Problematic Revisit." *American Journal of Clinical Nutrition* 91, no. 3 (March 2010): 497–499.

Stamler, Jeremiah, and Frederick H. Epstein. "Coronary Heart Disease: Risk Factors as Guides to Preventive Action." *Preventive Medicine* 1, no. 1 (1972): 27–48.

Staprans, Ilona, Xian-Mang Pan, Joseph H. Rapp, Carl Grunfeld, and Kenneth R. Feingold. "Oxidized Cholesterol in the Diet Accelerates the Development of Atherosclerosis in LDL Receptor- and Apolipoprotein E–Deficient Mice." *Journal of Arteriosclerosis, Thrombosis, and Vascular Biology* 20, no. 3 (March 2000): 708–714.

Stearns, Peter N. *Fat History: Bodies and Beauty in the Modern West.* New York: New York University Press, 1997.

Stefanick, Marcia L., Sally Mackey, Mary Sheehan, Nancy Ellsworth, William L. Haskell, and Peter D. Wood. "Effects of Diet and Exercise in Men and Postmenopausal Women with Low Levels of HDL Cholesterol and High Levels of LDL Cholesterol." *New England Journal of Medicine* 339, no. 1 (July 2, 1998): 12–20.

Stefansson, Vilhjalmur. *The Fat of the Land.* Enlarged Edition of *Not By Bread Alone,* first published in 1946. New York: Macmillan, 1956.

———. *The Friendly Arctic: The Story of Five Years in Polar Regions.* New edition (First edition: New York: MacMillan, 1921). New York: Greenwood Press, 1969.

Stehbens, William E., and Elli Wierzbicki. "The Relationship of Hypercholesterolemia to Atherosclerosis with Particular Emphasis on Familial Hypercholesterolemia, Diabetes Mellitus, Obstructive Jaundice, Myxedema, and the Nephrotic Syndrome." *Progress in Cardiovascular Diseases* 30, no. 4 (January–February 1988): 289–306.

Stein, Joel. "The Low-Carb Diet Craze." *Time,* November 1, 1999.

Steinberg, Daniel. "An Interpretive History of the Cholesterol Controversy: Part 1." *Journal of Lipid Research* 45, no. 9 (September 2004): 1583–1593.

———. "An Interpretive History of the Cholesterol Controversy. Part II. The Early Evidence Linking Hypercholesterolemia to Coronary Disease in Humans." *Journal of Lipid Research* 46, no. 2 (February 2005): 179–190.

———. "The Pathogenesis of Atherosclerosis: An Interpretive History of the Cholesterol Controversy, Part IV: The 1984 Coronary Primary Prevention Trial Ends It—Almost." *Journal of Lipid Research* 47, no. 1 (January 2006): 1–14.

Stemmermann, Grant N., Abraham Nomura, Lance K. Heilbrun, Earl S. Pollack, and Abraham Kagan. "Serum Cholesterol and Colon Cancer Incidence in Hawaiian Japanese Men." *Journal of the National Cancer Institute* 67, no. 6 (December 1981): 1179–1182.

Stender, Steen, and Jørn Dyerberg. "High Levels of Industrially Produced Trans Fat in Popular Fast Foods." *New England Journal of Medicine* 354, no. 15 (April 13, 2006): 1650–1652.

Stern, Linda, Nayyar Iqbal, Prakash Seshadri, et al. "The Effects of Low-Carbohydrate versus Conventional Weight Loss Diets in Severely Obese Adults: One-Year Follow-up of a Randomized Trial." *Annals of Internal Medicine* 140, no. 10 (May 18, 2004): 778–785.

Stout, Clarke, Jerry Morrow, Edward N. Brandt, Jr., and Stewart Wolf. "Unusually Low Incidence of Death from Myocardial Infarction: Study of Italian American Community in Pennsylvania." *Journal of the American Medical Association* 188, no. 10 (June 8, 1964): 845–849.

Sturdevant, Richard A. L., Morton Lee Pearce, and Seymour Dayton. "Increased Prevalence of Cholelithiasis in Men Ingesting a Serum-Cholesterol-Lowering Diet." *New England Journal of Medicine* 288, no. 1 (January 4, 1973): 24–27.

Sutherland, Wayne H. F., Sylvia A. de Jong, Robert J. Walker, et al. "Effect of Meals Rich in Heated Olive and Safflower Oils on Oxidation of Postprandial Serum in Healthy Men." *Atherosclerosis* 160, no. 1 (January 2002): 195–203.

Svendsen, Kristin, Hanne Naper Jensen, Ingvill Sivertsen, and Ann Kristin Sjaastad. "Exposure to Cooking Fumes in Restaurant Kitchens in Norway." *Annals of Occupational Hygiene* 46, no. 4 (2002): 395–400.

Takeya, Yo, Jordan S. Popper, Yukiko Shimizu, Hiroo Kato, George G. Rhoads, and Abraham Kagan. "Epidemiologic Studies of Coronary Heart Disease and Stroke in Japanese Men Living in Japan, Hawaii and California: Incidence of Stroke in Japan and Hawaii." *Stroke* 15, no. 1 (January–February 1984): 15–23.

Tanaka, Heizo, Yutaka Ueda, Masayuki Hayashi, et al. "Risk Factors for Cerebral Hemorrhage and Cerebral Infarction in a Japanese Rural Community." *Stroke* 13, no. 1 (January–February 1982): 62–73.

Tanaka, T., and T. Okamura. "Blood Cholesterol Level and Risk of Stroke in Community-Based or Worksite Cohort Studies: A Review of Japanese Cohort Studies in the Past 20 Years." *Keio Journal of Medicine* 61, no. 3 (2012): 79–88.

Tang, Jian, Qi Zhang Jin, Guo Hui Shen, Chi Tang Ho, and Stephen S. Chang. "Isolation and Identification of Volatile Compounds from Fried Chicken." *Journal of Agricultural and Food Chemistry* 31, no. 6 (1983): 1287–1292.

Tang, W. H. Wilson, Zeneng Wang, Bruce S. Levison, et al. "Intestinal Microbial Metabolism of Phosphatidylcholine and Cardiovascular Risk." *New England Journal of Medicine* 368, no. 17 (April 25, 2013): 1575–1584.

Tannenbaum, Albert. "The Genesis and Growth of Tumors. III. Effects of a High-Fat Diet." *Cancer Research* 2, no. 7 (July 1942): 468–475.

Taubes, Gary. "The Soft Science of Dietary Fat." *Science* 291, no. 5513 (March 2001): 2536–2545.

————. "What if It's All Been a Big Fat Lie?" *New York Times Magazine*, July 7, 2002.

————. *Good Calories, Bad Calories: Fats, Carbs, and the Controversial Science of Diet and Health.* New York: Alfred A. Knopf, 2007.

————. "Do We Really Know What Makes Us Healthy?" *New York Times Magazine*, September 16, 2007.

————. Letter to the Editor. "Eat, Drink and Be Wary." *New York Times*, October 28, 2007.

————. "The Science of Obesity: What Do We Really Know about What Makes Us Fat? An Essay by Gary Taubes." *British Medical Journal* 346 (April 16, 2013).

————. "What Makes You Fat: Too Many Calories, or the Wrong Carbohydrates?" *Scientific American* 309, no. 3 (September 2013): 60–65.

Teicholz, Nina. "Heart Breaker." *Gourmet,* June 2004, 100–105.

Teti, Vito. "Food and Fatness in Calabria." In *Social Aspects of Obesity #1.* Edited by Igor De Garine and Nancy J. Pollock. Translated by Nicolette S. James. Amsterdam: Gordon and Breach, 1995.

Thannhauser, S. J., and Heinz Magendantz. "The Different Clinical Groups of Xanthomatous Diseases: A Clinical Physiological Study of 22 Cases." *Annals of Internal Medicine* 11, no. 9 (March 1, 1938): 1662–1746.

Tillotson, Jeanne L., Hiroo Kato, Milton Z. Nichaman, et al. "Epidemiology of Coronary Heart Disease and Stroke in Japanese Men Living in Japan, Hawaii, and California: Methodology for Comparison of Diet." *American Journal of Clinical Nutrition* 26, no. 2 (February 1973): 177–184.

Tolstoi, Edward. "The Effect of an Exclusive Meat Diet Lasting One Year on the Carbohydrate Tolerance of Two Normal Men." *Journal of Biological Chemistry* 83, no. 3 (September 1929): 747–752.

————. "The Effect of an Exclusive Meat Diet on the Chemical Constituents of the Blood." *Journal of Biological Chemistry* 83, no. 3 (September 1929): 753–758.

Torrey, John C. "Influence of an Exclusively Meat Diet on the Human Intestinal Flora." *Proceedings of the Society for Experimental Biology and Medicine* 28, no. 3 (December 1930): 295–296.

"Trans Fatty Acids and Risk of Myocardial Infarction." Toxicology Forum Annual Summer Meeting, July 11–15, 1994.

"Trial of Clofibrate in the Treatment of Ischaemic Heart Disease. Five-year Study by a Group of Physicians of the Newcastle Upon Tyne Region." *British Medical Journal* 4, no. 5790 (December 25, 1971): 767–775.

Trichopoulos, Dimitrios. Letter to the Editor. "In Defense of the Mediterranean Diet." *European Journal of Clinical Nutrition* 56, no. 9 (September 2002): 928–929.

Trichopoulou, Antonia, Tina Costacou, Christina Bamia, and Dimitrios Trichopoulos. "Adherence to a Mediterranean Diet and Survival in a Greek Population." *New England Journal of Medicine* 348, no. 26 (June 26, 2003): 2599–2608.

Trichopoulou, Antonia, Antigone Kouris-Blazos, Mark L. Wahlqvist, et al. "Diet and Overall Survival in Elderly People." *British Medical Journal* 311, no. 7018 (December 2, 1995): 1457–1460.

Trichopoulou, Antonia, and Pagona Lagiou. "Healthy Traditional Mediterranean Diet: An Expression of Culture, History, and Lifestyle." *Nutrition Reviews* 55, no. 11, pt. 1 (November 1997): 383–389.

Trichopoulou, Antonia, Philippos Orfanos, Teresa Norat, et al. "Modified Mediterranean Diet and Survival: EPIC-Elderly Prospective Cohort Study." *British Medical Journal* 330, no. 7498 (April 28, 2005): 991.

Troiano, Richard P., Ronette R. Briefel, Margaret D. Carroll, and Karil Bialostosky. "Energy and Fat Intakes of Children and Adolescents in the United States: Data from the National Health and Nutrition Examination Surveys." *American Journal of Clinical Nutrition* 72, no. 5 suppl. (2000): 1343S–1353S.

Trowell, H. C., and D. P. Burkitt, eds. *Western Diseases: Their Emergence and Prevention.* London: Edward Arnold, 1981.

Truswell, A. Stewart. "Diet and Plasma Lipids—A Reappraisal." *American Journal of Clinical Nutrition* 31, no. 6 (June 1978): 977–989.

———. "Evolution of Dietary Recommendations, Goals, and Guidelines." *American Journal of Clinical Nutrition* 45, no. 5 suppl. (May 1987): 1060–1072.

———. "Problems with Red Meat in the WCRF2." *American Journal of Clinical Nutrition* 89, no. 4 (April 2009): 1274–1275.

Tunstall-Pedoe, Hugh, Kari Kuulasmaa, Markku Mähönen, Hanna Tolonen, Esa Ruokokski, and Phillippe Amouyel. "Contribution of Trends in Survival and Coronary-Event Rates to Changes in Coronary Heart Disease Mortality: 10-Year Results from 37 WHO MONICA Project Populations. Monitoring Trends and Determinants in Cardiovascular Disease." *Lancet* 353, no. 9164 (May 8, 1999): 1547–1557.

Turpeinen, Osmo, Martti Karvonen, Maija Pekkarinen, Matti Miettinen, Reino Elosuo, and Erkki Paavilainen. "Dietary Prevention of Coronary Heart Disease: The Finnish Mental Hospital Study." *International Journal of Epidemiology* 8, no. 2 (1979): 99–118.

Twain, Mark. *Life on the Mississippi.* 1883. Reprinted. Hollywood, CA. Simon & Brown, 2011.

Uauy, Ricardo, Charles E. Mize, and Carlos Castillo-Duran. "Fat Intake During Childhood: Metabolic Responses and Effects on Growth." *American Journal of Clinical Nutrition* 72, no. 5 suppl. (November 2000): 1345S–1360S.

Ueshima, Hirotsuga, Minoru Iida, and Yoshio Komachi. Letter to the Editor. "Is It Desirable to Reduce Total Serum Cholesterol Level as Low as Possible?" *Preventive Medicine* 8, no. 1 (January 1979): 104–111.

Ueshima, Hirotsugu, Kozo Tatara, and Shintaro Asakura. "Declining Mortality From Ischemic Heart Disease and Changes in Coronary Risk Factors in Japan, 1956–1980." *American Journal of Epidemiology* 125, no. 1 (1987): 62–72.

US Census Office. *Census Reports II: Twelfth Census of the United States, Taken in the Year 1900. Population. Part II.* Washington, DC. US Census Office, 1902.

US Congress. House. Committee on Agriculture. *National Academy of Sciences Report on Healthful Diets: Hearings before the House Subcommittee on Domestic Marketing, Consumer Relations, and Nutrition.* 96th Congress, 2nd Session, 1980.

———. House. Committee on Appropriations. *Dietary Guidelines for Americans: Hearings before the House Subcommittee on Agriculture, Rural Development and Related Agencies.* 96th Congress, 2nd Session, 1980.

———. Senate. Commmittee on Nutrition and Human Needs. *Diet Related to Killer Diseases.* 94th Congress, July 27 and 28, 1976.

———. Senate. Committee on Nutrition and Human Needs. *Obesity and Fad Diets: Hearings Before the Select Committee on Nutrition and Human Needs of the US Senate.* 93rd Congress. Washington, DC: US Government Printing Office, April 12, 1973.

US Department of Agriculture. *Nutrition and Your Health: Dietary Guidelines for Americans Home and Garden Bulletin* 228. Washington, DC: Science and Education Administration, 1980.

———. "Profiling Food Consumption in America." In *Agricultural Fact Book 2001–2002.* 13–21. Washington, DC: US Government Printing Office, 2003.

US Department of Agriculture and US Department of Health and Human Services. *Dietary Guidelines for Americans, 2010.* 7th Edition, Washington, DC: US Government Printing Office, December 2010.

Van Deventer, Hendrick, W. Greg Miller, Gary L. Meyers, et al. "Non-HDL Cholesterol Shows Improved Accuracy for Cardiovascular Risk Score Classification Compared to Direct or Calculated LDL Cholesterol in Dyslipidemic Population." *Clinical Chemistry* 57, No. 3 (2011): 490–501.

Vernon, Mary C., John Mavropoulos, Melissa Transue, William S. Yancy, and Eric C. Westman. "Clinical Experience of a Carbohydrate-Restricted Diet: Effect on Diabetes Mellitus." *Metabolic Syndrome and Related Disorders* 1, no. 3 (September 2003): 233–237.

Volek, Jeff S., Kevin D. Ballard, Ricardo Silvestre, et al. "Effects of Dietary Carbohydrate Restriction Versus Low-Fat Diet on Flow-Mediated Dilation." *Metabolism* 58, no. 12 (December 2009): 1769–1777.

Volek, Jeff S., Stephen D. Phinney, Cassandra E. Forsythe, et al. "Carbohydrate Restriction Has a More Favorable Impact on the Metabolic Syndrome than a Low Fat Diet." *Lipids* 44, no. 4 (April 2009): 297–309.

Volek, Jeff S., Matthew J. Sharman, and Cassandra E. Forsythe. "Modification of Lipoproteins by Very Low-Carbohydrate Diets." *Journal of Nutrition* 135, no. 6 (June 2005): 1339–1342.

Volek, Jeff S., Matthew Sharman, Ana Gomez, et al. "Comparison of Energy-Restricted Very Low-Carbohydrate and Low-Fat Diets on Weight Loss and Body Composition in Overweight Men and Women." *Nutrition & Metabolism* 1, no. 13 (2004): 1–32.

Volek, Jeff S., Matthew J. Sharman, et al. "Comparison of a Very Low-Carbohydrate and Low-Fat Diet on Fasting Lipids, LDL Subclasses, Insulin Resistance, and Postprandial Lipemic Responses in Overweight Women." *Journal of the American College of Nutrition* 23, no. 2 (April 2004): 177–184.

Von Noorden, C. *Clinical Treatises on Pathology and Therapy of Disorders of Metabolism and Nutrition, Part VIII. Diabetes Mellitus.* New York: E. B. Treat, 1907.

Vos, Eddie. "Modified Mediterranean Diet and Survival: Key Confounder Was Missed." *British Medical Journal* 330, no. 7503 (June 4, 2005): 1329.

Wade, Nicholas. "Food Board's Fat Report Hits Fire." *Science* 209, no. 4453 (July 11, 1980): 248–250.

Walden, Carolyn E., Barbara M. Retzlaff, Brenda L. Buck, Shari Wallick, Barbara S. McCann, and Robert H. Knopp. "Differential Effect of National Cholesterol Education Program (NCEP) Step II Diet on HDL Cholesterol, Its Subfractions, and Apoprotein AI Levels in Hypercholesterolemic Women and Men After 1 Year: The beFIT Study." *Arteriosclerosis, Thrombosis, and Vascular Biology* 20, no. 6 (June 2000): 1580–1587.

Wallace, A. J., W. H. F. Sutherland, J. I. Mann, and S. M. Williams. "The Effects of Meals Rich in Thermally Stressed Olive and Safflower Oils on Postprandial Serum Paraoxonase Activity in Patients with Diabetes." *European Journal of Clinical Nutrition* 55, no. 11 (November 2001): 951–958.

Wallace, Lance, and Wayne Ott. "Personal Exposure to Ultrafine Particles." *Journal of Exposure Science and Environmental Epidemiology* 21 (January–February 2011): 20–30.

Wallis, Claudia. "Hold the Eggs and Butter." *Time*, March 26, 1984.

Walvin, James. *Fruits of Empire: Exotic Produce and British Taste, 1660–1800.* New York: New York University Press, 1997.

Waterlow, John C. "Diet of the Classical Period of Greece and Rome." *European Journal of Clinical Nutrition* 43, suppl. 2 (1989): 3–12.

Wears, Robert L., Richelle J. Cooper, and David J. Magid. "Subgroups, Reanalyses, and Other Dangerous Things." *Annals of Emergency Medicine* 46, no. 3 (September 2005): 253–255.

Weld, Isaac. *Travels Through the States of North America, and the Provinces of Upper and Lower Canada, During the Years 1795, 1796, and 1797.* London: printed for John Stockdale, Piccadilly, 1799.

Werdelin, Lars. "King of Beasts." *Scientific American* 309, no. 5 (November 2013): 34–39.

Werkö, Lars. "Risk Factors and Coronary Heart Disease—Facts or Fancy?" *American Heart Journal* 91, no. 1 (January 1976): 87–98.

Wertheimer, E., and B. Shapiro. "The Physiology of Adipose Tissue." *Physiology Reviews* 28, no. 4 (October 1948): 451–464.

Westman, Eric C. "Rethinking Dietary Saturated Fat." *Food Technology* 63, no. 2 (2009): 30.

Westman, Eric C., Richard D. Feinman, John C. Mavropoulos, et al. "Low-Carbohydrate Nutrition and Metabolism." *American Journal of Clinical Nutrition* 86, no. 2 (August 2007): 276–284.

Westman, Eric C., John C. Mavropoulos, William S. Yancy, and Jeff S. Volek. "A Review of Low-Carbohydrate Ketogenic Diets." *Current Atherosclerosis Reports* 5, no. 6 (November 2003): 476–483.

Westman, Eric C., Jeff S. Volek, and Richard D. Feinman. "Carbohydrate Restriction Is Effective in Improving Atherogenic Dyslipidemia even in the Absence of Weight Loss." *American Journal of Clinical Nutrition* 84, no. 6 (December 2006): 1549.

Westman, Eric C., William S. Yancy, Joel S. Edman, Keith F. Tomlin, and Christine E. Perkins. "Effect of 6-month Adherence to a Very Low Carbohydrate Diet Program." *American Journal of Medicine* 113, no. 1 (2002): 30–36.

Westman, Eric C., William S Yancy, and Margaret Humphreys. "Dietary Treatment of Diabetes Mellitus in the Pre-Insulin Era (1914–1922)." *Perspectives in Biology and Medicine* 49, no. 1 (Winter 2006): 77–83.

White, Caroline. "Suspected Research Fraud: Difficulties Getting at the Truth." *British Medical Journal* 331, no. 7511 (July 30, 2005): 281–288.

White, Paul Dudley. "Heart Ills and Presidency: Dr. White's Views." *New York Times*, October 30, 1955.

Willett, Walter C. *Eat, Drink and Be Healthy: The Harvard Medical School Guide to Healthy Eating.* New York: Simon & Schuster, 2001.

———. "The Great Fat Debate: Total Fat and Health," *Journal of the American Dietetic Association* 111, no. 5 (May 2011): 660–662.

Willett, Walter C., and Alberto Ascherio. "Trans Fatty Acids: Are the Effects Only Marginal?" *American Journal of Public Health* 84, no. 5 (May 1994): 722–724.

Willett, Walter C., and David J. Hunter. "Prospective Studies of Diet and Breast Cancer." *Cancer* 74, no. 3 suppl. (August 1, 1994): 1085–1089.

Willett, Walter C., Frank Sacks, Antonia Trichopoulou, et al. "Mediterranean Diet Pyramid: A Cultural Model for Healthy Eating." *American Journal of Clinical Nutrition* 61, no. 6 (June 1995): 1402S–1406S.

Willett, Walter C., Meir J. Stampfer, Graham A. Colditz, et al. "Dietary Fat and the Risk of Breast Cancer." *New England Journal of Medicine* 316, no. 1 (January 1, 1987): 22–28.

Willett, Walter C., Meir J. Stampfer, JoAnn E. Manson, et al. "Intake of Trans Fatty Acids and Risk of Coronary Heart Disease Among Women." *Lancet* 341, no. 8845 (March 6, 1993): 581–585.

Williams, Roger R., Paul D. Sorlie, Manning Feinleib, et al. "Cancer Incidence by Levels of Cholesterol." *Journal of the American Medical Association* 245, no. 3 (January 16, 1981): 247–252.

Wood, Randall, Fred Chumbler, and Rex Wiegand. "Incorporation of Dietary *cis* and *trans* Isomers of Octadecenoate in Lipid Classes of Liver and Hepatoma." *Journal of Biological Chemistry* 252, no. 6 (March 25, 1977): 1965–1970.

Wood, Randall, Karen Kubena, Barbara O'Brien, Stephen Tseng, and Gail Martin. "Effect of Butter, Mono- and Polyunsaturated Fatty Acid-Enriched Butter, Trans Fatty Acid Margarine, and Zero Trans Fatty Acid Margarine on Serum Lipids and Lipoproteins in Healthy Men." *Journal of Lipid Research* 34, no. 1 (January 1993): 1–11.

Wood, Randall, Karen Kubena, Stephen Tseng, Gail Martin, and Robin Crook. "Effect of Palm Oil, Margarine, Butter and Sunflower Oil on Serum Lipids and Lipoproteins of Normocholesterolemic Middle-Aged Men." *Journal of Nutritional Biochemistry* 4, no. 5 (May 1993): 286–297.

Woodhill, J. M., A. L. Palmer, B. Leelarthaepin, C. McGilchrist, and R. B. Blacket. "Low Fat, Low Cholesterol Diet in Secondary Prevention of Coronary Heart Disease." *Advances in Experimental Medicine and Biology* 109 (1978): 317–330.

Wootan, Margo, Bonnie Liebman, and Wendie Rosofsky. "Trans: The Phantom Fat." *Nutrition Action Healthletter* 23, no. 7 (1996): 10–14.

World Cancer Research Fund and the American Institute for Cancer Research. *Food, Nutrition, Physical Activity, and the Prevention of Cancer: A Global Perspective.* Washington, DC: American Institute for Cancer Research, 2007.

World Health Organization. "Diet, Nutrition, and the Prevention of Chronic Diseases: Joint WHO/FAO Expert Consultation." *World Health Organization Technical Report Series* 916. Geneva, Switzerland: WHO, 2003.

Worth, Robert M., Hiroo Kato, George G. Rhoads, Abraham Kagan, and Sherman Leonard Syme. "Epidemiologic Studies of Coronary Heart Disease and Stroke in Japanese Men Living in Japan, Hawaii and California: Mortality." *American Journal of Epidemiology* 102, no. 6 (December 1975): 481–490.

Wrangham, Richard. *Catching Fire: How Cooking Made Us Human.* Philadelphia: Basic Books, 2009.

The Writing Group for the DISC Collaborative Research Group. "Efficacy and Safety of Lowering Dietary Intake of Fat and Cholesterol in Children with Elevated Low-Density Lipoprotein Cholesterol." *Journal of the American Medical Association* 273, no. 18 (May 10, 1995): 1429–1435.

Wu, She-Ching, and Gow-Chin Yen. "Effects of Cooking Oil Fumes on the Genotoxicity and Oxidative Stress in Human Lung Carcinoma (A-549) Cells." *Toxicology in Vitro* 18, no. 5 (October 2004): 571–580.

Yancy, William S., Maren K. Olsen, John R. Guyton, Ronna P. Bakst, and Eric C. Westman. "A Low-Carbohydrate, Ketogenic Diet Versus a Low-Fat Diet to Treat Obesity and Hyperlipidemia: A Randomized, Controlled Trial." *Annals of Internal Medicine* 140, no. 10 (May 18, 2004): 769–777.

Yang, Mei-Uih, and Theodore B. Van Itallie. "Composition of Weight Lost During Short-Term Weight Reduction. Metabolic Responses of Obese Subjects to Starvation and Low-Calorie Ketogenic and Nonketogenic Diets." *Journal of Clinical Investigation* 58, no. 3 (September 1976): 722–730.

Yano, Katsuhiko, George G. Rhoads, Abraham Kagan, and Jeanne Tillotson. "Dietary Intake and the Risk of Coronary Heart Disease in Japanese Men Living in Hawaii." *American Journal of Clinical Nutrition* 31, no. 7 (July 1978): 1270–1279.

Yellowlees, Walter W. "Sir James Mackenzie and the History of Myocardial Infarction." *Journal of the Royal College of General Practitioners* 32, no. 235 (February 1982): 109–112.

Yerushalmy, Jacob, and Herman E. Hilleboe. "Fat in the Diet and Mortality from Heart Disease; A Methodologic Note." *New York State Journal of Medicine* 57, no. 14 (July 1957): 2343–2354.

Yngve, Agneta, Leif Hambraeus, Lauren Lissner, et al. "Invited Commentary: The Women's Health Initiative. What Is on Trial: Nutrition and Chronic Disease? Or Misinterpreted Science, Media Havoc and the Sound of Silence from Peers?" *Public Health Nutrition* 9, no. 2 (2006): 269–272.

Yonge, C. D., ed. and trans. *The Deipnosophists, or, Banquet of the Learned, of Athenæus.* London: Henry G. Bohn, 1854.

Young, S. Stanley. "Gaming the System: Chaos from Multiple Testing." *IMS Bulletin* 36, no. 10 (2007): 13.

Young, Shun-Chieh, Louis W. Chang, Hui-Ling Lee, Lung-Hung Tsai, Yin-Chang Liu, and Pinpin Lin. "DNA Damages Induced by Trans, Trans-2, 4-Decadienal (tt-DDE), a Component of Cooking Oil Fume, in Human Bronchial Epithelial Cells." *Environmental and Molecular Mutagenesis* 51, no. 4 (February 2010): 315–321.

Yudkin, John. *Pure, White and Deadly.* New York: Penguin, 1972.

Zarkovic, Neven. "4-Hydroxynonenal as a Bioactive Marker of Pathophysiological Processes." *Molecular Aspects of Medicine* 24, no. 4–5 (August–October 2003): 281–291.

Zhang, Quing, Ahmed S. M. Saleh, Jing Chen, and Qun Shen. "Chemical Alterations Taken Place During Deep-Fat Frying Based on Certain Reaction Products: A Review." *Chemistry and Physics of Lipids* 165, no. 6 (September 2012): 662–681.

Zhong, Lijie, Mark S. Goldberg, Yu-Tang Gao, and Fan Jin. "Lung Cancer and Indoor Air Pollution Arising from Chinese-Style Cooking among Nonsmoking Women Living in Shanghai, China." *Epidemiology* 10, no. 5 (September 1999): 488–494.

Zhong, Lijie, Mark S. Goldberg, Marie-Élise Parent, and James A. Hanley. "Risk of Developing Lung Cancer in Relation to Exposure to Fumes from Chinese-Style Cooking." *Scandinavian Journal of Work, Environment and Health* 25, no. 4 (August 1999): 309–316.

Zimetbaum, Peter, William H. Frishman, Wee Lock Ooi, et al. "Plasma Lipids and Lipoproteins and the Incidence of Cardiovascular Disease in the Very Elderly. The Bronx Aging Study." *Arteriosclerosis, Thrombosis, and Vascular Biology* 12, no. 4 (April 1992): 416–423.

Zock, Peter L., and Martijn B. Katan. "Hydrogenation Alternatives: Effects of Trans Fatty Acids and Stearic Acid Versus Linoleic Acid on Serum Lipids and Lipoproteins in Humans." *Journal of Lipid Research* 33, no. 3 (March 1992): 399–410.

Zukel, William J., Robert H. Lewis, Philip E. Enterline, et al. "A Short-Term Community Study of the Epidemiology of Coronary Heart Disease: A Preliminary Report on the North Dakota Study." *American Journal of Public Health and the Nation's Health* 49, no. 12 (1959): 1630–1639.

Permissions

28 "Keys's 1952 Chart"
Copyright © Journal of Mt. Sinai Hospital, New York, 1953. This material is reproduced with permission of John Wiley & Sons, Inc.

34 "Yerushalmy and Hilleboe: Data from Twenty-Two Countries"
Reprinted with permission from the Medical Society of the State of New York.

51 "Ancel Keys on the Cover of *Time:* January 13, 1961"
From *TIME* Magazine, January 13, 1961 © 1961, Time Inc. Used under license.

52 "Cartoon of Risks vs. Benefits"
Reprinted with permission from S. Harris.

66 "Cartoon of the Changing Cholesterol Story"
Reprinted courtesy of Harley Schwadron.

83 "Consumption of Fats in the United States, 1909–1999"
The American Journal of Clinical Nutrition (2011:93, 954), American Society for Nutrition. Reprinted with permission.

85 "Take This Ad to Your Doctor," Mazola, 1975"
Reprinted with permission from ACH Food Companies, Inc.

115 "Meat Consumption In the United States, 1800–2007"
Reprinted with permission from Cambridge University Press.

116 "Meat Consumption in the United States, 1909–2007"
Reprinted with permission from Cambridge University Press.

132   "NIH Consensus Conference: *Time*, March 26, 1984"
      From *TIME* Magazine, March 26, 1984 © 1984, Time Inc. Used under license.

139   "Cartoon of Restaurant"
      Reprinted with permission from S. Harris.

172   "Cartoon on Low-Fat Dieting"
      Reprinted courtesy of Harley Schwadron.

175   "Antonia Trichopoulou"
      Reprinted with permission from Antonia Trichopoulou.

177   "Ancel Keys and Colleagues Touring the Archeological Site of Knossos"
      Reprinted with permission from Christos Aravanis.

180   "Anna Ferro-Luzzi"
      Reprinted with permission from Anna Ferro-Luzzi.

187   "Mediterranean Diet Pyramid, 1993"
      Copyright © Oldways (www.oldwayspt.org). Reprinted with permission from Oldways.

190   "Walter Willett and Ancel Keys, Cambridge, Massachussetts, 1993"
      Copyright © Oldways (www.oldwayspt.org). Reprinted with permission from Oldways.

229   "Sokolof Advertisement Appearing in the *New York Times*, November 1, 1988"
      Copyright © the National Heart Saver Association. Reprinted with permission.

231   "Vegetable Oil Consumption in the United States, 1909–1999"
      The American Journal of Clinical Nutrition (2011:93, 954), American Society for Nutrition. Reprinted with permission.

288   "Cartoon of Eskimo Diets"
      Reprinted with permission from S. Harris.

312   "*The New York Times Magazine* Cover July 7, 2002"
      From *The New York Times*, July 7, 2002 © 2002 *The New York Times*. All rights reserved. Used by permission and protected by the Copyright Laws of the United States. The printing, copying, redistribution, or retransmission of this Content without express written permission is prohibited.
      Photograph © by Lendon Flanagan. Reprinted with permission.

Index

Italicized page numbers indicate location of illustrations

American Dietetic Association, 289, 325
American Heart Association (AHA), 38, 74–75,
   90, 145, 255, 276*n*
   children and, 147, 152
   cholesterol and, 49, 52, 92, 162, 175, 317–18,
      321–23
   dietary recommendations of, 4, 13, 48–50,
      52, 83–84, 91–92, 103–5, 122, 136–37,
      146, 169, 171–73, 175, 198, 210*n*, 215,
      240–42, 276, 279, 286, 289, 306, 307*n*,
      310, 314, 319–23, 326, 328–29, 332
   diet-heart hypothesis and, 47, 49–50, 52, 68,
      70
   Eisenhower and, 48, 48*n*–49*n*, 68
   heart disease and, 47–50, 52, 68–69, 85, 103,
      146, 162, 241, 321–23, 326–28, 332
   hydrogenated oils and, 86, 241–42, 245
   Keys and, 47, 49–50, 68, 70, 122
   Krauss and, 316, 319–20, 323
   low-fat diet and, 4, 50, 92, 105, 136–38,
      146–47, 169, 171, 198, 210, 215, 240,
      306, 310, 329, 332–33
   Mann and, 67–68
   Mediterranean diet and, 198, 210*n*
   NHLBI and, 68–70, 133–34
   political issues and, 68, 103–5, 122, 127
   research funding of, 47–48, 68, 70, 91–92,
      137–38, 210*n*, 306, 307*n*, 309–10, 315*n*,
      329
   saturated fats and, 49–50, 240, 306,
      319–20
   trans fats and, 242, 244*n*
   vegetable oils and, 83–86, 241, 276, 284
   White and, 32, 48, 69–70
American Institute for Cancer Research, 111,
   143, 168
American Journal of Cardiology, 191, 211*n*
American Journal of Clinical Nutrition (AJCN),
   54, 61, *83,* 188, 197*n,* 211*n, 231,* 324–25,
   329
American Medical Association (AMA), 125,
   198, 290
American Oil Chemists' Society (AOCS), 241,
   247*n*–48*n,* 282–83
American Soybean Association (ASA), 231–33,
   235–37
Anderson, Clayton & Company, 91, 237,
   244
Anitschkow, Nikolaj, 22

Anti-Coronary Club trial, 73–75, 79
anti-inflammatory effects, 203, 205*n*
Applewhite, Thomas H.:
   Enig's conflicts with, 247–48, 250
   trans fats and, 245, 247–48, 250–51, 256
Aravanis, Christos, 192, 195, 217*n,* 222
Archer Daniels Midland (ADM), 268–69, 272,
   283–84
arteries, 15, 142*n,* 228, 273, 306, 317*n*
   children and, 146, 151, 155–56
   cholesterol and, 21–22, 53, 161–62
   heart disease and, 20–22, 30, 53, 62
   Ornish and, 141–43
   trans fats and, 240, 243
   see also arteriosclerosis and atherosclerosis
arteriosclerosis, 298–99
Associated Press, 69*n,* 253
atherosclerosis, 15, 20*n, 34,* 65, 75, 142*n,* 159,
   246, 281, 329*n*
   children and, 146, 148, 151
   cholesterol and, 21–22
   Keys and, 27–29, 36, 43
Atkins, Robert C., 6, 140, 145, 287–93
   death of, 291, 307*n*
   dietary supplement business of, 288, 291
   high-fat recommendations of, 287–89, 291,
      302–4, 306, 308–9, 311
   Ornish and, 289–90, 305
Atkins diet, 189, 197, 287–92, 291, 293*n,*
   302–11, 315
   research on, 290–91, 302–11, 322*n*
   weight loss and, 287, 290–91, 303, 305–6,
      310
Atkins flu, 305
Australia, 17, *28, 34,* 117, 155
Austria, *34,* 294–96, 311

bacon, 4, 10, 51, 53, 58, 64, 101, 132, *132,* 289,
   325, 335
Bacon, Francis, 56
baked goods, 173
   hydrogenated oils and, 226–27
   trans fats and, 251, 257
   trans-free alternatives and, 269–72
   vegetable oils and, 82, 88–89
Banting, William, 292–93, 298, 302, 306*n*
Bardi, 17
Barker, J. Ellis, 301
Beauchamp, Gary, 203

grains, 1, 16, 102, 112–13
  carbohydrates and, 4, 286–87, 315
  children and, 149, 153*n*, 157–58
  clinical trials and, 5, 169
  low-fat diet and, 5, 332
  Mediterranean diet and, 174, *187*, 199
  Ornish and, 140
  USDA and, 13, 135–36, 153*n*, 186
  whole, 5, 13, 105, 169, 174, 287, 315,
    332
  women and, 158, 169
Great Expectations (Dickens), 336
Greece, 138, 168, 205*n*–6*n*
  ancient, 107*n*, 200, 204, 219, 221*n*
  appeal of, 191–93
  heart disease and, 38–39
  Mediterranean diet and, 40, 174–76, *175*,
    178–80, 182–86, *187*, 190–95, 206–8,
    212, 217, 219–24
  olive oil and, 175–76, 195, 200–202, 204,
    233
  Seven Countries study and, 37–41, 176, 192,
    194–95, 216
Greenland, Sander, 217–18
Greenwald, Peter, 167, 192

Hall, Richard, 264
Hamilakis, Yannis, 204
Handler, Philip, 126–27
Harman, Denham, 279–80
Harper, Alfred E., 125–26
Harris, Ron, 237
Harvey, William, 292, 306*n*
Hawaii, 33, 98, 195*n*, 197*n*, 237
Hayes, K. C., 256
Health and Human Services, Department of,
  US (DHHS), 123*n*, 124
Healthy People goal, 5
heart disease, 16, 102, 164–67, 273, 307,
  336
  AHA and, 47–50, 52, 68–69, 85, 103, 146,
    162, 241, 321–23, 326–28, 332
  Ahrens and, 58–59, 122
  Atkins and, 287, 289–91, 306, 308, 310
  carbohydrates and, 24, 58–59, 125, 298–301,
    314, 326, 335
  children and, 21–22, 146, 146*n*–47*n*, 148,
    151, 154–56
  cholesterol and, *see under* cholesterol

clinical trials and, 5, 64–67, 74–80, 92–93,
  96, 102*n*, 127–30, 133, 138, 154, 161–62,
  170, 171*n*, 202–3, 209–10, 213–15, 276,
  306, 310
connection between fat and, 3, 11, 13, 19–20,
  27–40, *28, 34,* 42–45, 52, 54–56, 58, *132,*
  183, 297–98, 300, 302, 304, *312, 326*
Consensus Conference and, 132, *132*
deaths from, *see under* deaths
diagnosis of, 35–36, 38–39, 54*n*, 98, 119*n*,
  151, 171*n*
diet-heart hypothesis and, 54–57, 316
epidemics of, 19–20, 27*n*, 32, 47, 51, 78, 119,
  159, 294
epidemiological studies and, 37–39, 42, 55,
  97–99, 97*n*–98*n*, 178, 216, 219*n*, 223
high-fat diet and, 302, 304, 306, 330–31
history and, 113, 117–19
hydrogenated oils and, 228
Keys and, 19–21, 23, 27–37, *28,* 42–43, 47,
  50–51, *51,* 54, 58, 60, 62, 73, 85, 176,
  178, 181, 205, 216, 222, 239, 297, 316,
  327
Krauss and, 316–18, 319*n*, 324–25
Lancet and, 100–101
low-carbohydrate diet and, 294, 298, 331
low-fat diet and, 5, 39, 53, 54*n*, 73–74, 101,
  146, 150, 156, 166, 171–72, 213, 216,
  266, 289, 327, 332
Mann and, 12–13, 20, 30, 35, 49*n*, 62, 66,
  71, 142*n*
Masai and, 12–13, 20, 56, 62, 142*n*
meat and, 6, 31–32, 35, 38, 42, 52, 55,
  108–10, 112, 119, 300
Mediterranean diet and, 175, 179, 185, 205,
  207–10, 213–16, 221–23
Mediterranean region and, 30, 176, 178,
  191–92
Native Americans and, 15
NHLBI and, 68–70, 80, 159–60
nutrition science and, 13–14, 18
olive oil and, 38, 202–3, 333
Ornish and, 140–43
political issues and, 104, 112, 122–23, 125,
  323
prevention of, 12*n*, 20, 33, 39, 50, 52, 73, 85,
  97, 101, 127–28, 130, 133, 146, 179, 202,
  205, 241, 266, 289, 304, 323, 330
saturated fats and, *see under* saturated fats

hydrogenated oils (*cont.*)
    promotion of, 88, 231–32
    research on, 78, 239–40, 248–49, 254–56
    trans fats and, *8,* 87, 88*n,* 225, 226*n,* 236–39,
        241, 243–44, 248–49, 253–54, 269–70,
        275
    trans-free alternatives and, 269–72, 277
    tropical oils vs., 231–32, 236–37
    US consumption of, 83*n,* 232
    vegetable oils and, 87–91, 225, 228, 241, 243,
        246*n,* 249, 254, 273, 276
    versatility of, 226–27
4-hydroxynonenal (HNE), 280–83

ice cream, 42, 75, 91*n,* 154
Iliad, The (Homer), 219
In Defense of Food (Pollan), 13
India, 14, 54, 97
Indo-Mediterranean Heart Study, 211–13
Institute for Shortening and Edible Oils (ISEO),
    242, 245–48, 250–51, 253–54, 267
Institute of Medicine (IOM), 267
insulin, 213
    body fat and, 295–96
    carbohydrates and, 296, 311
    obesity and, 296*n,* 311, 314
interesterified fats, 273, 276
International Agency for Research on Cancer
    (IARC), 278–79
International Life Sciences Institute (ILSI), 257,
    265
International Olive Oil Council (IOOC),
    193–95, 197*n,* 226
Inuit, 9–11, 29, 86*n,* 293, 298–301, 308
    carbohydrates and, 10, 299–301
    high-fat diet of, 9–10, 13–14, 17, 63
    Schaefer on, 298–300
    Stefansson on, 9–10, 13–14, 17, 62–63,
        309*n*
Ireland, *34,* 54, 97
Israel, *34,* 117
    Atkins and, 309–10, 315, 322*n*
    Mediterranean diet and, 212–15, 309–10, 315
    vegetable oil consumption in, 82
Israel Civil Service Study, 97, 97*n*–98*n,* 100
Italian-Americans, 55–57, 97
Italy, 30, 33, *34,* 168, 331
    clinical trials and, 212–13
    heart disease and, *28,* 38

Mediterranean diet and, 174–79, *180,*
    181–82, 184–86, *187,* 190, 194–95,
    212–13, 219–21, 223–24
olive oil and, 186, 193*n,* 195, 200, 204–5
Seven Countries study and, 37–38, 40, 42,
    176–78, 216

Jacobson, Marc, 155
Jacobson, Michael, 227–28, 266
James, W. Philip T., 183
Japan, 30, 33, 129, 158, 206
    fat consumption of, 56
    heart disease and, *28, 34,* 35*n,* 94, 98–100,
        223
    oil oxidation and, 280
    Seven Countries study and, 37
    triglycerides and, 59
    women and, 166
Jenkins, Nancy Harmon, 197
Jolliffe, Norman, 73–74
Joseph, Stephen, 271–72
Journal of the American Medical Association
    (JAMA), 46, 55–56, 71, 130, 167, 290,
    324
    Ornish and, 141–42
    WHI and, 169–70
Judd, Joseph T., 239, 255–57
Jungle, The (Sinclair), 119

Kannel, William B., 65, 159*n*
Katan, Martijn B.:
    trans fats and, 252–57, 260–61
    trans-free alternatives and, 270
Keebler Company, *229,* 230, 235
Kellogg's, 137, 212*n, 229,* 230
Kenya, 62, 101, 144, 157*n*
    Mann's study in, 11–13
ketones, 304–5
Keys, Ancel Benjamin, 27–47, 86, 311, 315
    AHA and, 47, 49–50, 68, 70, 122
    Ahrens and, 32, 59
    and bias against meat, 106–7
    on body fat, 29–30
    cancer and, 94
    cholesterol and, 21, 23–24, 27, 30–33, 50, 53,
        73–74, 85, 94, 100, 106–7, 239, 316
    clinical trials and, 81, 96, 128
    comparisons between Willett and, 258–59,
        264

About the Author

Nina Teicholz wrote on food and nutrition science for *Gourmet* and *Men's Health* magazines. She was a reporter for National Public Radio for five years, covering Washington, DC, and Latin America. She also contributed, on a variety of topics, to *The New Yorker*, the *Economist*, the *Washington Post*, the *New York Times*, and *Salon*, among other publications. In addition, she served as the associate director for the Center for Globalization and Sustainable Development at Columbia University. Teicholz was a student of biology at Yale and Stanford Universities and earned a graduate degree from Oxford University. She lives in New York City with her husband and their sons.

IC 6-5-14
WH 8-7-14
OS 10-9-14
AG 12-11-14
ET 2-12-15
OM 4-13-15
PL 6-15-15
ST 8 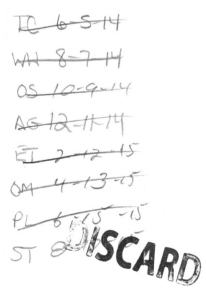DISCARD

ST8-2015KP